The Legal Aspects of Complementary Therapy Practice

For Judy

For Churchill Livingstone

Commissioning Editor: Inta Ozols
Project Manager: Valerie Burgess
Project Development Editor: Mairi McCubbin
Copy Editor: Tamsin Bacchus
Indexer: John Sampson
Project Controller: Valerie Burgess
Design Direction: Judith Wright
Sales Promotion Executive: Jason Clark

The Legal Aspects of Complementary Therapy Practice

A Guide for Health Care Professionals

Bridgit Dimond MA LLB DSA AHSM
Barrister-at-Law, Emeritus Professor of the University of Glamorgan

Foreword by

Hazel Courtenay
Health Journalist of the Year; Sunday Times Columnist

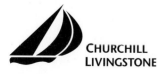

CHURCHILL
LIVINGSTONE

EDINBURGH LONDON NEW YORK PHILADELPHIA SYDNEY TORONTO 1998

Churchill Livingstone
A Division of Harcourt Brace and Company Limited

First published 1998

ISBN 0 443 056153

British Library Cataloguing in Publication Data
A catalogue record for this book is available from the British Library.

Library Congress Cataloging in Publication Data
A catalog record for this book is available from the Library of Congress.

Medical knowledge is constantly changing. As new information becomes available, changes in treatment, procedures, equipment and the use of drugs become necessary. The author and publishers have, as far as it is possible, taken care to ensure that the information given in this text is accurate and up to date. However, readers are strongly advised to confirm that the information, especially with regard to drug usage, complies with latest legislation and standards of practice.

Neither the publishers nor the author will be liable for any loss or damage of any nature occasioned to or suffered by any person acting or refraining from acting as a result of reliance on the material contained in this publication.

9901 647

WB 890

The
publisher's
policy is to use
**paper manufactured
from sustainable forests**

Produced by Addison Wesley Longman China Limited, Hong Kong
C&C/01

Contents

Foreword

During the past 10 years, interest in alternative remedies and therapies has grown enormously to the point where one in four people now use alternatives. In the West there is a tidal wave of chronic, degenerative illnesses which orthodox medicine in most cases cannot cure. Up to one million people annually are admitted to hospital suffering the side effects of prescription drugs. At last the medical establishment is realising that nutritional medicine and alternative therapies are not quackery. Aromatherapy, osteopathy, homeopathy, herbalism, even healing, are in some areas available on the NHS, and private alternative clinics are springing up all over the UK. There are now over half a million positive research papers on nutritional medicine, alternative therapies and remedies, and the public are beginning to realise that in many cases they can help themselves towards better health.

I am not decrying orthodox medicine which daily saves many lives; but it also takes lives, and I firmly believe the time has come to offer the public integrated medicine, an amalgam of orthodox and alternatives, as the medicine of the future.

But many doctors, NHS fund managers, therapists and members of the public are confused by certain claims that are being made for these 'new' therapies and remedies. People are asking where they stand in law if things go wrong.

For the most part virtually every alternative therapist, doctor and practitioner I have met has enormous integrity; however, as in every walk of life, there are good and bad practitioners, and patients.

In this book, Professor Dimond clearly explains the laws regarding complementary therapies. Her aim is to provide the information for clients to understand their legal rights and for therapists to know the laws which apply to their practice.

Therapists also wish the law to provide protection for those who have undergone considerable training and experience against the false and sometimes overstated claims of those who have not. Therapists also need to be clear on what claims they can or cannot make for their treatments.

Also, of course, there are vexatious litigants who make complaints which are often entirely unjustified. They try to exploit the legal system to get compensation to which they may not be entitled. Claims for back injuries whilst at work are a classic example.

It is essential in this area of rapid development and interest, that both therapists and their clients, and also the practitioners and managers within the NHS who may purchase their services, have a well-defined understanding of the law. This book provides a clear explanation of the legal framework for alternative therapies. In addition Professor Dimond looks at each of the main therapies and explores the specific laws which apply to them, analysing through case histories some of the legal issues which often arise.

For those of us who would like to see changes to some of the present restrictions, this book also gives an understanding of the current laws regarding alternative health issues. I have always found the law a very complex subject and can easily see how it creates barriers. But in this book Professor Dimond explains the complexities of the law in an easy-to-read and understandable manner, enabling us all to contribute towards a more informed debate about an area of increasing importance to the nation's health.

1998   Hazel Courtenay

Preface

'Counsellors should work within the law. Counsellors should take all reasonable steps to be aware of current law affecting the work of the counsellor. A counsellor's ignorance of the law is no defence against legal liability or penalty including inciting or "counselling", which has a specific legal sense, the commission of offences by clients.'[1]

These words from the Code of Ethics and Practice of the British Association for Counselling are echoed in many of the codes for complementary therapists.

This therefore is a book to meet that need. The book has three audiences in mind: first, those who practise or hope to practise in a field of complementary or alternative medicine or therapy and who therefore need to know the constraints provided by the laws in the context of which they practise; second, those clients or patients who are interested in obtaining the services of such practitioners, who want to know what their rights are and what protections the law provides for them; and third, those who work in the field of health care as a health professional or manager who may be purchasing the services of those working in the field of complementary therapy, or who are caring for patients and who, as well as obtaining the services of orthodox medicine, are also in receipt of the services of a complementary therapist and therefore need to have an understanding of the legal aspects relating to the interface of each.

The purpose is to set out the legal context of the environment in which they work in clear, jargon-free language so that those who have no legal knowledge can come to an understanding of the legal principles which apply and affect their practice or which support them.

The number of those practising in complementary or alternative therapies has expanded considerably in recent years in parallel to increasing interest from the general population in the use of their services instead of, or in addition to, orthodox medicine. At present there are not many examples of litigation being brought against individual therapists, but there would appear to be no reason for complacency in assuming that there will not be an expansion in the numbers of therapists being held accountable for their practice and being required to pay compensation to clients.

The book is therefore written from the perspective of the non-lawyer, the lay person who wishes to have a readable explanation of the laws which apply across a wide area. It is perhaps therefore a book to dip into rather than to be read from cover to cover. Initial reading of the first two chapters will however be of value in explaining how the book is set out and giving a general introduction to the legal system which applies in this country. Where possible legal jargon has been avoided but a glossary is provided to give an explanation of the various legal terms which are in common use. The provision of addresses and a bibliography for most of the therapies considered also make this both a work of reference and of introduction.

From a negative perspective as a researcher into the topic I was amazed at the naivety of some members of complementary therapies who took the view that the public could not be harmed by their practices, that no formal regulation was necessary and that people providing services in their chosen field could only be prompted by the highest motives. There are of course, many examples of altruistic, unselfish practice of the highest standards. There are also examples of fraudulent exploitative activities. In addition, examples are available from the medical protection societies of potential claims in relation to harm suffered as a result of the practice of complementary therapies.

The difficult topic of definitions and use of language; how should all these therapies which are outside conventional medicine be described? I have used the term complementary therapy to cover both therapy and medicine and also alternative. The book uses the term 'complementary therapy and complementary therapist' to cover all these various health and self-promoting services. I appreciate that under this term will be included therapists who do not necessarily see themselves as practising alongside orthodox medicine and would prefer to use the word alternative. In addition osteopathy and chiropractic are also included whilst some may consider that, having achieved state registration, they have now ceased to be complementary and are part of orthodox medicine. The term will also cover those who would prefer to see themselves as practising a complementary medicine rather than a therapy. The inadequacies of the term 'complementary therapy' in covering the wide variety of organisations included in this book are recognised. However it makes for easier reading to use one term to cover all these diverse practices rather than to attempt to use 'complementary medicine', 'complementary therapy', 'alternative therapy' or other terms in specific instances. I hope that those individuals and organisations who consider that they have been wrongly included under the umbrella term 'complementary therapy' will understand the reasons and therefore pardon me.

It is impossible to cover the hundreds of different therapies and their organisations which claim to provide a service in health care or the promotion of good health. I have been compelled to limit discussion to the most popular ones. Clearly the legal issues which apply to these will also be relevant to those therapies which I do not cover and certainly the general chapters in Part One should be of assistance to those practitioners who are creating a business or who are concerned with their liability in law or with identifying the rights of the client. Nor have I been able to identify all the organisations under which the therapists are grouped. I have chosen those who appear to be typical of some of the main areas which are central to the aork of this book. Again I ask the indulgence of those individuals and organisations who consider that their view point has been omitted or neglected in this book. If they are prepared to let me know then hopefully any future new editions can remedy the oversight.

Without the unstinting help of the many organisations representing the therapists, this book could not have been written and I am indebted to them for the information they provided for their constitution, Codes of Conduct and membership regulations. Other valuable reference material were the *Fundamentals of complementary and alternative medicine* edited by Marc Micozzi.[2] *The natural family doctor* by Dr Andrew Stanway,[3] Denis Rankin-Box's edited work on the *The nurses' handbook for complementary therapies.*[4] The updated *Which Guide to Complementary Therapies* written by Barbara Rowlands[5] is excellent in its crisp succinctness and a useful resource. Other books of reference are included in the bibliography.

The aim of the core chapters in Part One is to set out the basic principles of law which apply across the field of complementary therapies and to follow up some of the themes raised above. There then follows in Part Two a short chapter on each of the main specialities within complementary therapy. Each of these short chapters will cover where relevant, the following topics:

- brief history and membership numbers, links with traditional medicine, controlling body
- registration (if applicable), membership, admission qualifications, examinations
- definitions of standards of competence
- rules on professional misconduct, control and disciplines
- insurance cover and professional indemnity
- special situations with legal significance.

The overall objective is to provide a handbook for those with no legal knowledge to understand the context within which they practise or use complementary therapies, so that their own professional practice is promoted and their clients protected.

1998   Bridgit Dimond

REFERENCES

1. Paragraphs B2.7.1 and 2.7.2 from the Code of Ethics and Practice of the British Association of Counselling May 1996.
2. Micozzi M (ed) 1996 Fundamentals of complementary and alternative medicine. Churchill Livingstone, NY
3. Stanway A 1987 The natural family doctor. Gaia Publications
4. Rankin-Box D (ed) 1995 The nurses' handbook of complementary therapies. Churchill Livingstone, Edinburgh
5. Rowlands B 1997 The Which? guide to complementary therapies. Consumers Association

Acknowledgements

Very many people have assisted me in the writing of this book and the collection of relevant material and I can only mention the principal ones here. They include: Andrew Vickers of the RCCM, Anthony Baird of the Institute of Complementary Medicine, Sylvia Baker of the Aromatherapy Organisations Council, Richard Booth of the College of Healing, Barry Devlin of the National Federation of Spiritual Healers, David Repard of the Confederation of Healing Organisations, David Sutton (Devitt Insurance Services Ltd), Ken Woodward (LCSP), Dr Paul Williams (BCP), Theo Gimbel of the Hygeia College of Colour Therapy, Jill Reeves-Bond (APNT), Don Harrison of the Institute of Allergy Therapy and many, many others who have sent me helpful information about their therapies.

I thank also Tessa Shellens of Bevan Ashford (solicitors) Catherine Cotterill, librarian at Bevan Ashford, Isobel Puscas, librarian of the Bro Taf Health Authority, Pat Evans (Llandough), Jean Timmins (RCN), Lynne Yeates, Diana Wright and Ann Saer.

My thanks finally to my indulgent family and especially to Bette who read through the typescript. Above all my appreciation is due to my sister Judy whose interest in allergy therapy first brought my attention to the field of complementary therapies and to whom this book is dedicated.

Disclaimer

Many examples are given in this book where writers and therapists have recommended certain therapies or products for specific conditions. Readers should not use such examples as a recommendation by the author of this book. The author of this book is a lawyer and is not in any way making any recommendations of any therapy, product (natural or synthetic), oil or technique to readers. Professional advice should be sought from the appropriate person or organisation before any therapy, product or technique is used.

Where situations with a legal significance are discussed, these are entirely fictitious and do not relate to any living person. In contrast where cases are discussed, these relate to actual incidents.

Table of cases

Table of statutes and regulations

SECTION 1

General Principles of Law

SECTION CONTENTS

Introduction

INCREASE IN POPULARITY OF COMPLEMENTARY MEDICINE

All the evidence shows an increasing interest in and use of complementary medicines over the past ten years. Examples of some of the evidence is given below.

In 1985 a Consumers Association survey found that one in seven members (total members 28,000) had visited a non-conventional practitioner in the previous 12 months.[1] In 1991 in an unpublished survey this number was found to have increased to one in four members.[2] Since these surveys are based on their membership it is not possible to state that this increase would apply to the population as a whole. However other evidence such as that published by Thomas[3] and the British Holistic Medical Association[4] indicate a growing interest by patients, not necessarily as an alternative to conventional health care but complementary to it. Figures on the numbers of those practising in the area of non-conventional medicine have shown a similar increase with the British Holistic Medical Association suggesting that the number of therapists is increasing by about 11% a year. It was reported in the BMJ in July 1996,[5] quoting from a survey by the Research Council for Complementary Medicine, that one in ten people in Britain consults a practitioner of complementary medicine each year. Of the 160 different treatments which the Council identifies, six account for three quarters of those used.

Registered medical practitioners have not been indifferent or unaffected by these developments and the British Medical Association concludes from its review of the evidence 'that there is growing interest among medical practitioners in various non-conventional therapies; this is particularly marked in younger doctors and in women doctors'.

ACCESS VIA THE NHS

One of the results of this growth in interest is the extent to which access to complementary therapies has been via the NHS. In 1993 the National Association of Health Authorities and Trusts (NAHAT) published the report of a survey undertaken on the use of complementary therapies within the NHS.[7] The survey of DHAs, FHSAs and GP fundholders of their attitudes towards the availability of complementary therapies in the NHS was supplemented by a questionnaire to the royal colleges, medical organisations and patient representative organisations, and also complementary therapy bodies, on their view of the role of complementary therapies within the NHS.

Over 50% of respondent DHAs, FHSAs and GP fundholders considered that some complementary therapies should be available on the NHS. Those who did not were influenced by:

- lack of proven effectiveness;
- lack of proven cost effectiveness;
- resource constraints and priorities;
- fears about uncontrolled demands on NHS resources;
- lack of demand from the public or from GPs.

Acupuncture received the greatest support from those responding, almost 100% of FHSAs considering that it should be available on the NHS; osteopathy was the next most popular, then homeopathy, chiropractic and aromatherapy with less than 25% and reflexology with less than 5%.

Figures on availability within the NHS showed that 15% of the FHSAs had approved a policy about complementary therapies and 44 of the FHSAs had given approval to health promotion clinics which used wholly or partly complementary therapies. Acupuncture was the most common therapy to have been given approval and was mainly used in smoking cessation and pain relief clinics. In the main DHAs were funding complementary therapies on an individual basis as extra-contractual referrals. 43% had contracts for complementary therapies with either NHS providers or providers in the private sector. Some authorities refused to fund extra-contractual referrals (ECRs) for complementary therapies whilst others would only fund them if the conventional therapies had failed to produce satisfactory results. The survey of GP fundholders showed that complementary therapies could be used in the following conditions:

- chronic back pain
- osteo arthritis
- rheumatoid arthritis
- hay fever
- anxiety
- insomnia
- obesity
- smoking

- peptic ulcer
- maturing onset diabetes.

The report concludes that well over £1 million was spent on complementary therapies in 1992. In general, however, funding complementary therapies is not given a high priority. There is a lack of agreement about the effectiveness of individual therapies compounded by a general lack of information about such therapies, appropriate training and qualifications, cost effectiveness and the current regulations on commissioning them. The report recommends the action shown in Box 1.1.

Box 1.1 Action recommended in NAHAT report

---

1. Research into the effectiveness of complementary therapies.
2. Evaluation of complementary therapy services currently available within the NHS.
3. Research into the cost/benefit of complementary therapies.
4. The development of standards for training and qualification.
5. Guidelines, research findings, and general information to be disseminated widely.

The Medical Care Research Unit at Sheffield University conducted a national survey of access to complementary health care via general practice in 1995.[8] Its tentative conclusions based on a response rate of 62% are shown in Box 1.2.

Box 1.2 Results of Sheffield survey

---

1. 39.5% of all practices currently provide access to complementary therapies for their NHS patients.
2. An estimated 21.4% are offering access via the provision of treatment by a member of the primary health care team.
3. An estimated 6.1% employ an 'independent' complementary therapist.
4. An estimated 24.6% of partnerships make NHS referrals for a complementary therapy.
5. The most frequently cited type of provision is NHS referral, reported by one in four practices, mostly for homeopathy or acupuncture at NHS hospitals.
6. The most frequently employed independent practitioners were osteopaths.
7. Fundholding practices are significantly more likely to offer complementary therapies via a member of the primary health care team than non-fundholding practices.
8. Single handed GPs are significantly less likely to offer this service.

The survey undertaken by Sheffield University concluded that:

Access to complementary therapies in general practice is widespread amongst practices, but appears to affect a relatively small number of patients.

There is every sign that this increase in access to complementary therapies via the NHS is likely to continue and the British Medical Association, following its own survey of complementary therapies, recognised the need to ensure that there is better information in the use and practice of non-conventional therapies. Even where registered medical practitioners do not wish to practice complementary therapies themselves, they need to be aware of the implications of any referral, which their patients are increasingly likely to request.

Everett Koop, former Surgeon General of the United States, says in his introduction to *Fundamentals of complementary and alternative medicine*[9]

In the opinion of most doctors, there is not a definite answer on the value of complementary and alternative medicine. I would like to see us undertake the study and research that could provide definitive answers to prudent questions about the usefulness of complementary and alternative medicine for society at large.

One proponent of an integrative approach between orthodox and complementary therapy is Dr Andrew Weil, a Harvard graduate in medicine who is described as advocating a combination of conventional treatment and alternative therapies called 'integrative medicine'.[10] Dr Weil's prescription is shown in Box 1.3.

Box 1.3 Dr Weil's prescription for optimum health

1. Walk at least 45 minutes a day.
2. Take vitamin C.
3. Practise breathing deeply.
4. Avoid excessive radiation from computers.
5. Eat more broccoli and ginger, and less animal fat.
6. Remember there are times when only modern drugs and high-tech medicine will do.

OPPOSITION TO COMPLEMENTARY THERAPIES

In comparison to these encouraging signs of interest and involvement of registered medical practitioners in complementary therapies, there are those whose opposition has been firmly stated. Dr Barry Beyerstein of Simon Fraser University in British Columbia and Dr Wallace Sampson of Standford University are quoted as denouncing alternative therapies as quackery at the American Association for the Advancement of Science in Seattle February 1997.[11]

A fertile climate for quackery has been created by a number of social and psychological factors, which are convincing both the purveyors and the consumers of alternative therapies that the treatments are valid.

They stated that there was no credible evidence for most of the claims that were made.

COMPLEMENTARY OR ORTHODOX MEDICINE?

There is no clear understanding as to what is or is not complementary as opposed to orthodox medicine but this book has followed the accepted conventional distinctions in deciding what to include. There is possibly a danger that some of the skills of basic medical and nursing care may be hived off and a specialism created around them and then they are defined as 'complementary'. Thus Denise Rankin-Box[12] in her book on complementary therapy for nurses includes a separate section on humour which many would have held to be a basic skill in nursing.

At what point can it be said that a therapy is no longer complementary but has become orthodox?

- When it acquires state registration? (e.g. osteopaths and chiropractors)
- When it can be purchased through the NHS? (e.g. aromatherapy)
- When it is practised by a registered medical practitioner? (e.g. homeopathy and acupuncture)
- When it is included in the basic syllabus of medical or nursing students?

Perhaps all of these developments must take place before a therapy can be described as part of orthodox medicine. For this reason, osteopathy and chiropractic are included in this book although they are now both state registered.

RESULTS OF INCREASING ACCEPTANCE

Difficulties of terminology

There is no clear acceptance of the distinction between the terms 'alternative' and 'complementary'.

Complementary therapies are defined in a pamphlet produced by the BCMA[13] as:

completing: together making up a whole, ... of medical treatment, therapies, etc ... (1. Complementum – *com-*, intents, and *plere* to fill)[12]

Alternative therapies can be seen as those which operate instead of orthodox medicine rather than as complementary to it. It would follow that, in the case of alternative therapies, the therapist would not see any necessity to work in conjunction with the registered medical practitioner of the client.

Walter Wardwell[14] stated that since the term 'alternative medicine' is defined residually as anything not regular medicine, it is not a useful category. It needs further specification as it includes primitive medicine, folk medicine, herbal medicine, homeopathy, chiropractic, naturopathy, faith healing, New Age Healing, etc. Wardwell originally classified health professions into ancillary, limited, marginal, and quasi-practitioners. This categorisation he suggests offers a fruitful set of categories for investigating relationships between these groups and organised medicine, and the movement of these groups from one status to another. Within the quasi-professional group, further subclassification distinguishes between folk and primitive healers, faith healers, and quacks; also between those who heal using natural forces and those who frankly invoke supernatural forces or entities. Wardwell points out that

The main advantage of the term 'alternative' is that it aggrandizes the status (and egos) of orthodox practitioners who then disparage all other healing practices as inferior, if not totally false, and it provides attractive topics for anthropologists to study as esoteric curiosities or for medical historians to use to show how far medicine has advanced from its pre-scientific origins.

The difficulty with accepting Wardwell's revised classification is that it is value laden and would not necessarily be accepted by those who practise the various therapies.

Baroness Trumpington when Parliamentary Under Secretary of State in her lecture to the 7th Colloquium on Conventional Medicine and Complementary Therapies on 13 June 1986[15] stated:

I prefer the term 'alternative', not for dogmatic reasons, but because I feel a little uneasy about the idea of herbal or homeopathic medicines 'complementing', say, an antibiotic. One has to recognise that within the so-called umbrella term of alternative therapies is a wide range of possible treatments. Many procedures are only regarded as 'alternative' when the claims for their use are greatly extended; for example manipulative therapy for a severely deformed rheumatoid joint.

Baroness Trumpington would also like to confine the term 'medicines' to homeopathy and herbalism and use 'therapies' in relation to the others.

Claire Monod Cassidy[16] distinguishes between:

- professionalised systems which tend to be found in an urban setting, are taught in colleges with the aid of written texts, and demand, from a usually legal standpoint, criteria for practice, examinations, licensing by the state, one to one practitioner/patient care, and that practitioners are in members' organisations; and
- community based systems, or folk or tribal systems, found in both urban and rural settings, where training is by apprenticeship and ends when the teacher considers that the apprentice is ready to practice, rather than on completion of written examinations; students are tested by practising medicine under guidance and essentially the community itself determines if a student is 'good enough'.

Orthodox health professionals practising complementary therapies

Perhaps one of the most interesting developments is the extent to which state registered doctors and nurses are increasingly developing interest and expertise in complementary therapies. This is leading to increasing pressure on the existing state registration bodies such as the GMC, the UKCC and the CPSM to lay down rules of conduct in relation to their registered practitioners working in spheres which are not recognised as part of their state registered practice. These matters are considered in more detail in Chapter 6.

This in turn places new responsibilities upon employers to define what is expected of the health professional they employ e.g. would a midwife be expected or allowed to practise reflexology?

Society's concern with regulation

This is specifically considered in Chapter 6. There is a narrow line to be drawn between the right of a citizen to practise in an area where he or she feels that a benefit can be offered to other people and the requirement that society protects those who are vulnerable to exploitation. For the most part the usual criminal laws against fraud, obtaining a pecuniary advantage by deception, and the Trade Descriptions Acts (see Chapter 5) and the civil laws relating to breach of contract (see Chapter 4) and other civil wrongs such as negligence (see Chapter 3) or defamation should protect the public and at the same time ensure that there is freedom to practise in a sphere which could provide benefit.

Increasingly, however, members of the different associations and organisations involved in complementary therapies have sought state recognition for two distinct reasons:

- to ensure that the public is protected against those who do not have the same examination standards and membership qualifications; and
- to protect the rights of those who have achieved certain levels of competence against those who are unqualified.

The constraints upon the organisations and associations of those providing complementary therapies are considered in Chapter 6.

A survey for BBC2[17] reported that of the 688 out of 1521 GPs who responded 80% had referred patients to complementary therapies. However 87% considered that there should be more regulation and 52% reported adverse reactions, including four deaths which were purported to arise from the use of complementary therapies. Evidence given on the programme showed this naive assumption amongst members of the general public, and those vulnerable to suggestion and unsupported claims, that natural is 'green' and must be healthy. There is evidence that our existing general laws and the self-regulation of the responsible practitioners may not be sufficient to protect the susceptible.

INDIVIDUAL PURSUIT OF HEALTH AND FULFILMENT

Ultimately this book is therefore about the legal tight rope between the role of the law in preventing harm to individuals and the role of the law in preserving the freedom of others to experiment in a wide variety of ways. We all face death. Good health cannot always be bought, but where money can, sometimes, postpone the inevitable end, people are vulnerable to any offers that health could be improved and diseases cured. From the earliest evidence of Chinese medicine thousands of years ago, one of mankind's major concerns has been the postponement of death and the improvement of health.

The current growth of interest in complementary medicine is possibly linked with a cynicism about orthodox medicine, especially in treating chronic conditions, and the increasing evidence of its iatrogenic effects.

COMPLEMENTARY THERAPIES AND THE EUROPEAN COMMUNITY

In 1996 the report of Paul Lannoye,[18] the Belgiun deputy prime minister and MEP was published. It calls for the recognition, regulation and harmonisation of complementary medicine throughout the EU and significantly increases the likelihood of an enhanced position for complementary medicine within health care provision.[19] The report is to be debated by the Committee of the Environment, Public Health and Consumer Protection of the European Parliament and, if approved, could form the basis of an EC Directive by 1999. This would result in recognition across the EU of specified complementary therapies. The report also emphasises the need to rationalise training and define a common minimum curriculum for complementary therapists. His earlier interim report in April 1996 called for member states social security systems to fund non-conventional therapies without discrimination. The report has been strongly criticised in France, where the practice of any therapy is restricted to registered medical practitioners.

The response by the EU to the Lannoye Report and any resulting Directive may have profound implications for the organisation and expansion of complementary therapies in this country.

REFERENCES

1. Magic or Medicine? Which? October 1986: 443
2. Consumers Association Survey Research Group 'Supertrawl' Survey 1991
3. Thomas K J et al 1991 Use of non-orthodox and conventional health care in Great Britain. British Medical Journal 302: 207–10
4. British Holistic Medical Association 1991 Response to the Government's Green Paper Health of the Nation BHMA, London
5. 1996 News item. British Medical Journal 313: 131–3
6. British Medical Association 1993 Complementary Medicine: New Approaches to Good Practice. Oxford University Press, Oxford
7. Cameron-Blackie G 1993 Complementary Therapies in the NHS National Association of Health Authorities and Trusts, Birmingham
8. Thomas K, Fall M, Parry G, Nicholl J 1995 A National Survey of Access to Complementary Health Care via General Practice in 1995. The Medical Care Research Unit Sheffield University, Sheffield
9. Micozzi M (ed) 1996 Fundamentals of complementary and alternative medicine. Churchill Livingstone, New York
10. Driscoll M Trust me I'm a guru. The Sunday Times 18 May 1997 p 15
11. Editorial Alternative therapies derided as Quackery. The Times 15 February 1997
12. Rankkin-Box D (ed) 1995 The nurses' handbook of complementary therapies. Churchill Livingstone, New York
13. Pamphlet of the British Complementary Medicine Association.
14. Wardwell W I 1994 Alternative medicine in the United States. Social Science & Medicine 38(8): 1061–8
15. Trumpington 1987 Alternative medicine and therapies and the DHSS. Journal of the Royal Society of Medicine 80: 336–8
16. Monod-Cassidy C 1996 Cultural context of complementary and alternative medicine systems. In Marc M (ed) Fundamentals of Complementary and Alternative Medicine. Churchill Livingstone, New York
17. Home ground. BBC2: 15 July 1997
18. Lannoye P 1996 Initial report on complementary medicine in the EU. EN/PR/289/289543
19. News item 1996 Medical law monitor November: 6–7

An introduction to the legal system

This chapter sets out to explain the legal system, including the sources of law, the courts system, differences between civil and criminal law and some of the basic legal terminology.

SOURCES OF LAW

Law derives from two main sources: Acts of Parliament (known as statute law) and judge made law (known as the common law or case law).

Statute law

Acts of Parliament take supremacy over all other laws apart from those made by the European Community, because, as a result of the UK signing the Treaty of Rome, it is now bound by the laws made by the European Community.

    An Act of Parliament must be passed through the two Houses of Parliament and then signed by the Queen before it becomes law. It may be effective the day it is signed or a later date (or dates) may be given for different sections or the whole act to come into force. Sections of some acts are still not in force many years after they were passed. (For example there are several sections of the Disabled Persons (Services, Consultation, and Representation) Act 1986 which are still not in force.)

Statutory Instruments (SIs)

Sometimes the Act of Parliament gives power to a Minister of State or another specified person or body to draw up Statutory Instruments covering detailed points. These would be placed before the Houses of Parliament for approval before they come into force.

European laws

Since the acceptance by the UK of the Treaty of Rome and membership of the European Community, the laws of the European Community are part of the law of this Country. There is a Council of Ministers and the European Commission which have the power to make laws. Each member state is represented on the Council of Ministers. Secondary legislation is issued in the form of Regulations, Directives and Decisions.

Regulations are automatically binding on each member state.

Directives, whilst binding in terms of purpose, require each individual member state to choose how the content of the Directive will be implemented. Thus the European Directives in relation to health and safety were implemented by means of regulations being passed through Parliament (see Chapter 13).

Decisions are made by the European Commission and take the form of rulings on individual cases. They can be addressed to a state, an organisation or an individual.

The European Parliament does not have the power to make legislation, but essentially fulfils a consultative and debating function.

Interpretation of statutes and SIs

There are rules relating to the interpretation of statutes and statutory instruments to ensure some consistency in their implementation. Sometimes there may be uncertainty over the interpretation and this could lead to a case being heard in the courts when the judge or judges may have to rule on how the specific section or subsection should be interpreted.

It is also the case that, where there is doubt, English legislation has to be interpreted in conformity with European law on the matter.

The common law

Judges hear cases where disputes arise between individuals or institutions or where a prosecution is brought in the criminal courts. Their decisions create 'precedents' which are binding upon judges hearing subsequent cases depending upon a hierarchy of courts. The cases they hear may centre on an uncertainty in the interpretation of an Act of Parliament or statutory instrument. They may also be concerned with an area where there is no statutory provision but the situation is governed by the common law. Judges may also have to determine what the law should be in areas where there is no precedent or statute. Thus for many years there was no statute law which defined the duty of the occupier of land to trespassers who were injured on the land. The duty of the occupier in relation to non-trespassers, or visitors, was defined by the Occupiers' Liability Act 1957. The duty of the occupier to trespassers was defined in a series of court decisions culminating with the leading case of *British Railways Board* v. *Herrington* (1971). It was not until 1984 that a further Occupiers' Liability Act was passed which filled the statutory gap and laid down by Act of Parliament the occupier's duty towards trespassers. Similarly the definition of the reasonable standard of care to be exercised by a professional is not set out in statute but by the common law in a case decided by a judge in 1957.[1] From the name of the case it has been called 'The Bolam Test' and its implications are discussed in Chapter 3 on civil accountability and the laws of negligence.

The Court of Justice of the European Community meets in Luxembourg and should not be confused with the European Court of Human Rights which meets in Strasbourg (see below). Each member state has one judge in the Court of Justice. Where it makes a ruling on European law, the courts in each member state must recognise and enforce it.

Court hierarchy and court reports

The following questions arise about the common law:

- How is it decided which decision of which court should be followed if there is a conflict in the decisions from different courts?
- Who decides what the court laid down in each case?

The first question is answered by understanding the hierarchy of courts and the system of precedence. This is covered later in this chapter. The second question is answered by the system of court reports.

The details of the cases including the facts of the dispute, the arguments put before the court and the speeches of the judges are recorded in official reports of the court, which each judge will read and agree that it forms a correct record of what took place. These reports are available in any law library. In 1865 a Council was established to ensure that the reports were reliable and accurate. In 1870 this Council became known as the Incorporated Council of Law Reporting for England and Wales. Reporters, who must be barristers, are employed to record the facts and the judgments of the cases. Thus authorised series of reports are published. Each case can be identified by its own reference details. Other series have developed covering medical law and other specialist topics.

For example '[1993] 1 All ER 821' means volume 1 of the All England Reports for 1993 at page 821, 'Med LR' stands for Medical Law Reports, and 'WLR' stands for Weekly Law Reports.

Codes of practice and professional conduct

Many associations enact Codes of ethical practice and professional conduct for their members. These are not part of the law of the land, so they cannot be used as the basis of a prosecution. However they can be used in evidence in the event of any professional conduct proceedings to show that there was failure by a member to comply with the standards set by the association. In cases where harm has occurred, failure to follow the Code of professional practice may be evidence that the reasonable standards of the profession have not been followed and this may be used as evidence of a breach of the duty of care owed to a client.

The Codes are not law in themselves, but guidance which the associations strongly recommend should be followed. They form part of ethical practice (see below). In certain circumstances it may be possible to show why there were special reasons why the guidelines of the Code could not be followed. This argument would not, however, be available where an Act of Parliament or Statutory Instrument has been broken. Failure to obey the law of the land could be followed by criminal prosecution or other proceedings. Ignorance of the law is no defence.

DIFFERENT KINDS OF LAW

There are different ways of classifying kinds of law. One is the distinction between criminal law and civil law. The former relates to an act or omission which can be followed by criminal proceedings. Usually these are brought in the name of the crown and are the state bringing an action against a private citizen. However it is possible for a private individual to bring a private prosecution alleging that the accused is guilty of the offence with which he is charged. (Criminal law is explained in more detail in Chapter 5.)

Civil relates to those proceedings between private citizens or private and public bodies in which specific harm or civil wrong is alleged. The largest category of civil wrongs are known as 'torts'. These cover such civil wrongs as:

- negligence,
- trespass,
- nuisance,
- defamation and
- breach of a statutory duty.

Breach of contract cases are civil cases but do not come under the name of torts. (The law of negligence is explained in Chapter 3, the law of contract in Chapter 4.)

Many actions or omissions may be both criminal and civil wrongs. Thus to assault a person would be a criminal act as well as a trespass to the person, which is a civil wrong. The law makers can decide at any time if an act should become or cease to be regarded as a criminal wrong. For example under the Suicide Act 1961 it ceased to be a criminal act to attempt to commit suicide. However it remains a criminal act for a person to aid, abet or in any way assist another person to commit suicide.

A BILL OF RIGHTS

Unlike the United States of America, the UK has not had a Bill of Rights to which all judges must refer, and which can only be amended by following a special procedure. Great Britain is a signatory of the European Convention on Human Rights, but this has not been incorporated into English law. However, under proposals now being placed before Parliament, people who consider that their rights have not been respected in this country will, instead of appealing to the Court of Human Rights in Strasbourg, be able to raise with a court in this country the fact that there would appear to be a breach of the European Convention on Human Rights. Judges will be able to declare if an Act of Parliament is in conflict with the Convention and there will be a fast track procedure through Parliament for the clash to be discussed and possibly removed.

THE DIFFERENT COURTS AND THEIR FUNCTION

We mentioned above the system of court hierarchies. Figure 2.1 shows the civil courts and indicates that the decisions of the House of Lords are binding on all lower courts on similar facts. Figure 2.2 illustrates the courts which deal with criminal cases. Again any decisions by the House of Lords will bind all courts below it on similar facts.

Other courts and forums

There are other courts and forums which a practitioner might encounter professionally.

Coroner's court

The coroner holds inquests into unexplained deaths to determine the identity of the deceased, the place, time and cause of death, and the particulars required for the death to be registered. This is an example of a court which is inquisitorial not accusatorial. This means that the coroner summons the witnesses and may do most of the questioning. In contrast, a civil or criminal hearing is based on an accusatorial system, where one party is attempting to prove a case against another and the judge sits to determine the outcome with intervention only when necessary to ensure that justice is done and seen to be done.

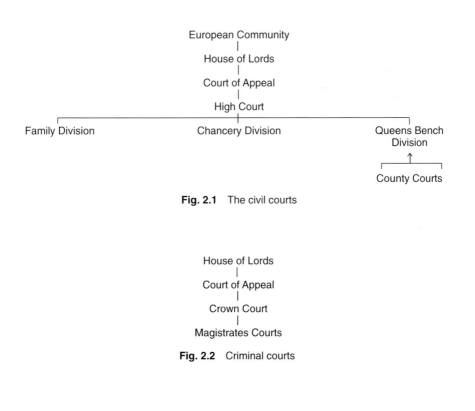

Fig. 2.1   The civil courts

Fig. 2.2   Criminal courts

Industrial tribunal

This forum will hear applications for unfair dismissal and other issues relating to employment. It is intended to be speedy, informal and cheap, where the man in the street could present his application or defend himself. Unfortunately, as employment law has become more complex, it is likely that most parties will be legally represented thus increasing the costs and adding to the complexity of the cases.

Other tribunals

Many tribunals have been created for specific purposes such as Planning Tribunals, Rent Tribunals, Social Security Tribunals. Mental Health Review Tribunals.

LEGAL PERSONNEL

There are two distinct professions for lawyers: barristers and solicitors. They used to have more distinctive roles but gradually the distinction is weakening. They now have a common first part of training: a law degree or the successful completion of the common professional examination. Then solicitors take the Legal Practice Course, study in articles with a firm of solicitors and take the Professional Skills Course, whilst barristers take the examinations of the Council for Legal Education and become pupils in a set of chambers where barristers work on a self-employed basis. It used to be the rule that barristers took the case in court, being briefed by a solicitor to undertake the case and clients would not approach a barrister direct but only through a solicitor. However the rights of solicitors to present cases in court has gradually been extended to cover most cases and courts providing they have a recognised status and training as a solicitor advocate.

In addition there are the judges who decide on issues of fact and law in civil cases and magistrates courts and issues of law in crown court cases and, servicing the court functions and ensuring they run smoothly, a host of clerks and ushers.

THE PROCEDURE

There are significant differences between the progress of a civil case and a criminal case.

In a criminal prosecution the burden of proof is on the prosecution to establish beyond reasonable doubt that the accused is guilty of the criminal offence with which he has been charged.

In civil proceedings it is usually the task of the person bringing the claim to prove, on a balance of probabilities, that the elements of the civil action which is being brought are established.

It is possible for an action to be both a civil wrong and a criminal act. If criminal proceedings are being brought, there are advantages to a plaintiff (the person bringing a civil action) to await the outcome before initiating the civil action. For example, if a therapist was injured in a road accident and the police made it known that criminal charges were being brought against the other driver, then, if they succeed, there is unlikely to be any necessity for civil proceedings: the insurance company will accept liability in the civil action. (If it is shown beyond all reasonable doubt that the accused was guilty of careless or dangerous driving, then it follows that he or she must, on a balance of probabilities, have been in breach of a duty of care (see Chapter 3) owed to the plaintiff.)

THE LEGAL LANGUAGE

Many different terms are being used which have a special legal significance. Often the law appears to be forbidding because of this unfamiliarity with the language. Every effort must be made to become familiar with some of the terms so that the language is not allowed to become a hurdle to a full understanding of the law. Most of the legal terms which are used in this textbook can be found in the Glossary. Readers might find it helpful to add to this list where necessary.

LAW AND ETHICS

One of the most perplexing issues for the practitioner is the distinction between law and ethics: where one begins and one ends and where do practitioners stand if they hold ethical views which are contrary to the law.

The law as we have seen from the first section above is based on the statute law or common law. Ideally it should conform to moral views of what is right and wrong. However there will be situations where the law is narrower than what is considered morally correct. For example there is no law which makes it illegal for a therapist to have an affair with a client who is a mentally competent adult. Such a liaison could not therefore be followed by criminal proceedings. Most therapists would, however, see such conduct as being unethical and not acceptable practice and most organisations involved in complementary therapy with self-regulating provisions would consider it contrary to their Codes of Ethical Practice. Professional conduct proceedings could be brought against a member transgressing in this way who could be removed from the membership.

In contrast to park on double yellow lines is illegal but not everyone would see this act as immoral or unethical. Indeed some therapists may see it as justified in certain emergency circumstances.

What is ethically right to an individual depends upon their cultural and ethnic background and their upbringing and religious views. It is a very personal matter.

There could be occasions where the law permits an activity which is seen by some to be immoral. One example of this is a termination of pregnancy. In this instance the law itself recognises the dilemma and the Abortion Act 1967 provides a conscientious objection clause which enables a practitioner to refuse to participate in a termination. This does not, however, apply in an emergency situation where serious harm to the mother may occur if the termination is not carried out. There is a similar conscientious objection clause in the Human Fertilisation and Embryology Act 1990.

Two books discuss the dual dimension of law and ethics by looking at specific themes, sometimes taking case studies and comparing them from an ethical and legal perspective. Whilst neither is specifically directed to complementary therapy practice, some of the topics discussed are relevant to the complementary therapy practitioner. The books are:

- *Ethics, Law and Nursing* by Nina Fletcher and Janet Holt (consultant editors Margaret Brazier and John Harris) Manchester University Press, 1995: and
- *Nursing Law and Ethics* (edited by John Tingle and Alan Cribb) Blackwell Science, 1995.

They both cover some of the general chapters to be found in this book, e.g. the law relating to consent to treatment and the law relating to confidentiality.

Professional issues, ethics and the law

The Codes issued by the various complementary therapy associations are not the law (see above), but they are part of what would be considered to be ethical practice. Complementary therapy practitioners might find that there is a conflict in instructions which they receive from their clients and the standards they are expected to follow in complying with their professional association code of practice. There may be special circumstances but generally failure to conform to the Code could lead to disciplinary action being brought against that member, and this could ultimately lead to dismissal from the association and from any register of members held by that association.

Questions and Exercises

1. Draw up a list of legal jargon which you encounter in your reading. Use the Glossary and/or a dictionary to familiarise yourself with the meanings. Refresh your memory from time to time.
2. Using a reasonably informative newspaper, identify the cases which are reported, noting what is the nature of the court (civil, criminal, tribunal etc.), who is conducting the case, who are the parties to the case, and what is the point at issue.
3. What would be the advantages and disadvantages of having a single legal profession combining both barristers and solicitors?
4. Major reforms of the legal process are being discussed to ensure justice is done and also seen to be done. The debate is on-going. Keep a file of cuttings relating to the proposals for change.
5. What rights do you consider should be given primary status in a Bill of Rights?

REFERENCES

1. Bolam *v.* Friern Hospital Management Committee [1957] 2 All ER 118

3

Negligence

A SAFE PRACTICE?

It is a claim of many practitioners and therapists in complementary therapies that, in contrast with orthodox medicine, their activities are safe and they do not have side effects. Many consider that negligence actions are extremely unlikely and it is true that at present insurance premiums are low reflecting the fact that few legal actions for negligence are commenced in relation to complementary therapy practice. However this may be only a temporary phenomenon and, as interest and practice in an ever widening sphere of complementary therapy grows, so will litigation. In addition, those who praise the lack of harm caused by the practice of their particular sphere of complementary therapy would emphasise that this is when a competent practitioner is providing the service. There is always scope for harm to be caused by non-competent persons and for competent persons to act negligently or even recklessly thereby causing harm to the client. One of the features of complementary therapy is that there are few laws which prevent an unqualified person setting up practice as a complementary therapist.

CIVIL ACTIONS

These include those actions which are brought in the civil courts by an individual or organisation, usually with the aim of obtaining compensation or other remedy which the court is able to order. The main group of civil actions are called torts i.e. civil wrongs excluding breach of contract. Within the group of civil actions called torts are included: negligence, trespass, breach of statutory duty, defamation, nuisance and others. In each case the burden will usually be upon the person bringing the action (known as the plaintiff) to establish on a balance of probabilities the elements which must be established in that cause of action. Thus in an action for trespass to the person (see Chapter 9) the plaintiff must show that there was

- a direct interference or touching of his/her person,
- without his/her consent or other lawful justification.

PRINCIPLES OF NEGLIGENCE

Negligence is the most common civil action, brought in situations where the plaintiff alleges that there has been personal injury (mental as well as physical) or death, or damage to or loss of property. Compensation is sought for the loss which has occurred. To succeed in the action, the plaintiff has to show the following elements:

- that the defendant owed to the person harmed a duty of care
- that the defendant was in breach of that duty
- that the breach of duty caused reasonably foreseeable
- harm to the plaintiff.

These four elements, duty, breach, causation and harm, are discussed below.

Duty of care

The law recognises that a duty of care will exist where one person can reasonably foresee that his or her actions and omissions could cause reasonably foreseeable harm to another person. A duty of care will always exist between the therapist and the client, but it might not always be easy to identify what it includes. For example, would a complementary therapist have a duty of care to advise a client that her daughter may be suffering from a specific disorder which required attention by an orthodox medical practitioner.

Situation 1   The extent of the duty of care

A complementary therapist is visiting a client who has just been discharged from hospital and is told that the neighbour has not been seen for a few days and there are concerns about her health. Does the therapist have a duty of care to the neighbour?

Could the therapist in Situation 1 say, 'That person is not my client and so I am not going to take any further action'? It could happen that the neighbour died and the relatives, on hearing that the therapist had been told of possible problems, commenced a civil action for failure to fulfil the duty of care. Would the allegation that a duty of care existed be upheld? There is no decided case on the point, but it is not likely that the courts would recognise the duty of care as existing in relation to potential clients such as the neighbour. The basic principle is that no person has a duty to volunteer help. Legally it is therefore lawful to pass a road accident. It may not, of course, be ethical or moral practice.

If, however, an individual takes on the duty, the law requires him or her to follow a reasonable standard of care in carrying out that duty.

In the leading case of *Donoghue* v. *Stevenson*[1] the House of Lords defined the duty of care owed at common law (i.e. judge made law) as follows:

You must take reasonable care to avoid acts or omissions which you can reasonably foresee would be likely to injure your neighbour. Who then in law is my neighbour? The answer seems to be persons who are so closely and directly affected by my act that I ought reasonably to have them in contemplation as being so affected when I am directing my mind to the acts or omissions which are called in question.

The point at which a duty of care arises for a person practising in complementary therapy would normally be the point at which a referral is accepted or there is an agreement between practitioner and client for services to be provided. However there may be special circumstances where the courts may hold that the duty arises at an earlier point. It is essential in cases of doubt that the complementary therapist should ensure that there is an orthodox health professional who is assuming responsibility for a client in need, particularly where there are doubts over the capacity of the client.

If a complementary therapist visits a client in what circumstances does the therapist have a duty of care to the carer of that client? This would be answered in law on the basis of the principles set out above laid down in the *Donoghue* v. *Stevenson* case. The answer is likely to be that there would be no duty in law to volunteer help. It may, however, be part of the advice and the care offered to the client that the needs of any carer are taken into account and met.

Breach of duty

In order to determine whether there has been a breach of the duty of care, it will first be necessary to establish the required standard. The courts have used what has become known as the 'Bolam test' to determine the standard of care required by a professional. In the case from which the test took its name[2] the court laid down the following criteria to determine the standard of care which should be followed:

The standard of care expected is the standard of the ordinary skilled man exercising and professing to have that special skill (McNair, page 121)

The Bolam test was applied by the House of Lords in a case[3] where negligence by an obstetrician in delivering a child by forceps was alleged:

When you get a situation which involves the use of some special skill or competence, then the test as to whether there has been negligence or not ... is the standard of the ordinary skilled man exercising and professing to have that special skill. If a surgeon failed to measure up to that in any respect (clinical judgment or otherwise) he had been negligent and should be so adjudged.

The House of Lords found that the surgeon was not liable in negligence and held that an error of judgment may or may not be negligence. It depends upon the circumstances.

This standard of the reasonable professional man following the accepted approved standard of care can be used to apply to any professional person, architect, lawyer or accountant, as well as any health professional. The standard of care which a complementary therapist should have provided would be judged in this way. Expert witnesses would give evidence to the court on the standard of care they would expect to have found in the circumstances of the case. These experts would be respected members of the same profession as the defendant whose practice is under attack, possibly the president or chairman of the association, a lecturer from an educational institution, or another person well established in that particular area of practice.

In a civil action, the judge would decide, in the light of the evidence which has been given to the court, what standard should have been followed. There is therefore, in a sense, a peer review subject to the overall approval of the judge. Clearly it would not be appropriate to judge an osteopath, for example, by the standard of a registered medical practitioner. An osteopath would be judged by the standard of an osteopath.

Case 1   An abscess after ear piercing[4]

A woman went to a jeweller to have her ears pierced, and 12 days after the piercing she felt a pain in her neck. An abscess developed which had to be operated upon and the operation left a small scar. She claimed compensation.

The court held that:

If a person wants to ensure that the operation of piercing her ears is going to be carried out with that proportion of skill and so forth that a Fellow of the Royal College of Surgeons would use, she must go to a surgeon. If she goes to a jeweller, she must expect that he will carry it out in the way that one would expect a jeweller to carry it out. One would expect that he would wash his instruments. One would expect that he would take some means of disinfecting his instrument, just in the same way as one knows that the ordinary layman, when he is going to use a needle to prick a blister or prick a little gathering on a finger, generally takes the precaution to put the needle in a flame...

The jeweller was held not to have been negligent.

This was a case in 1938; clearly the standards of care, including those of jewellers and those practising complementary therapies, will rise over time.

Differing experts

Experts can, of course, differ and a case may arise where the expert giving evidence for the plaintiff (i.e. the person bringing the action) states that the accepted approved standard of care was not followed by the defendant or, it being sued vicariously (see below), the employees. In contrast the expert evidence for the defendant states that the defendant or the employees followed a reasonable standard of care. Where such a conflict arises the House of Lords has laid down the following principle:

> It was not sufficient to establish negligence for the plaintiff to show that there was a body of competent professional opinion that considered the decision was wrong, if there was also a body of equally competent professional opinion that supported the decision as having been reasonable in the circumstances.[5]

Other difficulties

Once it has been established what the reasonable standard of care should have been, the next stage is to decide whether what took place was in accordance with that reasonable standard, i.e. has there been a breach of the standard. Evidence will be given by witnesses of fact as to what actually took place. The role of witnesses is considered in Chapter 14.

What if the particular field of practice is not considered to have professional status? What if the therapy is a holistic one, where treatments are given subjectively on the basis of a wide range of criteria including emotional as well as physical factors. Some therapies such as homeopathy do not necessarily have a 'standard practice', intuitive factors would determine what the individual therapist would recommend. In such circumstances can there be any standard that matches up with the Bolam test?

This absence of clear objective standard setting in some therapies would make it very difficult to establish any breach of the duty of care by the therapist. In contrast in other therapies such as acupuncture or aromatherapy standards, for example in relation to hygienic practice, may be more easily determined.

Difficulties could also arise where there are different schools covering a particular therapy. It would be reasonable, however, for the practice of individual therapists to be measured against the stated standard of the school which they professed to follow. Experts from that school should be able to advise the parties on the standard that they would expect to have been followed.

Specific examples of possible negligence by individual therapists are given in Section 2 of this book describing the specific therapies.

Causation

Plaintiffs must show that not only was there a breach of the duty of care, but that this breach of duty caused them actual and reasonably foreseeable harm. This requires both:

- factual causation to be shown, and also
- evidence that the type of harm which occurred was reasonably foreseeable.

Factual causation

There may be a breach of the duty of care and harm but there may be no link between them. The classic case which illustrates this point is that of *Barnett* v. *Chelsea Hospital Management Committee*.[6]

Case 2 Arsenic poisoning

Three night watchmen drank tea which made them vomit. They went to the casualty department of the local hospital. The casualty officer, on being told of the complaints by a nurse, did not see the men, but told them to go home and call in their own doctors. Some hours later one of them died from arsenical poisoning. The hospital was sued for negligence by the widow of one of the men.

The court held that:

1. The casualty department officers owed a duty of care in the circumstances.
2. The casualty doctor had been negligent in not seeing them.
3. However, even if he had seen them, it was improbable that the only effective antidote could have been administered in time to save the deceased.
4. Therefore the defendants were not liable. The patient would have died anyway.

The onus is on the plaintiff to establish that there is this causal link between the breach of the duty of care and the harm which occurred.

The case of *Wilsher* v. *Essex Area Health Authority*[7] tragically illustrates the difficulties associated with causation.

Case 3 Problems of proving causation

A premature baby was being treated with oxygen therapy. A junior doctor mistakenly inserted the catheter to monitor the oxygen intake into the vein rather than an artery. A senior registrar when being asked to check what had been done failed to notice the error. The baby was given excess oxygen. The parents claimed compensation for the retrolental fibroplasia that the baby suffered.

The parents failed to prove that it was the excess oxygen which had caused the harm. They therefore failed to prove their claim outright. It was agreed that there were several different factors which could have caused the child to become blind and the negligence was only one of them. It could not been have presumed that it was the defendant's negligence which had caused the harm. Ten years after the event the House of Lords ordered the case to be reheard on the issue of causation.

It has also been difficult for claimants to establish causation when suing for compensation for harm which it is claimed has resulted from vaccine damage. In the case of *Loveday* v. *Renton and another*[8] a case was brought against the Wellcome Foundation who made vaccine against whooping cough, and against the doctor who administered it, seeking compensation for brain damage which was alleged to have been caused by the vaccine. The case failed because the judge held that the plaintiff had not established, on a balance of probabilities, that the pertussis vaccine had caused the brain damage.

Subsequently however in an Irish case brought against the Wellcome Foundation and others for vaccine damage[9] it has been held that causation as well as breach was established and this enabled the plaintiff in this case to obtain compensation. The facts were that the High Court had dismissed the plaintiff's claim because of the lack of proof of causation. However the Irish Supreme Court held that the Wellcome Foundation was liable for the negligent manufacture and release of a particular batch of triple vaccine and that the brain damage was caused as a result. It referred the case back to the High Court on the amount of compensation. On May 11 1993 the High Court approved an award of £2.75 million as compensation for the brain damage sustained in September 1969, an unusually large compensation payment because it covered the costs of keeping a brain damaged person for life.

Reasonably foreseeable harm

The harm which might arise may not be within the reasonable contemplation of the defendant so that, even though there is a breach of duty and there is harm, the defendant is not liable.

For example a therapist may have failed to check on certain sensitivities of a patient to essential oils, but the client may have been harmed because she failed to notify the aromatherapist that she was also taking some orthodox medication which contraindicated the essential oils. In such a case the complementary therapist may have been in breach of the duty of care, but the client might have suffered the harm because of the medication of which she failed to inform the therapist.

New intervening cause

It may also happen that any causal link between the therapist's breach of duty and the harm suffered by the client is interrupted by an intervening event. For example, a therapist may have failed to undertake an appropriate assessment prior to treating the client, but, following the session, the client drives her car negligently thus causing harm to herself. The negligent driving has interrupted any causal effect of the therapist's failure to carry out an appropriate assessment.

Causation in complementary therapy

Whilst in some fields a causal connection can be established between the activities of the therapist and the impact on the client, e.g. aromatherapy and hypnotherapy, in others, such as healing, it is more difficult to establish a causative element. It would therefore be difficult for plaintiffs to prove that any harm they suffered is the result of a breach of duty of such a therapist.

Harm

To succeed in an action for negligence plaintiffs or their representatives must establish that they have suffered harm which the court recognises as being subject to compensation. Thus personal injury, death, loss or damage to property are the main areas of recognisable harm. In addition the courts have ruled that nervous shock (known as post traumatic stress syndrome), where an identifiable medical condition exists, can be the subject of compensation within strict limits of liability. A test of proximity to the defendant's negligent action or omission has been set by the House of Lords.[10]

Some of the types of harm that can be considered the effects of personal injury are illustrated below in the section showing how compensation is calculated.

Again, as it is not always easy to show benefit from a complementary therapy, so it may also be difficult for plaintiffs to establish that any harm which they suffer is the result of the actions of the therapist.

VICARIOUS LIABILITY

Vicarious liability is the principle whereby the employer of a negligent person can, in certain circumstances, be sued for injury caused by their employee's negligence. To establish the vicarious liability of the employer the plaintiff must show that:

- the employee
- was negligent (or was guilty of another wrong)
- whilst acting in course of employment.

Therapists as employees/independent contractors

All complementary therapists who are self-employed are responsible personally if any harm should befall the client as the result of their activities. However, where a therapist is employed by a GP for example, or by another therapist or organisation, then that employer would be considered to be vicariously liable for the fault of the employee. It is therefore very important to identify the nature of the relationship between such persons. A GP may refer patients to an aromatherapist (as an example, but the same principles apply to all other therapists) on two different bases:

1. The aromatherapist may remain an independent practitioner and the referral will therefore come to him or her as a contract for services with the GP. The GP will pay for the service on the basis of so many treatments and the aromatherapist will provide those services as an independent contractor. Should harm befall the client as the result of the activities of the aromatherapist, then the aromatherapist would be liable as a self-employed independent contractor. Such independent contractors must therefore have their own professional indemnity insurance cover.

2. The GP may employ the aromatherapist on a sessional basis. The aromatherapist undertakes the care of clients, having that work delegated to him or her. In this case the GP would be vicariously liable for any harm arising from the work of the aromatherapist.

It is usually clear whether a contract of service (i.e. a contract of employment exists) or whether there is a contract for services (i.e. the individual is a self-employed independent contractor), but there are advantages in a therapist clarifying this at the beginning of any contract. Recently, as an example, the courts have held that the doctor to the Tottenham Hotspur football club was not an employee, since he was engaged as an independent contractor supplying medical expertise who was paid fees rather than a salary.[11]

Therapists as employers

Independent practitioners have to accept personal liability for their actions but they may also be vicariously liable for the harm, caused during the course of employment, by anyone they employ. Each of the elements shown above must be established so that:

- The employer is not liable for the acts of his independent contractors, i.e. self-employed persons who are working for him on a contract for services, unless he is at fault in selecting or instructing them.
- The employer may challenge whether the actions in question were performed in the course of employment.

In the course of employment

If a complementary therapist is employed on a sessional basis by an NHS trust there may be a dispute as to whether the activities were all undertaken as a consequence of that employment or whether some of the activities, and specifically those which caused harm to the client, were incurred as a result of activities outside the course of employment.

The therapist may also undertake additional therapies which are not part of the employment and there may be doubt as to whether these activities would be considered to be in the course of employment so that, if the therapist were negligent, the employer would be vicariously liable for this negligence.

It is not possible to generalise since each case depends upon its particular circumstances. Some help would be provided from the contract drawn up between the employer and the therapist over the provision of services. It does not follow, however, that disobeying instructions of the employer would automatically take the work outside the contract of employment.

Liability of referring doctors

Does the referring doctor remain vicariously liable and responsible for the actions of the complementary therapist?

Stephen Dorrell, then Parliamentary Secretary for Health, emphasised in a press statement in December 1991 that

The GP remains clinically accountable for the care offered by the complementary therapist. It is not a 'referral' system, whereby one registered practitioner refers a patient for treatment by another. It is a 'delegation' system, where the GP asks another professional to provide care for which he remains clinically accountable. It is therefore for the individual GP to decide in the case of each individual patient whether the alternative therapist offers the most appropriate care to treat that patient's condition.[12]

This statement is subject to dispute and is contrary to the principles of vicarious liability. It is submitted that GPs would be directly liable if they act negligently in referring a patient either to a specific therapist, e.g. one known to be removed from a list of approved practitioners, or to an inappropriate therapy. GPs would be indirectly or vicariously liable if they actually employed the therapist whose negligence caused harm to a patient. Where, however, a GP acts appropriately in referring a patient to a therapist for that particular therapy and that individual is self-employed, then there is no direct liability and in law the principle of vicarious liability would not apply.

DEFENCES TO AN ACTION

The main defences to an action for negligence are shown in Box 3.1.

Box 3.1   Defences to an action for negligence

- Dispute on facts and allegations
- Denial that all elements of negligence are established
- Contributory negligence
- Exemption from liability
- Limitation of time
- Voluntary assumption of risk

Dispute on facts and allegations

Many cases will be resolved entirely on what facts can be shown to exist. Thus the effectiveness of the witnesses for both parties in establishing the facts of what did or did not occur will be a determining factor in who wins the case. Reference should be made to Chapter 14 on record keeping and on witnesses in court for further discussion on the nature of evidence and the role of the witnesses.

Denial that negligence is established

The plaintiff must establish that all the elements required to prove negligence are present, i.e. duty, breach, causation and harm. If one or more of these cannot be established then the defendant will win the case.

As explained above the plaintiff may have considerable difficulty in establishing what should have been the standard of care in a particular complementary therapy and that this standard was not followed, and also in establishing a causal link between any breach of such a duty of care and harm suffered.

Contributory negligence

If the client is partly to blame for the harm which has occurred then there may still be liability on the part of the professional but the compensation payable might be reduced in proportion to the client's fault. In extreme cases such a claim may be a complete defence if 100% contributory negligence is established. In determining the level of contributory negligence, the physical and mental health and the age of the client would be taken into account.

> **Situation 2** Contributory negligence
>
> A therapist in taking a personal history asks a client about her family but does not specifically ask if she is pregnant. The therapist also asks if the client is suffering from any specific health problems. The client states that she is not. The therapist gives the client treatment which is contraindicated for pregnant women. The client suffers a miscarriage.

In this situation, there has probably been a failure of the duty of care in that the therapist failed to ask if the client was pregnant. If the client knew of this fact, and failed to make the therapist aware of it, it could be argued that there is contributory negligence on the part of the client. If she were therefore to sue the therapist for negligence in causing the miscarriage, any compensation she claimed may be reduced according to her responsibility for that loss.

The Law Reform (Contributory Negligence) Act 1945 enables an apportionment of responsibility for the harm which has been caused which may result in a reduction of damages payable. The Court can reduce the damages 'to such extent as it thinks just and equitable having regard to the claimant's share in the responsibility for the damage' (section 1(1)).

One of the most frequent examples of contributory negligence being taken into account is in road traffic accidents where the injuries sustained by the plaintiff are the greater because the plaintiff was not wearing a seat belt.

If the therapist has given specific instructions to the client on any follow-up action or treatment to be taken and the client fails to observe those instructions then there will be a clear case of contributory negligence. However the therapist may have difficulty in establishing that this information was in fact given. There are strong arguments in favour of written information being given to the client and for a record to be kept that this was done (see Chapter 9).

Exemption from liability

It is possible for people to exempt themselves from liability for harm arising from their negligence but the effects of the Unfair Contract Terms Act 1977 mean that this exemption only applies to loss or damage to property. A defendant cannot exclude liability for negligence which results in personal injury or death, either by contract or by a notice.

Where exemption from liability for loss or damage to property is claimed by the defendant, it must be shown by the defendant that it is reasonable to rely upon the term or notice which purported to exclude liability. The provisions of the Unfair Contract Terms Act 1977 are shown in Box 3.2.

The significance of this provision for complementary therapists is that, if a therapist acts negligently and causes harm to a client, the therapist cannot rely on any document which he had asked a client to sign whereby the client agreed that any treatment would be at the client's own risk. On the other hand if the therapist places a notice in a waiting room that any possessions are left at the owner's risk and the

---

Box 3.2 Unfair Contract Terms Act 1977

Section 2
   (1) A person cannot by reference to any contract term or to a notice given to persons generally or to particular persons exclude or restrict his liability for death or personal injury resulting from negligence.
   (2) In the case of other loss or damage, a person cannot so exclude or restrict his liability for negligence except in so far as the term or notice satisfies the requirement of reasonableness.

Section 11
   (3) In relation to a notice (not being a notice having contractual effect) the requirement of reasonableness under this Act is that it should be fair and reasonable to allow reliance on it, having regard to all the circumstances obtaining when the liability arose or (but for the notice) would have arisen.
   (5) It is for those claiming that a contract term or notice satisfies the requirement of reasonableness to show that it does.

---

client subsequently loses a briefcase, then it may be reasonable for the therapist to rely on that notice to deny responsibility for the missing object. It would be for the therapist to show that it was reasonable to rely on the exclusion notice.

Limitation of time

Actions for personal injury or death should normally be commenced within three years of the date of the event which gave rise to the harm or three years from the date on which the person had the necessary knowledge of the harm and the fact that it arose from the defendant's actions or omissions. There are however some major qualifications to this general principle and these are shown in Box 3.3.

Box 3.3 Situations where time limits can be extended

---

1. Those suffering from a disability.
   - Children under 18 years – the time does not start to run until the child is 18 years.
   - Those suffering from a mental disability – time does not start to run until the disability ends.
   In the case of those who are suffering from severe learning disabilities this may not be until death.
2. Discretion of the judge. The judge has a statutory power to extend the time within which a plaintiff can bring an action for personal injuries or death, if it is just and equitable to do so.

   The implications of the rules relating to limitation of time is that, in those cases which might come under one of the exceptions to the three year time limit, records should be kept and not destroyed. This is particularly important in the case of children and those with learning disabilities. For example in the case of *Bull* v. *Wakeham*[13] the case was brought 18 years after the birth. In a news item report in 1995[14] a man, then 33 years old, obtained compensation of £1.25 million because of a failure to diagnose severe dehydration a few weeks after birth. Like the vaccine case referred to above, the compensation may seem to be for a large sum but this is because of the cost of care (see on quantum below).

Voluntary assumption of risk

Volenti non fit injuria is the Latin tag for the defence that the person willingly undertook the risk of being harmed. It is unlikely to succeed as a defence in an action for professional negligence since the professional cannot contract out of liability where harm occurs as a result of her negligence (see the Unfair Contract Terms Act which is considered above). However it may be relevant to the therapist who undertakes risky activities with a client, such as new treatments or physical activities. Such activities may have an element of danger about them and, if the risks are explained to the client and the client has the competence to take upon themselves the risk of harm arising, then this may be a successful defence. However where the client lacks the mental competence to make such a decision, then there is a duty of care placed upon the therapist to take all reasonable care according to the Bolam test that harm would not occur.

CALCULATION OF COMPENSATION (QUANTUM)

In some cases of negligence, liability might be admitted (i.e. the defendant accepts responsibility for a negligent act or omission causing harm), but there might be disagreement between the parties over the quantum of damages (i.e. the amount of compensation). In other cases, there might be agreement over the amount of compensation that would be payable but liability is denied. In others, liability and quantum might both be in dispute.

Expert witnesses are frequently required to give evidence of assessment in cases where there is a dispute over quantum. This is further discussed in Chapter 14.

The principle which the courts apply in trying to assess the amount of compensation due to a victim who has suffered personal injuries as a result of negligence on the part of another is to attempt, so far as possible, to put the victim into the position she would have been in had the negligent act not occurred. The money compensation paid is calculated under two categories, 'general damages' and 'special damages'.

General damages

The general damages represent an attempt, so far as it is possible, to compensate a person who has suffered personal injury for their pain and suffering and any continuing loss of amenity and pleasure in life. Judges are guided in this impossible task by precedent – looking at what has been awarded in similar cases (see Chapter 2) – and in recent years by tariff tables published by the Lord Chancellor's Department. Each case is, however, still judged very much on its individual facts. A keen young amateur sportsman left with a limp would be awarded more for loss of amenity than would a more elderly sedentary person.

Special damages

Special damages are intended to reimburse and make future provision for the additional costs and loss which the victim has incurred and will continue to incur as a result of the injuries. They require special proof and will not be presumed to follow from the magistrate. Factors to be taken into account are loss of earnings (both past and future, taking into consideration any disadvantage on the job market resulting from the injuries) and the cost of special equipment and care.

As seen from the cases mentioned above, ensuring adequate compensation can give rise to awards in excess of £1 million and in contested cases experts ranging from accountants to occupational therapists will be called to assist the parties with their arguments before the court.

Deductions are made from damages in respect of payments from the Social Security.

SPECIAL SITUATIONS

Failure in communication

Failures in communication can also give rise to liability in negligence should the therapist fail to pass on information or if she has failed to communicate with other health professionals or the client and carers appropriately. An understanding of practitioner/client and practitioner/practitioner interaction is therefore essential to ensure real communication.

This principle also applies where the therapist gives advice expecting it to be relied upon. Should the person receiving that advice act upon it, and as a consequence suffer harm, then the therapist could be held liable for that harm.[15]

Failure to obtain the full information about a referral can cause many problems for the therapist, but it would not always be possible to adhere rigidly to a rule which states that the referral will be refused if the full information is not supplied. This is an issue which is covered by individual Codes of ethics and practice of specific complementary therapy organisations.

What is the situation in the case of a self-referral where the client is not prepared either to allow the therapist to make contact with her doctor or to give full information about her previous history to the therapist? In such circumstances, the therapist should make it clear to the client, that unless there is contact with the client's doctor over pre-existing medical conditions and existing treatment the therapist cannot fulfil the duty of care owed to the client according to the approved standard of care. Ultimately the therapist could advise that it would be hazardous to treat the client without the full information and therefore may have to refuse the referral. The therapist should of course make every effort to discover what the reasons are for the client's objection to the information being passed on. The therapist should also be able to reassure her over the standards of confidentiality.

Not all complementary therapies covered in this book would see themselves as related to orthodox medical practice in the way discussed above. For these a Code of practice would impose no necessity to ensure any contact with an orthodox medicine practitioner.

Negligent advice

There can be liability for negligence in giving advice but plaintiffs would have to show that it was clear at the outset they that would rely upon the advice, that they had done so and that in so doing they had suffered reasonably foreseeable loss or harm.

Therapeutic advice

The therapist has a duty to take care in advising the client. Failure to give proper and full advice (including discussion of any risks involved) can invalidate the client's consent to treatment and give rise to liability (see Chapter 9).

References

Liability for advice is not limited to the obvious therapist/client relationship and duty of care; a different example can be seen from the following situation.

Situation 3   Negligent reference
A therapist is asked to provide a reference for a patient who has a mental health problem. The patient asks the therapist not to refer to the history of mental illness. What is the position if the therapist gives the reference without mentioning the mental illness, the patient obtains the post and then the employer blames the therapist for an inaccurate reference which has led to harm?

If the mental health of the patient should have been mentioned in a reference the therapist could be liable to the employer for negligent advice. In such circumstances, she should either have refused to give a reference, or should have told the patient that if she gave a reference it would have to include a mention of the mental illness. This is a difficult area since many persons who have suffered mental ill-health may find that they are discriminated against without justification.

On the other hand, there can also be liability to the person on whose behalf the reference is given, if the reference is written without reasonable care and if financial loss occurs to the person as a result of potential employers relying upon the reference.[16] Thus a person who has been asked to provide a reference has a duty of care to both the subject of the reference and also the recipient of the reference. Every care should be taken to ensure that it is written accurately in the light of the facts available.

Supervision and delegation

Exactly the same principles of care apply to the delegation and supervision of tasks as to the therapist carrying out the activities directly. The therapist delegating a task, should only do so if she is reasonably sure that the person to whom she is delegating is reasonably competent and experienced to undertake that activity safely for the care of the patient. At the same time, she must ensure that the person undertaking that activity has the level of supervision which is sufficient to ensure that she is reasonably safe in carrying out that delegated activity.

Should harm befall a client because an activity was carried out by a junior member of staff, a student or an assistant, it is no defence to the client to argue that the harm occurred because that person did not have the ability, competence or experience to carry out that task reasonably safely.[17]

Liability of a volunteer

Where a therapist is volunteering services and not charging for them there would not be a contract. However, the therapist would still owe a duty of care to any client who suffers harm as a result of negligence on the part of the therapist. It is therefore important for therapists to obtain insurance cover, even for voluntary activities.

Care of property

Failure to look after another person's property could lead to a civil action for negligence in causing harm to property. In an action for negligence, the person who has suffered the loss or damage of property must as plaintiff establish the same four elements which must be shown in a claim for compensation for personal injury, i.e. duty, breach, causation and harm.

Where, however, property is specifically left in the care of a particular person (the bailee) then, should the property be lost or damaged, the burden would be on the bailee to establish how that occurred without fault on his or her part. It should be noted that liability for loss or damage to property can be excluded if such an exclusion is reasonable (see the Unfair Contract Terms Act above).

Documentation

In every area of practice it is essential to ensure that comprehensive clear records are kept in the interests of client care and also for the defence of the therapist in the event of any dispute or complaint. Reference should be made to Chapter 14 on record keeping.

WEAKNESSES OF THE PRESENT SYSTEM

The potential plaintiff faces several difficulties. Some of the problems in establishing the standard of care or causation in complementary therapies have already been pointed out. In addition a would-be litigant faces all the other hurdles and obstacles faced by any patient pursuing a case involving orthodox health care practice.

Financial problems

The plaintiff may not meet the legal aid criteria for having financial assistance to bring a case. The Government has recently approved the system of conditional fees being introduced into the UK. The plaintiff is able effectively to negotiate with a solicitor payment on a 'no win – no fee' basis, i.e. if the plaintiff loses the solicitor does not charge any fees. Costs of the successful defendant would still be owing, and suggestions are being made for insurance protection to meet these and other costs not covered by the agreement with the solicitor.

Although litigation in relation to personal injury and death is increasing in this country, the Woolf Report (see below) showed the difficulties faced by many litigants in achieving success. Cost, complexity, slowness, and time delays caused by the system of expert witnesses all deter potential claimants.

Problems of proof

These are numerous. There may simply be the difficulty of establishing the facts of the case if it becomes a matter of the patient's word against that of the therapist. Even if a breach of a duty of care is established there are the further problems of proving that the harm that has arisen was actually caused by the negligent act or omission on the part of the defendant (see the Wilsher case above). At all stages, moreover, the court may be faced with the difficulty of receiving conflicting expert evidence in which case, as mentioned above, the doubt is resolved in favour of the defendant.[18]

SOURCES OF ADVICE FOR AN AGGRIEVED CLIENT

Formal complaints procedures Most therapists who belong to recognised organisations are required to abide by a Code of Practice or Conduct and this will set out a complaints procedure. Chapter 12 considers complaints procedures generally and details of the individual organisations are covered in Section 2 of this book. There is often considerable value in the client pursuing a complaint through the established procedure, including the use of mediation, before beginning litigation. However, should this process prove tardy, the time limits for issuing a writ must not be forgotten.

Community Health Councils Where the services complained about are NHS services, then help is available from the secretary of the local community health council (see Yellow Pages).

Action for Victims of Medical Accidents This well established association which assists several thousand patients who have suffered harm as the result of alleged negligence will also advise persons who have suffered as a result of the activities of complementary therapists. These are at present extremely small in number compared with the orthodox medicine claims, but are likely to increase in line with the growth in popularity of complementary therapies.

Prevention of Professional Abuse Network This organisation provides advice and support for those who have suffered as a result of the conduct of therapists (see Chapter 35).

Citizens' Advice Bureaux Advice can be obtained on how to choose a solicitor and in some districts arrangements with local colleges and student lawyers can enable some basic legal advice to be given about any complaint and potential cause of action.

Government bodies Officers from Trading Standards, Environmental Protection or Health and Safety organisations can provide assistance if there is an allegation of criminal wrong (see Chapters 6 and 13).

THE FUTURE

The Pearson Report and no-fault liability

The present system of obtaining compensation for personal injuries is extremely unsatisfactory. It is slow, expensive, uncertain and by no means ensures that justice is done or seen to be done. However the Royal Commission,[19] which reported in 1978 (the Pearson Report), recommended that we should on the whole retain our present system of proving liability by establishing fault (except in some specific circumstances, e.g. vaccine damage and volunteers in medical research.

Attempts to introduce a no-fault liability system have failed. In this system, as the result of an arrangement between insurance companies, employers and the state, a compensation fund exists from which payment is made to people injured in certain circumstances without needing to prove anyone at fault. The Pearson Report did not recommend no-fault liability in the case of medical accidents, but there are strong calls for its introduction. Sweden, Finland and New Zealand have systems where compensation is paid on the basis of no-fault liability.

An alternative which is being considered by the Department of Health is the introduction of an alternative form of dispute resolution (ADR) such as mediation or arbitration. This would have the advantage of a cheaper, speedier, resolution and there would be much to recommend any system which ensures that money paid out is to the benefit of the person who has suffered the harm, rather than in fees for lawyers, experts and the like.

The Woolf reforms

In June 1995 Lord Woolf, a Lord Justice of Appeal appointed Master of the Rolls in 1996, issued an interim report on *Access to Justice*.[20] This reported on recommendations to change our system of obtaining compensation for personal injuries. It was followed in January 1996 by a consultation document[21] with papers covering the following issues:

1. Fast track
2. Housing
3. Multi-party actions
4. Medical negligence
5. Expert evidence
6. Costs.

Lord Woolf's interim report contained a new procedural framework for civil litigation of which the central feature is a new system of case management with the courts rather than the parties taking the main responsibility for the progress of cases. The fast track paper suggested that defended cases would be allocated for the purposes of case management by the courts to one of three 'tracks':

- small claims (up to £3 000)
- a new fast track with limited procedures and reduced costs (up to £10 000)
- a new multi-track (for more complex cases over £10 000).

However certain exceptions to the fast track were recommended and these included medical negligence cases. The consultation paper on medical negligence cases considers that these should nevertheless benefit from Lord Woolf's proposed reforms on the following grounds:

- More informative pleadings should help to define the real issues at an earlier stage and speed up the progress of cases.
- Case management should encourage a less adversarial approach and enable cases to settle on appropriate terms at an earlier stage.
- Extended summary judgment provisions may help prevent unmeritorious cases being pursued or defended too long.
- Improved training and greater specialisation should help judges to identify weak cases, narrow and determine issues and limit the scope of evidence.
- More use of split trials will limit unnecessary work on quantum in cases where liability is in issue and may not be proved.
- Greater emphasis on early definition of issues between experts should encourage a less adversarial approach and reduce cost and delay. The recommendations relating to expert witnesses are discussed in Chapter 14.

The final report from Lord Woolf,[22] following consultation, was published in the summer of 1996. The changes are expected to be implemented in October 1998. Any further new legislation should consider the extent to which the present tort system of obtaining compensation is appropriate to the field of complementary therapy or whether alternative systems should be encouraged.

The NHS litigation authority

In the meantime a new litigation authority has been set up for the NHS.[23] From the 20 November 1995 the NHS litigation authority is responsible for the establishment and the administration of the scheme for meeting liabilities of health service bodies to third parties for loss, damage or injury arising out of the exercise of their functions. The NHS litigation authority does not cover liabilities for practitioners in complementary therapies unless the alleged harm arose from their work as employees within the NHS. It may be that if litigation amongst complementary therapists increases, then new schemes of cooperation between the various organisations and associations may be of value.

Questions and Exercises

1. Explain the difference between vicarious liability and personal liability.
2. Take any situation where harm nearly occurred to a client, and work out what the client would have had to prove to obtain compensation if he had suffered an injury.
3. How would you define the reasonable standard of care in relation to any chosen treatment provided by yourself?
4. Prepare a protocol to ensure safe delegation to and supervision of an assistant.

REFERENCES

1. Donoghue *v.* Stevenson [1932] AC 562
2. Bolam *v.* Friern Hospital Management Committee [1957] 1 WLR 582
3. Whitehouse *v.* Jordan [1981] 1 All ER 267
4. Phillips *v.* William Whitelely Ltd [1938] 1 All ER 566
5. Maynard *v.* W Midlands Regional Health Authority HL [1985] 1 All ER 635
6. Barnett *v.* Chelsea Hospital Management Committee [1968] 1 All ER 1068
7. Wilsher *v.* Essex Area Health Authority HL [1988] 1 All ER 871
8. Times Law Report 31 March 1988
9. Best *v.* Wellcome Foundation and others [1994] 5 Med LR 81 (discussed 1993 Medico Legal Journal 61(3): 178)
10. Alcock *v.* Chief Constable of the South Yorkshire Police [1991] 4 All ER 907
11. Horsnall M Spurs team doctor loses job claim. The Times 18 July 1997
12. Press release Department of Health 3 December 1991
13. Bull *v.* Wakeham Transcript 2 February 1989
14. Laurance J Man handicapped as a baby 33 years ago wins £1.25m. The Times 15 November 1995 p 5
15. Hedley Byrne & Co Ltd *v.* Heller [1964] AC 465
16. Spring *v.* Guardian Assurance PLC and others Times Law Report 8 July 1994
17. Wilsher *v.* Essex Area Health Authority CA [1986] 3 All ER 801
18. Maynard *v.* West Midlands Regional Health Authority HL [1985] 1 All ER 635
19. Pearson 1978 Royal Commission on Civil Liability and Compensation for Personal Injury. HMSO, London (The Pearson Report)
20. Woolf 1995 Interim report on access to justice inquiry. Lord Chancellor's Office, London
21. Woolf January 1996 Access to civil justice inquiry consultation paper. Lord Chancellor's Office, London
22. Woolf July 1996 Access to justice final paper. Lord Chancellor's Office, London
23. National Health Service Litigation Authority (Establishment and Constitution) Order 1995 SI 1995/2800

4

Contract law

In the last chapter, we discussed the law of negligence which is one of a group of civil wrongs known as 'torts'. In this chapter we look at another civil action known as contract which is outside the law of 'torts'.

THE LAW OF CONTRACT

A contract has been defined as 'a legally binding agreement made between two or more persons, by which rights are acquired by one or more to acts or forbearances on the part of the other or others.'[1]

An enforceable contract contains three main elements:

- an agreement
- consideration and
- an intention to create legal relations.

39

Agreement

Invitation to treat

There are several distinct stages which lead to the agreement of a contract. A complementary therapist may, for example, advertise services in the press. This in law would constitute an 'invitation to treat'. It invites persons to make contact to consider whether they could become clients. The therapist would usually (depending on the wording of the advertisement) be completely free to either ignore any response or to follow up any interested persons. This might involve inviting the potential client to the examination rooms, again without obligation. Similarly a therapist may have had a stall at a health fair. Leaflets may be displayed. These leaflets would be part of an invitation to treat, not an offer to provide services. If this were not so, then individuals who pick up leaflets could state that they accepted the offer to provide services and the therapists would then find themselves under a binding agreement since once an offer is accepted the contract comes into being. Therapists would then not be in a position to refuse to provide services to a person they did not trust or had other adverse feelings towards. The fact that the display on the counter or the advertisement (depending on its wording) would be regarded in law as part of the invitation to treat, rather than an offer, is therefore of some protection to the therapist.

Offer

At some subsequent stage the therapist may offer a course of treatment to the client, who then has the opportunity to accept this offer. Alternatively, the client may offer to undertake certain treatment sessions and the therapist agrees to this. It might appear that this lacks any significance. However if there are disputes over whether in fact a contract exists and what has been agreed, it is extremely important in law to establish what was part of the invitation to treat, what constituted the offer and when, if at all, there was an acceptance of the offer. The following legal principles apply to the different stages:

- A request for further information is not an offer.
- An offer can be withdrawn at any time before it is accepted unless it is made subject to being kept open for a specified time.

Acceptance

The following rules apply to an acceptance:

- An acceptance must be on the same terms as that set out in the offer, otherwise it would be regarded as a counter-offer.
- An acceptance must be unconditional and unequivocal.
- The acceptance must be communicated to the offeror (i.e. the person making the offer) unless it is sent by post, in which case the rule is that acceptance takes place as soon as the letter is validly posted.

Once an offer is accepted an agreement comes into existence and this will constitute an enforceable contract if the other elements are present (i.e. consideration and an intention to create legal relations – see below).

An offer cannot be withdrawn once it has been accepted.

The significance of these legal principles can be seen in the following situation.

Situation 1   A binding agreement?

A health centre for complementary therapies advertised its services including aromatherapy. Mrs B wrote asking for a series of aromatherapy sessions. The aromatherapist responded inviting her to come to visit on a specific day. In the meantime the aromatherapist discovered from colleagues at the centre that Mrs B was well known to them and had several unpaid bills outstanding. The aromatherapist when she met Mrs B stated that she would be prepared to undertake aromatherapy on a sessional basis but would require payment before each session commenced. Mrs B stated that she was not prepared to pay in advance and considered that she had a right to receive aromatherapy immediately.

The stages would be seen in law as the following:

- The advertisement by the health centre would be seen as an invitation to treat.
- The request by the aromatherapist for Mrs B to visit would also be part of the invitation to treat.
- The visit by Mrs B could be seen as part of the invitation to treat although Mrs B could argue that it was an offer.
- In this case the aromatherapist would say that the offer was neither acceptable to her nor accepted.
- The aromatherapist's statement that she would provide sessions on payment in advance would be a counter-offer, which was not acceptable to Mrs B.

The conclusion is that there is no binding agreement and therefore no contract between the parties.

Consideration

To create a legally enforceable agreement, there must be consideration. This has been legally defined:

A valuable consideration in the sense of the law, may consist either in some right, interest, profit or benefit accruing to one party, or some forbearance, detriment, loss or responsibility given, suffered or undertaken by the other.[2]

It is important to note that it is not necessary for the consideration to be payment in money. It could therefore be payment in kind: an allergy therapist could agree the exchange of sessions with a reflexologist and this would be seen as consideration for the agreement.

On the other hand if a therapist agreed to give sessions to a neighbour and the neighbour understood that this would be a gift, the neighbour could not enforce the provision of the gift since there was no consideration for this. This would not be so if the therapist drew up a document, signed and witnessed, which undertook to provide the sessions without payment: a promise can be enforced if it is made by way of such a deed. Where a therapist says to a neighbour, 'Since I appreciate your being prepared to provide baby sitting cover for my children, I will give you some sessions without payment', then this would be enforceable, since the baby sitting would count as the consideration. This does not apply if the baby sitting was undertaken in the past: past consideration does not count as consideration for the promise. (NB it may be argued that in a friendly situation there is no intention to create legal relations so an enforceable contract does not come into being in any event – see below.)

Other rules which apply to consideration are:

- The consideration must be recognisable in law as such.
- The consideration does not necessarily have to equate in economic value to the benefit being obtained.
- An already binding obligation cannot constitute consideration.

It must be understood that whilst the lack of consideration may prevent a binding contract arising, this does not mean that there is no duty of care in the law of negligence (see Chapter 3). Thus therapists may provide services for friends without charging but, if harm arises, they (and through them their insurers) could still be sued by those friends).

An intention to create legal relations

This final element necessary for an agreement in law to be recognised as binding, means that both parties must see the agreement as one which has a legal significance. There is a presumption in social and domestic matters that there is no intention to create legal relations: thus, if I promise to give my children pocket money if they tidy their bedrooms, the children cannot take me to court if I fail to pay them the money even when the bedrooms are tidied since the law would presume that there is no intention to create legal relations in such a domestic matter. In contrast in business affairs there is a presumption in favour of the intention to create legal relations and it would be presumed that, where a therapist is offering services to a client, then both would have the intention of creating legal relations. However in both sets of circumstances the presumption can be replaced: thus in domestic matters the parties could provide evidence that the agreement was intended to create legal relations and in business matters the parties could declare that the agreement is not intended to create legal relations.

Where therapists are using their domestic premises to carry on a service, it must be made clear to clients who may be friends or neighbours that, if it is indeed the case, there is an intention to create legal relations.

OTHER FEATURES OF A VALID CONTRACT
Doctrine of privity

Once a contract has been agreed between parties, then the doctrine of privity applies. This is that only the parties to the contract can sue or be sued under the contract, unless one party is acting as the agent of another person. This is the legal background to the case *Donoghue* v. *Stevenson*.[3] The person who suffered shock by seeing the decomposed remains of a snail in the bottle of ginger beer she had been drinking and was ill afterwards, was not the purchaser of the ginger beer, so she could not bring a claim of breach of contract: she had no contract with the seller or manufacturer. This is why she brought her claim in negligence because the duty owed under the law of negligence is wider than that owed under contract law which applies only to the parties to the contract. This case itself extended and redefined the law of negligence.

Formalities

There is no legal obligation for a contract (which is not for the sale of land or an interest in land) to be in writing. Agreements made by word of mouth can, if the essential elements are present, be binding upon the parties. However difficulties can be caused over what was the actual content of the agreement and it may be one party's word against another. There are considerable practical advantages in putting any contract in writing and Box 4.1 sets out a suggested list of what could be included in the agreement.

Box 4.1 List of suggested contents for the agreement

1. Names of the parties
2. Description of the services to be provided
3. Payment to be made and intervals or time of payment, e.g. in advance, arrears, at each session
4. Payment in the event of non-attendance
5. Date for performance
6. Rights to end the agreement
7. Date of the agreement
8. Location of the services
9. Duty of confidentiality
10. Other rights of the client and responsibilities of the therapist set out in any Code of Ethics and Practice of the organisation to which the therapist belongs

---

Obviously it is important that therapists do not frighten clients by placing before them a complex legal document. The list shown in Box 4.1 could be set out in a very simple, easily understood form, with a carbon copy so that both parties have a record. The document could also mention any specific aspects of the therapy of which it is essential that the client is aware (see Chapter 9).

Capacity

To be valid a contract must be agreed between persons who have the capacity to make that agreement. The following categories of persons will be considered: children and mentally ill and those with learning disabilities.

Children

Under the Family Law Reform Act 1969 a person below the age of 18 years is classed as a minor, sometimes known in law as 'an infant'. The law divides agreements entered into by minors in two: contracts which are binding and contracts which are voidable.

Contracts for necessaries The basic principle is that where a minor contracts for necessaries then this is binding upon the minor. Section 3(3) of the Sale of Goods Act 1979 requires an infant to pay a reasonable price for necessaries. Necessaries are goods which are necessary, and this can relate to the income and the way of life of the infant. Could complementary therapy sessions be regarded as necessaries? In practice there is no reason why they could not be so defined, but this would depend upon the infant's circumstances and the reasons why the therapy was recommended. The absence of any legal decision on the point means that the question remains open.

If complementary therapy sessions are defined as necessaries, then the implications are that if a person under 18 years old contracts for and receives the services, then the therapist could bring a legal action to recover a reasonable price for the services.

The difference between capacity to contract and the capacity to give a valid consent to treatment must be emphasised. In Chapter 9 the ability of a person of 16 and 17 to give valid consent to treatment under the Family Law Reform Act 1969 is discussed together with the right of a person below 16 years to give consent if 'Gillick competent'. Whether complementary therapies are covered by the definition of medical and dental treatment under section 8(2) of the Act is also discussed. In this chapter we are considering the capacity of an infant to be bound by contract and therefore to pay for services provided. Different tests are used to decide competence in the law of consent and the law of contract.

Contracts for non-necessaries Where the contract is not for necessaries, then the infant cannot be bound by the contract if he repudiates the contract whilst he is under 18 years or within a reasonable time of becoming 18.

Mentally ill and those with learning disabilities

Contracts made by mentally disordered persons are not binding upon the person in the following circumstances:

1. Where the person is defined under the Mental Health Act 1983 by two doctors as being incapable by reason of mental disorder of managing his own affairs and property. In this case the contract is not binding unless it has been made on behalf of that person by the Court of Protection.

2. Where the other party to the contract is aware of the person's mental disorder and the mentally disordered person did not understand the nature of the transaction. Those acting for the mentally disordered person will have the burden of proving both these elements in a dispute.

In other circumstances, the person suffering from mental disorder would be bound by the contract.

> **Situation 2**   Aromatherapy for learning disabilities
>
> Glen lives in a community home, having been discharged from long term accommodation for those with learning disabilities. He has sufficient funds from social security to pay for aromatherapy sessions. The sessions are considered to be in his best interests.

In this situation, it is not clear if Glen has the mental capacity to agree a contract with the aromatherapist or to give consent to the treatment. If the sessions are considered to be in his best interests, and it is considered that he lacks the mental capacity to form a contract, then the agreement would be made with Glen's carer on his behalf. The therapist could recover the fees from the carer.

The therapist however could not obtain consent from the carer for the treatment to proceed since no person has the power to give consent to treatment on behalf of a mentally incompetent adult. The therapist could nevertheless proceed with the therapy if she reasonably believed the treatment to be in the best interests of the client (see Chapter 9).

CONTRACTS OTHER THAN WITH CLIENTS

Provision in the NHS

A recent development in the field of complementary therapy is the purchasing of therapies by NHS purchasers or providers. Thus a therapist may agree a contract with a GP practice or with an NHS trust. There is a difference between the contracts. The contract with the GP practice will either be with a partnership or with a single handed practitioner; the contract with the NHS trust will be with a corporate body. In these situations within the NHS, the client does not have a contract with the therapist, the contract is between the purchaser and the therapist and the client has no direct rights against the therapist other than through the law of negligence and trespass to the person.

Other providers

Similarly the therapist may agree a contract with a private health organisation such as a private hospital or health centre. Nevertheless in private health care, whilst the private hospital or centre may set up an agreement for the provision of complementary therapy services, there may in practice be a contract between the client and the therapist for the provision of the therapy. A similar situation may exist in some hotels and leisure centres, where a therapist has an agreement with the occupiers/managers for services to be provided but the individual clients make their own agreement with the therapist. The managers of the premises may specifically exclude liability for any breach of contract or negligence by the therapist.

In contrast, in some nursing or residential homes or private hospitals the therapist may provide services as an employee of the owner of the home or hospital. It is essential that wherever these services are provided therapists are clear as to the nature of the agreement which they have with the organisation inviting them in.

FACTORS RENDERING CONTRACTS VOID OR VOIDABLE

After an apparently valid contract has been concluded it may be claimed that it is not binding for one of the following reasons:

- Misrepresentation
- Mistake
- Duress
- Illegality.

Misrepresentation

It may be that a client has been induced to agree to pay for sessions of complementary therapy on the understanding that it would achieve a specific outcome: for example a person might agree to have acupuncture in order to give up smoking.

Only if the client can prove that there has been a false statement of fact made with the intention of inducing another to enter into a contract, could it be argued in law that there has been a misrepresentation. To establish a misrepresentation the client would have to show that:

- the false statement was sufficiently important to influence him into entering the contract, and
- he did in fact rely upon it,
- not knowing it to be a false statement.

In some circumstances failure of the contracting party to perform the undertaking or fulfil the contractual obligation could be treated as a breach of contract rather than as a misrepresentation which induced the contract, the necessary elements being easier to prove.

If misrepresentation can be established, then the remedies depend upon the nature of the misrepresentation. The law recognises the following categories: fraudulent, innocent and negligent. Rescission (i.e. ending the contract) is available for all types of misrepresentation but only if

- the victim of the misrepresentation has not affirmed the contract,
- the victim elects to rescind the contract within a reasonable time, and
- it is still possible to restore the parties to their precontract position.

Fraudulent misrepresentation Where a misrepresentation has been made fraudulently, then the contract can be rescinded (i.e. ended) and damages can be claimed for all losses resulting from the misrepresentation.

Innocent misrepresentation Where the person making the statement genuinely believed it to be true the contract can be rescinded; but damages are not recoverable unless the court exercises its discretion under section 2(2) of the Misrepresentation Act 1967 and awards damages in lieu of rescission.

Negligent misrepresentation Rescission is available, and damages are awarded on the basis of reasonably foreseeable consequences, either on the basis of the common law leading case of *Hedley Byrne* v. *Heller*[3] or on the basis of section 2(1) of the Misrepresentation Act 1967 which is shown below in Box 4.2.

Box 4.2 Misrepresentation Act 1967 section 2

(1) Where a person has entered into a contract after a misrepresentation has been made to him by another party thereto and as a result thereof he has suffered loss, then, if the person making the misrepresentation would be liable to damages in respect thereof had the misrepresentation been made fraudulently, that person shall be so liable notwithstanding that the misrepresentation was not made fraudulently, unless he proves that he had reasonable ground to believe and did believe up to the time the contract was made that the facts represented were true.

(2) Where a person has entered into a contract after a misrepresentation has been made to him otherwise than fraudulently, and he would be entitled, by reason of this misrepresentation, to rescind the contract, then, if it is claimed, in any of the proceedings arising out of the contract, that the contract ought to be or has been rescinded, the court or arbitrator may declare the contract subsisting and award damages in lieu of rescission, if of the opinion that it would be equitable to do so, having regard to the nature of the misrepresentation and the loss that would be caused by it if the contract were upheld, as well as to the loss that rescission would cause the other party.

(3) Damages may be awarded against a person under subsection (2) of this section whether or not he is liable to damages under subsection (1) thereof, but where he is so liable any award under the said subsection (2) shall be taken into account in assessing his liability under the said subsection (1).

Mistake

A mistake might be mutual or else one sided (i.e. unilateral). A mutual mistake might relate to facts prior to the contract being agreed or to the actual content of the contract. The mistake will only affect the validity of the contract if it is fundamental. At common law a fundamental mistake by both parties can lead to the contract being held void from the beginning (void *ab initio*). The basis of this is that it means that there was no meeting of minds in relation to the agreement. In equity the result of a mistake can lead to the contract being voidable and, in certain circumstances, the contract can be rescinded or the court may rectify the terms of the contract so that it expresses the wishes of the parties.

Duress

It is essential that a contract is the result of the willing agreement of the parties: evidence that one party has been illegally coerced by another into forming the contract will lead to the contract being regarded as voidable. Undue influence will only affect the validity of the contract if it can be shown that one person has exploited the relationship between the parties to obtain an unfair advantage. The law distinguishes between actual undue influence and presumed undue influence; the latter arises where there is a relationship of trust or confidence between the victim and the party exerting the undue influence.

Illegality

A contract may be illegal because it is prohibited by Act of Parliament or is illegal at common law. Contracts which ignore these statutory or common law provisions may be void or voidable.

Situation 3   An illegal contract

Under hypnosis, a client agreed to perform a criminal act in exchange for free hypnotherapy. Such an agreement would not be binding upon the client since it would be illegal as against public policy. In addition it is doubtful if the agreement could be seen as being based upon the free will of the client.

The effect of the illegality can be overcome if the illegal terms can be severed from the contract whilst still leaving the basic contract intact. This is known as the 'blue pencil rule', the illegal terms being notionally crossed out with a thick blue pencil leaving the rest of the contract in place. If, however, the illegality is central to the contract, as it would be in the situation described above, the contract is void.

Examples of contracts which are illegal at common law include:

- Contracts to commit an illegal act
- Contracts which are contrary to public policy
- Contracts calculated to oust the jurisdiction of the court
- Contracts tending to corrupt the public service
- Contracts prejudicial to the status of marriage and the family
- Contracts in restraint of trade.

The last is most relevant to the therapist and will be considered in detail, taking an imagined situation to describe the significance of the law.

Situation 4   Restraint of trade

A partnership between therapists practising in aromatherapy came to an end and the one partner, Mrs Thorn, sought to set up a new practice in premises a few miles away. The other partner, Miss Robinson, tried to prevent the new practice being established by relying upon a clause in the partnership agreement which stated that in the event of a break up the outgoing partner could not set up as an aromatherapist for at least 20 years within an area of 500 miles, or provide a service to any persons who had been clients of the partnership in the last ten years. Mrs Thorn claimed that this term of the contract was invalid on grounds of restraint of trade. What is the legal situation?

A contract in restraint of trade is defined as 'one by which a party restricts his future liberty to carry on his trade, business or profession in such manner and with such persons as he chooses'.[4] The basic principles are that:

- All contracts in restraint of trade are prima facie void.
- Special factors can be taken into account to determine whether the restraint is justified.

- In determining the reasonableness of the restraint the interests of the public as well as the interests of the parties to the contract can be taken into account.
- It is the person who alleges that the restraint is unreasonable who has the burden of proving that allegation.

In determining the reasonableness of the restraint of trade term which the partnership agreement placed upon Mrs Thorn, the court would look at the duration of the restraint in terms of time, the geographical area, and the restriction in terms of clients. Account would be taken of the journeys which clients would be expected to travel in order to see an aromatherapist. The conclusion could well be that, whilst the limit in relation to former clients was reasonable, the geographical area and the duration of the restraint were both unreasonable since they would effectively prevent Mrs Thorn practising as an aromatherapist in this country. The restraint would therefore be void to that extent, applying a similar 'blue pencil' process to that referred to above.

CONTRACT TERMS AND PERFORMANCE

Implied terms

We have noted that a contract does not have to be in writing, but can be agreed by word of mouth. In addition certain terms not considered by the parties may be implied into the contract by operation of the law. Some terms, for example, are implied by the Sale of Goods and Services Act (see below). The terms which are implied into a contract of employment are considered in Chapter 7.

Terms may also be implied into a contract by common law if it is obvious that such a term would have been intended and it is necessary to make commercial sense of the contract. In such circumstances, the courts apply a test known as the 'officious bystander' test.

Situation 5   An officious bystander
A client and psychotherapist discuss a series of sessions and it is agreed that the client will come twice a week for six months. No mention is made of whether the client should pay if she fails to attend. The client fails to turn up on several occasions, the psychotherapist is unable to fill the time allotted to the client and charges for the session. The client refuses to pay. The psychotherapist maintains that such a clause is essential to make business sense of the contract.

Since there was no mention of payment for missed sessions in the agreement, the psychotherapist would have to argue that the law should imply into the contract a term that missed sessions should be paid for. The test which would be applied is as follows: if an official bystander listening to the two persons discussing the contract were to say 'What about payment for sessions missed by the client?' to which the parties would reply, 'Of course that must be a requirement', then such a term would be implied into the contract.

Conditions and warranties

Performance is usually required in accordance with the terms of the contract, but not all the terms are of equal effect. Some terms would be seen as major terms (conditions) i.e. terms which are fundamental to the contract and breach of which could lead to the innocent party electing to see the contract at an end (see below). Other minor terms (warranties) would, if broken give rise only to a claim for compensation rather than a right to treat the contract as at an end.

Exclusion clauses

The Unfair Contract Terms Act 1977

This Act regulates the extent to which persons can opt out of liability for personal injury, death or loss or damage to property. It is discussed in relation to exemption from liability arising from negligent acts in Chapter 3. Here we are concerned about exemption from liability in relation to contractual obligations. The relevant sections of the Act are shown in Box 4.3.

Box 4.3   Unfair Contract Terms Act 1977

Section 1
    (1) For the purposes of this Part of this Act, 'negligence' means the breach —
    (a) of any obligation, arising from the express or implied terms of a contract, to take reasonable care or exercise reasonable skill in the performance of the contract;
    (b) of any common law duty to take reasonable care or exercise reasonable skill (but not any stricter duty);
    (c) of the common duty of care imposed by the Occupiers' Liability Act 1957 or the Occupiers' Liability Act (Northern Ireland) 1957.

Section 2
    (1) A person cannot by reference to any contract term or to a notice given to persons generally or to particular persons exclude or restrict his liability for death or personal injury resulting from negligence.
    (2) In the case of other loss or damage, a person cannot so exclude or restrict his liability for negligence except in so far as the term or notice satisfies the requirement of reasonableness.
    (3) Where a contract term or notice purports to exclude or restrict liability for negligence a person's agreement to or awareness of it is not itself to be taken as indicating his voluntary acceptance of any risk.

Exemption from liability for loss or damage to goods can be excluded if it is reasonable. The definition of reasonableness is set out in section 11 of the Act and is shown in Box 4.4.

Box 4.4   Unfair Contract Terms Act 1977, section 11

    (1) In relation to a contract term, the requirement of reasonableness for the purposes of this Part of this Act... is that the term shall have been a fair and reasonable one to be included having regard to the circumstances which were, or ought reasonably to have been, known to or in the contemplation of the parties when the contract was made.

Box 4.4 *Cont'd*

---

(2) Where by reference to a contract term or notice a person seeks to restrict liability to a specified sum of money, and the question arises (under this or any other Act) whether the term or notice satisfies the requirement of reasonableness, regard shall be had in particular ... to —
  (a) the resources which he could expect to be available to him for the purpose of meeting the liability should it arise; and
  (b) how far it was open to him to cover himself by insurance.
(3) It is for those claiming that a contract term or notice satisfies the requirement of reasonableness to show that it does.

The 1977 Act defines business as including 'a profession and the activities of any government department or local or public authority'.

The basic principles from the 1977 Act are:

Firstly
- In a contract in the course of a trade or business
- liability for death or personal injury to any person resulting from negligence cannot be excluded whether that person deals as consumer or not.

Secondly
- Where the loss or damage relates to property, it is possible to exclude liability for any negligence which has resulted in this loss or damage,
- provided that the exclusion satisfies the test of reasonableness,
- which must be proved by the individual who is relying upon the exemption.

Unfair Terms in Consumer Contracts Regulations 1994

The above came into force on 1 July 1995 as the result of European Community Directive 93/13. The Regulations cover contracts between sellers or suppliers and consumers and make unfair and therefore unenforceable any contract term which has not been individually negotiated.

Regulation 4 is shown in Box 4.5.

Box 4.5 Unfair Terms in Consumer Contracts Regulations 1994, regulation 4

An unfair term is one which, contrary to the requirement of good faith, causes a significant imbalance in the parties' rights and obligations to the detriment of the consumer.

Criteria to be used in interpreting whether a term is in good faith are given in Schedule 2 and shown in Box 4.6.

Box 4.6 Criteria for good faith

- The strength of the bargaining positions of the parties
- Whether the consumer had an inducement to agree to the term
- Whether the goods or services were sold or supplied to the special order of the consumer
- The extent to which the seller or supplier has dealt fairly and equitably with the consumer

---

Regulation 3(4) enables a view to be taken of the whole contract even when terms are individually negotiated to assess whether it is a pre-formulated standard contract and if it can be considered as unfair within the meaning of the Regulations.

Under regulation 5 if a term is unfair then the consumer is not bound by it, but the rest of the contract will remain valid if that is possible. It is the seller or supplier who has the burden of proving that a term was individually negotiated (regulation 3(5)).

Powers are given to the Director General of Fair Trading, on receipt of a complaint, to apply for an injunction to restrain the use of any contract term(s) considered to fall outside the criteria for fairness and good faith (regulation 8).

Another consequence of the EC Directive is the power given to the Director General of Fair Trading to take action on behalf of individuals with complaints relating to fair trading. An injunction or other action before the courts can be taken against those in breach of the Regulations (see also Chapter 5 on the criminal law).

ENDING THE CONTRACT

Performance

Most contracts for complementary therapy services will come to an end when the agreed number of sessions have been provided. The client has transferred the consideration to the therapist and the therapist has provided the service. Unless they agree that there should be a new contract the legal relationship between them is ended.

Agreement

It may be that after starting on a series of therapy sessions, the client changes his mind and instead of receiving six sessions wishes to end the contractual relationship after two. The basic principle of law is that one party cannot unilaterally change the terms of the contract without the agreement of the other person. Therefore if he has agreed to have six sessions he may well be obliged to pay for the ones he no longer wishes to take, unless the therapist is prepared to waive the outstanding fees. The therapist could not of course insist on providing the service, since this may involve a trespass to the person (see Chapter 9 on consent). The client wishing to change the terms of the contract in this way must seek to obtain agreement from the therapist to the change.

Notice

Some contracts, especially those of employment, include provision for either side to give notice of their intention to end the contract. This may be the situation between a non-NHS purchaser and the therapist, where the therapist is permitted to provide services on the premises subject to the right of either party to give a specified time of notice to end the contract.

Breach

As has been seen above, if a party fails to comply with certain terms of the contract which are known as conditions, then the innocent party has the right to elect to see the contract as at an end. Such a decision to see the contract as at an end must be made within a reasonable time of the breach occurring and must be made clearly to the other party. Actions which suggest that the innocent party is electing to affirm the contract may be interpreted as an election not to see the contract as ended. In this case the innocent party is bound by the contract but can seek damages (compensation) for the breach.

Frustration

If an event occurs, which is completely outside the contemplation of the parties at the time the contract was agreed, which is not provided for within the contract terms, and which renders the performance of the contract very different from that intended by the parties, then it may in law be held that the contract is 'frustrated'. The result is that it comes to an end by operation of law.

Situation 6   Legal frustration

A hypnotist becomes blind and is unable to provide therapy; the contract would come to an end through frustration at law. Similarly if a client was imprisoned and therefore unable to attend for therapy, a contract for the supply of services would be brought to an end by operation of law i.e. the contract would be ended by frustration.

The Law Reform (Frustrated Contracts) Act 1943 sought to remedy the injustice which could arise from the automatic ending of a contract by the doctrine of frustration. It enables the recovery of moneys which have been paid in advance under the contract, allows for the payment of compensation for expenses which have been incurred in the performance of the contract and remedies any injustices where one party has received benefits under the contract without having made any payment. The Act need not apply if express provision has been made in the contract for the frustrating event.

REMEDIES FOR BREACH OF CONTRACT

It should be noted that remedies for breach of contract are in addition to any remedies for negligence by the supplier to the purchaser under the principle of *Donoghue* v. *Stevenson*[5] case where it was held that a duty of care was owed by the manufacturer to the ultimate consumer. Rights under the law of negligence are considered in Chapter 3.

Rescission

As has been seen above, breach of contract could lead to the ending of the contract or only the right of the innocent party to seek damages. This depends upon the nature of the term of the contract which has been broken – whether it is a condition or only a warranty.

Damages

Where damages are awarded, the amount is calculated on the basis of being the sum necessary to place the innocent party in the position he would have been in had the term of the contract not been broken. Compensation is not payable if loss or the harm which has been suffered is considered to be too remote, or not within the contemplation of the parties. It will be expected too that the innocent party will take reasonable steps to minimise (mitigate) any loss or harm which has occurred as the result of the breach. In determining the amount of compensation there is controversy as to whether account would also be taken of any contributory negligence by the innocent party. The Law Commission in 1993[6] recommended that there should be an apportionment of damages on the lines of the Law Reform (Contributory Negligence) Act 1945 (see Chapter 3).

The contract itself may seek to limit the amount of damages payable or specify the way in which they should be calculated. Where the parties make an attempt to calculate the actual losses (liquidated damages) the court would usually support such payments. However excessive sums in relation to the likely losses, which could be regarded as being in the nature of a penalty, would not be supported by the courts.

Specific performance

The court will seldom order the specific performance (i.e. ordering one party to perform his part of the contract) of a contract if damages are a reasonable alternative. This is particularly so in contracts for personal service, where it is considered inappropriate to order one person to provide services for another.

Situation 7   Personal service not specifically enforceable

An osteopath had agreed to provide 10 sessions for a client. He then became much in demand following a programme which proclaimed his work in sports injuries. He changed his mind about providing the remaining sessions. The client sought an order for specific performance requiring the osteopath to complete the contract.

In these circumstances, the osteopath is clearly in breach of contract. It would, however, be extremely unusual for the court to order specific performance of the contract. Damages would normally be sufficient compensation for the client. If, however, that particular osteopath had qualities which could not be purchased elsewhere the court might prohibit the osteopath providing services for others during the time he should have been treating the aggrieved client.

Injunction

This is available to enforce a negative stipulation in the contract.

Situation 8	Breach of confidentiality

A client discovers that his therapist is intending to use his case at a conference without his permission and he fears that he may be recognised, and the duty of confidentiality would not be kept. He considers that compensation would not be an adequate remedy for the intended breach of contract.

The client could apply to the court for an injunction to restrain the therapist from breaching the duty of confidentiality (see Chapter 10 on confidentiality). If the therapist goes ahead in spite of the injunction she is in contempt of court punishable in extreme cases by imprisonment.

TIME LIMITS IN CLAIMS FOR BREACH

The basic principle is that an action for breach of contract must be commenced (i.e. the writ issued) within six years from the date on which the cause of action accrued. This is set out in section 5 of the Limitation Act 1980. However where the breach relates to personal injuries, the action must be brought within three years from the date on which the cause of action accrued (section 11 of the Limitation Act 1980). The time limits do not start to run in the case of fraud, deliberate concealment or where the claim arises from a mistake, until the plaintiff has discovered (or could reasonably have been expected to have discovered) the fraud, concealment or mistake.

If the cause of action relates to the payment of a debt, each time the debt is acknowledged the limitation period begins to run afresh.

SALE OF GOODS AND SUPPLY OF SERVICES

Sale of Goods Act 1979

Goods provided by complementary therapists are covered by the Sale of Goods Act 1979 which implies certain terms in the contract for sale to protect the purchaser. Sometimes complementary therapists or others sell goods, books or equipment which promote their particular therapy. Such offers and sales contracts would be caught by the consumer protection legislation (see Chapter 13) and the Sale of Goods Act 1979. For example an *Innovations* catalogue[7] advertised for sale the 10 tape set from Paul McKenna called the 'Success for Life' tapes. Other hypnotherapy audio tapes called 'How to use the Power of your Mind' are stated to be of use in giving up smoking, slimming, sleeping, eliminating stress and in developing confidence, passing examinations etc. Purchasers would be able to claim compensation in the event of the tapes failing in their advertised purpose and, should harm befall the user (whether purchaser or not) as a consequence of their use, the manufacturer would be liable for any harm on the principles of *Donoghue* v. *Stevenson*[8] (see above and Chapter 3). Such goods are also subject to the Trade Descriptions Act (see Chapter 5). The Trading Standards Department of the local authority can give advice on any alleged breach of the legislation.

Supply of Goods and Services Act 1982

Usually complementary therapists provide services and (if there is a contract and they are paid for (see above)) these would be covered by the Supply of Goods and Services Act 1982. This Act was passed to give protection to consumers who were covered by the Sale of Goods Act 1979 in respect of goods which they purchased but not in relation to services which they received. Section 12 of the 1982 Act defines the supply of services covered by the Act as 'a contract under which a person ("the supplier") agrees to carry out a service'. This therefore would cover professional services carried out by architects, lawyers and doctors as well as those of builders, carpenters, plumbers etc. However section 12(2) excludes a contract of employment or apprenticeship from being the supply of services within Part II of the Act.

This thus creates a distinction. A complementary therapist who provides services to a client on the basis of a contract with that client would be subject to the provisions of the Supply of Goods and Services Act 1982. Where, however, the complementary therapist is employed, e.g. by a GP practice and provides services to the client on that basis as an employee, then the Supply of Goods and Services Act does not apply. Moreover if the client receives the services within the NHS there is no contract for payment and therefore the Act does not apply.

Whether a contract is for the sale of goods (and therefore comes under the 1979 Act) or one for the supply of services (and comes under the 1982 Act) depends upon what is the predominant purpose.

The 1982 Act implies specific terms into the contract for the supply of services:

- Section 13 an implied term about care and skill
- Section 14 an implied term about time for performance
- Section 15 an implied term about consideration.

Section 16 makes provision about the exclusion of these implied terms.

Implied term about care and skill

Box 4.7 Supply of Goods and Services Act 1982, section 13
In a contract for the supply of a service where the supplier is acting in the course of a business, there is an implied term that the supplier will carry out the service with reasonable care and skill.

The effect of section 13 is to incorporate into the contract for the supply of services the reasonable standard of care which the court applies to the duty of care in the law of negligence. This is considered in Chapter 3. In the common law the test is known as the Bolam test. The section enacts the common law position which was discussed by the Court of Appeal in a case in 1975.[9] In this case Lord Denning made the following statement:

The law does not usually imply a warranty that the professional man will achieve the desired result, but only a term that he will use reasonable care and skill. The surgeon does not warrant that he will cure the patient. Nor does the solicitor warrant that he will win the case. But, when a dentist agrees to make a set of false teeth for a patient, there is an implied warranty that they will fit his gums...

It seems to me that in the contractual employment of a professional man, whether it is a medical man, a lawyer, or an accountant, an architect or an engineer, his duty is to use reasonable care and skill in the course of employment.

However where complementary therapists make specific undertakings in relation to the services which they have agreed to supply, failure to supply the services may well constitute a breach of contract, even though there is no breach of section 13 of the Act.

Situation 9   An unfulfilled undertaking

An aromatherapist, somewhat unwisely, promised the client that two courses of therapy per week for six weeks would remove the stress and tension from which the client was suffering. At the end of the time the client found that the tension was still present. Could she claim a breach of an express term in the contract for services?

The answer is that the aromatherapist would appear to be in breach of her contract but not in breach of section 13. However if the aromatherapist had made no such undertaking but had just practised the reasonable standard of care expected of an aromatherapist, there would be no breach of contract or of section 13.

Implied term about performance

Box 4.8   Supply of Goods and Services Act 1982, section 14

(1) Where, under a contract for the supply of a service by a supplier acting in the course of a business, the time for the service to be carried out is not fixed by the contract, left to be fixed in a manner agreed by the contract or determined by the course of dealing between the parties, there is an implied term that the supplier will carry out the service within a reasonable time.
(2) What is a reasonable time is a question of fact.

The application of section 14 is seen from the following situation.

Situation 10   A reasonable time

A client requests acupuncture sessions in order to give up smoking. The acupuncturist agrees to provide six sessions and takes the money in advance. Unfortunately the acupuncturist then becomes ill and is unable to carry out the sessions immediately. Six months later, the client had still not received the therapy and asked for the money to be returned. The acupuncturist refused on the grounds that he would be able within two weeks to provide the sessions.

In the application of section 14 it could be argued that six months was an unreasonable time to wait for the supply of the service and therefore the acupuncturist was in breach of the implied term to provide the services within a reasonable time. The money should be refunded.

Implied term about consideration

Box 4.9   Supply of Goods and Services Act 1982, section 15

---

(1) Where, under a contract for the supply of a service, the consideration for the service is not determined by the contract, left to be determined in a manner agreed by the contract or determined by the course of dealing between the parties, there is an implied term that the party contracting with the supplier will pay a reasonable charge.
(2) What is a reasonable charge is a question of fact.

It is unlikely that complementary therapists will not have agreed with clients in advance of the amount of fees to be charged and in fact failure to agree this in advance with clients may constitute professional misconduct according to the Code of Ethics of some therapists. However, where there has been a failure in this respect, section 15 enables the therapist to recover a reasonable amount. This would relate to the nature of the therapy, the standing of the therapist and the area in which the service was provided.

Exclusion of the implied terms

Section 16 of the Act enables an implied term to be excluded in certain circumstances if there is express agreement between the parties.

Criminal aspects

The Trade Descriptions Act 1968, which makes it a criminal offence to apply a false trade description, and advertising offences under the Medicines Act 1968 are considered in Chapter 5.

INSURANCE CONTRACTS

An insurance contract is one in which one party (the insurer) agrees for payment of a consideration (the premium) to make monetary provision for the other (the insured) upon the occurrence of some event or against some risk. The insured must have an insurable interest in the subject matter of the contract. Brokers would negotiate the insurance contract with insurance companies or Lloyds underwriters on a commission basis and usually handle claims on their client's behalf. In the event of a claim an independent insurance assessor may be used to agree the sum due.

Need for insurance cover

The public at large are becoming increasingly aware of their rights and the potential to enforce them through litigation and so, irrespective of the requirements of any code of practice, all therapists offering services to the public, whether they subscribe to any such formal code or not, should ensure that they take out and maintain adequate insurance cover. If they fail to do so a successful claim against them could render them bankrupt and would also be grossly unfair on the injured client who could end up inadequately recompensed.

Claims for compensation are not limited to therapeutic matters (see Chapter 15 for occupiers liability in respect of premises).

Most therapists will ensure that they have public liability indemnity insurance which is now obtainable at reasonable rates from specialist insurance companies. In many therapies the Code of Ethics and Practice of the organisation requires the therapist to take out professional indemnity insurance. In addition it should be noted that the Osteopaths Act is the first statutory provision which requires a therapist to take out professional indemnity insurance cover (see Chapter 33).

One firm which provides a significant number of complementary therapists with insurance cover is SMG (Smithson Mason Group). It offers a scheme known as 'the Altmed Scheme'. This specifically covers alternative medicine practitioners and related disciplines. At the present time they have over 120 different therapies on their approved list. (See below for the bands of the more popular therapies.) At present the limit of indemnity is £1 000 000.

A member of SMG has described risks, liability and insurance cover for psychologists in a journal article.[10]

Uberrimae fidei

Whilst contracts for insurance cover follow the basic principles of contract law set out above, they have some special features. In particular they are known as contracts of the utmost good faith (*uberrimae fidei*). This means that if the insured person fails to disclose a fact material to the risk being covered, then the contract can be ended (i.e. is voidable) at the instigation of the other party. The insurer could also refuse to pay out compensation if this failure to disclose information later becomes known. This is so even if this missing information has no direct relevance to the claim which is being made.

Questions asked on a typical proposal form include those set out in Box 4.10.

Box 4.10 Standard questions in insurance proposal form
1. For which therapies is cover required?   2. Relevant qualifications?   3. Professional organisations of which the individual is a member?   4. Have you ever been refused insurance cover?   5. Declaration of truth and completeness of the information given.

However a footnote to the form reminds individuals that it is necessary

to inform us of all the facts which are likely to influence us in the acceptance of your insurance. Failure to do so could invalidate this insurance. If you are in doubt whether any fact may influence us you should disclose it.[11]

Risks covered

In this particular scheme therapies are ranged in three bands based on risk.

Band 1 with the lowest premium includes acupressure, the Alexander technique, counselling, hypnotherapy, kinesiology, massage – various techniques, polarity therapy, psychology, psychotherapy, reflexology, Reiki sound therapy and yoga.

Band 2 includes allergy therapy, Bach flower remedies, diathermy, electro-encephalography, herbal medicine, homeopathy, iridology, medigen, nutritional medicine, oriental medicine and vitamin therapy.

Band 3 with the highest premium includes acupuncture, aromatherapy and physiotherapy (some types only).

Coverage under the Altmed Scheme includes:

- professional indemnity
- public liability
- malpractice insurance
- product liability
- libel and slander insurance.

Matters not covered by typical insurance

The proposal points out that the policy covers liability arising out the practice of the therapy, not the running of training courses and separate advice should be sought for that. The exceptions to the policy also include any liability in respect of bodily injury to any employees arising out of or in the course of their employment by the insured. Endorsements on the policy might further restrict its coverage. Thus one typical endorsement is shown in Box 4.11.

Box 4.11 Endorsement restricting cover

The Company shall not indemnify the insured against liability:
  caused by or arising from medical diagnosis or prognosis or failure to medically diagnose other than in circumstances where the client is recommended by the therapist to consult a medical practitioner.

Another endorsement may exclude liability caused by or arising from any treatment knowingly provided to eczema sufferers, or the use of anaesthetics, ECG, X-Rays, surgical operations etc.

Another endorsement is as follows:

The Company shall not indemnify the Insured against liability caused by or arising from the failure of any treatment or therapy to achieve its desired object.

An endorsement may exclude HIV:

The Company shall not indemnify the Insured against liability for causing or failing to cure or alleviate any condition directly or indirectly caused by or associated with Human T-Cell Lymphotropic Associated Virus Type iii (HLTV iii) or Lymphadenopathy Associated Virus (LAV) or the mutants, or derivatives thereof or in any way related to Acquired

Immune Deficiency Syndrome (AIDS) or any condition of a similar kind howsoever it be named.

In the light of exceptions to cover or endorsements, all therapists need to read the small print to ensure that the cover concerned protects them from the work they are doing and that there are no areas where insurance protection does not exist. The advice and information they give to the client must therefore be correct. If, for example, a patient is seeking assistance for an eczema condition and the therapist knows that this is excluded from the cover the patient should be so advised.

Could the therapist tell the client, 'I am not covered for that so if you suffer harm, you cannot sue me?' The answer is that this is unlikely to be a successful line to take. Under the Unfair Contract Terms Act 1977 a person cannot exclude, by reference to a contract term or notice, liability for negligence which has resulted in personal injury or death. The therapist may still be liable, but may not have the assets to meet the claim.

Another point to note is the endorsement where the therapy is not successful. Therapists should always beware of promising more than they can guarantee as an outcome for an individual in using their services. Failure to achieve a promised outcome could be seen as a breach of contract if achieving success could be interpreted as a term of the contract. If an endorsement exists excluding failure to achieve a given outcome, then therapists may find that they are being sued for breach of contract but do not have the insurance cover for that particular risk.

Situation 11   An excluded condition

An allergy therapist obtains insurance cover for her practice. She fails to notice that treatment provided to eczema sufferers is excluded. She treats a client suffering from eczema, recommending a strict diet. Unfortunately the client suffers a severe reaction. The client demands compensation and when the therapist refers the claim to the company, she is told that she does not have cover for that.

In this situation, the therapist may still be liable to the client, and compensation would therefore have to be paid for out of the therapist's own personal funds, unless the allergy therapist has incorporated a company with limited liability for which she works. In this situation, liability ends with the company and her own private resources are not at risk.

Role of insurance in self-regulation

This field of professional indemnity insurance cover for therapists is potentially of extreme significance. Given the fact that there is minimal state regulation of individual therapies, then voluntary self-regulation is extremely important in maintaining standards of practice and in protecting the public. Those companies which provide the insurance cover can have an important role in setting the standards for the individual therapies and in determining what conduct will forfeit the right to insurance cover (see Chapter 6 on regulation).

Medical Defence Union and Medical Protection Society

Some registered medical practitioners who are covered by the above defence organisations will have indemnity cover for their work in complementary therapy from these organisations. The defence organisations are not, however, insurance companies and the protection they provide for their members is not therefore that of an insurance contract.

The Medical Protection Society provides the full range of benefits of membership to the members who practise alternative or complementary medicine. It does not, however, accept into membership practitioners who do not have a medical or dental qualification. It has paid out in respect of the following claims relating to complementary medical practice:

• pneumothorax, following the insertion of acupuncture needles
• adverse skin reactions following homeopathic treatments
• omissions of treatment for certain conditions (e.g. underlying breast lumps, bowel neoplasms, etc.) for which inappropriate remedies were given[12]

The Medical Defence Union also only provides protection for registered doctors and dentists, but will provide cover in respect of the activities of its members in the field of complementary therapies. It is evident that there are an increasing number of claims against doctors in respect of their work in complementary therapy.

The work of the Medical Defence Union and Medical Protection Society is discussed in Chapter 6 on the regulation of complementary therapies.

Questions and Exercises

1. Review your contractual pro formas for your clients. Are the forms clear? Do they contain all the information set out in this chapter? Are they easy to read and without legal jargon?
2. What does your contract require if a client misses an appointment? Is there a difference between a client failing to turn up, and a client telephoning to apologise for not being able to keep an appointment?
3. What provisions relate to the payment of fees?
4. Examine your contract of insurance. What is the significance of the small print in respect of your obligations and your rights? In what circumstances would your cover be forfeited?
5. What are the main differences between a contract of service and a contract for services (refer also to Chapter 7)?

REFERENCES

1. Guest (ed) 1984 Anson's Principles of the law of contract 26th edn. Oxford University Press, Oxford
2. Currie v. Misa [1875] LR 10 Ex 153
3. Hedley Byrne & Co Ltd v. Heller [1964] AC 465
4. Richards P 1995 Law of contract 2nd edn. Pitman Publishing, London
5. Donoghue v. Stevenson [1932] AC 562

6. Law Commission Report No. 219 1994 Contributory negligence as a defence in contract. HMSO, London
7. Explore August–December 1996 Innovations Mail Order
8. Donoghue *v.* Stevenson [1932] AC 562
9. Greaves & Co (Contractors) Ltd *v.* Baynham Meikle and Partners [1975] 3 All ER 99
10. BPS 1995 Professional Liability Insurance. The Psychologist 8(2)
11. SMG Proposal Form for Altmed Insurance
12. Personal communication to the author from the Secretary and Medical Director of the MPS. 9 May 1997

5

Criminal law

A feature of complementary therapies is that by and large they are not state regulated. They are free to organise and regulate themselves. This does not however mean that they do not have to operate within a legal context. Like any other citizens, therapists must be aware of the criminal law and how it applies to their practice. Ignorance of the law is no defence if an offence is committed.

DEFINITION OF A CRIMINAL OFFENCE

In Chapter 2 the difference between criminal law and civil law was explained. Although many criminal offences are based on a notion of what is morally wrong, this is not the criteria for determining what is criminal. In practice the only realistic definition is that a criminal act is one which could be followed by criminal proceedings. As discussed in Chapter 2 any government can decriminalise an act, e.g. to attempt to commit suicide, so that it ceases to be a criminal offence, just as it can pass legislation which creates a new criminal offence as was done with stalking (see below).

There can therefore be a mismatch between what an individual would regard as immoral or unethical and what is actually a criminal offence. Furthermore there is an overlap between the criminal law and the civil law. One incident could give rise to both forms of proceedings. For example if a therapist were to examine a client without consent, by touching him, that could constitute both a trespass to the person in the civil law (see Chapter 9) and also it could be grounds for a criminal charge of assault under section 39 of the Criminal Justice Act 1988.

Criminal offences are defined both by Act of Parliament, such as theft, and also by common law (judge made law) such as murder. The definition of the offence in either the Act of Parliament or the decision of the judge sets out the elements or ingredients of the offence.

Individual statutes are considered below and their elements or ingredients discussed. These elements are known as objective elements (*actus reus*) or mental elements (*mens rea*).

The *mens rea*

The *mens rea* is the mental element which, in most crimes, must be shown by the prosecution to exist before a prosecution can succeed. There are only a few crimes, known as offences of strict liability, where *mens rea* does not have to be proved.

Situation 1 An absence of *mens rea*

A client leaves her purse behind in a therapist's consulting room. When the therapist leaves to return home she fails to notice that the purse has fallen into her brief case. When she arrives home and opens her brief case she discovers the purse.

The therapist could not be successfully prosecuted for theft by reason of her taking the purse home. She lacked any mental intention to steal the purse from the client. Nor was there any intention to deprive the client of it permanently, which is a necessary ingredient of the offence of theft (see below). However, once at home, were she to use it for her own purposes then the offence of theft would be committed.

A defence of automatism or absent mindedness may succeed if it prevents the accused having the mental state to form the intention to carry out the relevant activity. Thus, if a client was involved in a car accident following treatment with hypnosis, it may be difficult for the prosecution to prove that the client had the necessary *mens rea* to support a prosecution for dangerous driving. On the other hand, if the client drives knowing that he suffers from an illness that renders him unfit to drive, this could constitute a criminal offence.

The *actus reus*

The *actus reus* (the deed element) is the objective requirements necessary to constitute an offence. Thus the *actus reus* of the offence of dangerous driving is driving a mechanically propelled vehicle on a road or other public place. Harm does not have to be established. In contrast, in causing death by dangerous driving it must be established that the dangerous driving as defined above actually caused the death.

PROCEDURE IN THE CRIMINAL COURTS

Offences are classed as 'indictable only', 'summary' or 'triable either way'. Indictable only offences are serious matters which must be tried in the crown court. Summary offences are less serious which must be tried before magistrates. Offences triable either way, by far the largest number of offences, can be serious or less so depending on each case (shoplifting a packet of sweets or stealing the Crown Jewels are both theft) and can be heard either before the magistrates or before the crown court. If the accused opts for a magistrates hearing in an offence which is triable either way the magistrates have the power to transfer the accused, if found guilty, to the crown court for sentencing. This is because the sentencing powers of the crown court are greater than those of magistrates.

Examining justices

Before a crown court hearing can take place, the accused must be committed (sent) to the crown court by the magistrates who act as examining justices in deciding whether there is sufficient evidence for the committal to take place.

Magistrates

Magistrates are either Justices of the Peace, i.e. unpaid lay persons who sit in groups of three to hear a case (hence the word 'bench'), or stipendiary magistrates, i.e. paid (hence stipend) lawyers who often sit alone. Magistrates act as judge and jury being advised on legal matters by a legally qualified court clerk. This is in practice a speedy, effective and extremely cheap form of criminal justice, dealing completely with the vast majority of criminal cases.

Crown court

The crown court is presided over by a judge whose seniority will depend upon the nature of the offence being heard. The proceedings are adversarial/accusatorial; lawyers for the Crown Prosecution Service seek to establish the defendant's guilt while lawyers for the defence try to undermine that evidence and maintain their client's innocence. The issues of fact, whether or not particular witnesses are to be believed, are decided by the jury; the judge decides issues of law and clarifies these (if necessary) for the jury. The accused is charged against an indictment which sets out each element of the offence. The accused is arraigned and the offence on the indictment put to them. The accused can either plead guilty or not guilty to the offences. Where a not guilty plea is made, a jury is empanelled from members of the public who can be challenged, for cause, by either prosecution or defence. The hearing will then take place.

Witnesses are called in turn to be examined 'in chief' (i.e. by the side calling them), cross examined (by the other side) and then re-examined on any point raised in the cross-examination. After the jury has considered its verdict the foreman will announce it to the court and if there is a verdict of 'guilty', the judge will give sentence. This may take place at adjourned proceedings in order that reports can be prepared. The lawyer (usually a barrister, though solicitors now have rights of audience) for the defendant may make a plea in mitigation before the judge sentences, giving reasons why, although the defendant is guilty, the sentence should be a light one. Except in cases of murder, the judge has considerable discretion over the sentence which could range from an absolute discharge to a lengthy term of imprisonment, subject to any limitations set in the statute which defined the offence.

THE THEFT ACTS

The Theft Act 1968 covers many separate offences which are associated with theft.

Obtaining property/services by deception

The *actus reus* for obtaining property by deception (section 15(1)) is:

- by making a false statement
- obtaining
- property belonging to another.

The *mens rea* is dishonesty with the intent to permanently deprive, and deliberately or recklessly deceiving the victim. Thus if a therapist were to suggest that a client should pay a sum of money for a session of complementary therapy, knowing that she had no skills or abilities in this field and simply in order to obtain the client's money, the offence would be committed. The prosecution would have to show all the ingredients of the *actus reus* and the *mens rea*.

The Theft Act 1978 section 1 added a new offence to cover a gap in the 1968 Act: the offence of obtaining services by deception. Thus if a client dishonestly pretended that he had the money to pay for a therapy session, and obtained that session as a result of this deception, he could be committing an offence under the 1978 Act.

Obtaining pecuniary advantage

The *actus reus* for obtaining a pecuniary advantage by deception (section 16 of the 1968 Act) is that the victim was misled and the perpetrator obtains, for himself or another, pecuniary advantage. The *mens rea* is deliberate or reckless dishonesty, and setting out to deceive.

Under section 3 of the 1978 Theft Act an offence is committed by a person who, knowing that payment on the spot for any goods or services done is required or expected of him, dishonestly, and with intent to avoid payment of the amount, makes off without having paid as required or expected.

TRADE DESCRIPTIONS ACT 1968

This act makes it a criminal offence to apply a false description to the supply or offer of goods.

Box 5.1 Trade Descriptions Act 1968, section 1

(1) Any person who, in the course of a trade or business—
  (a) applies a false trade description to any goods; or
  (b) supplies or offers to supply any goods to which a false trade description is applied;
  shall, subject to the provisions of this Act, be guilty of an offence.

Section 3 defines the word false in relation to a trade description as one which is false to a material degree. Also included in the definition of false is a trade description which is misleading, i.e. likely to be taken as an indication of such characteristics as quantity, size or gauge, fitness for purpose, strength, performance, behaviour or accuracy, approval by any person etc.

The Act also applies to services. Section 14 makes it a criminal offence for any person in the course of any trade or business to make a statement which he knows to be false; or recklessly to make a statement which is false on any of the matters listed in Box 5.2.

Box 5.2 Trade Descriptions Act 1968, section 14

Matters covered by section 14(1):
  (i) the provision ... of any services, accommodation or facilities;
  (ii) nature of any services, accommodation or facilities...;
  (iii) the time at which, manner in which or persons by whom any services, accommodation or facilities are so provided;
  (iv) the examination, approval, or evaluation by any person of any services, accommodation or facilities so provided;
  (v) the location or amenities of any accommodation so provided.

Thus under section 14 if a complementary therapist were to advertise that she had been approved by a specific Association or Organisation, knowing that this was not true, this would be a criminal offence under the 1968 Act. 'False' in section 14 means false to a material degree and 'services' does not include anything done under a contract of service. Thus statements under a contract of employment are excluded from the ambit of section 14. The statements are not confined to those which induce the making of the contract, they also include statements made after the contract is concluded.

An example of a prosecution under the Trade Descriptions Act is that of Larkhall Natural Health which was fined £1000 and ordered to pay £3500 prosecution costs after being found guilty on three charges under the Trade Descriptions Act over the packaging of its vitamin and mineral supplement, Tandem IQ.[1] Shropshire trading standards department, which brought the case, alleged that the packaging of Tandem IQ showing two children reading gave the impression that the product could improve the intelligence of all children, not just those who were poorly nourished. The stipendiary magistrate accepted that the company's packaging was not a deliberate hoax. Its chairman genuinely believed the product could enhance children's IQs. The company's offence lay in not taking sufficient care to limit the claims for its product. The magistrate said he was satisfied that there was reliable evidence that only children with a dietary deficiency were likely to benefit from vitamin and mineral supplements. Earlier two other manufacturers, Seven Seas and Raw Powder, pleaded guilty and were each fined £4000 for making false claims about their respective products 'Boost IQ' and 'Vitachieve'.

Another example of a successful prosecution under the Trade Descriptions Act is that of Elaine Smith who ran slimming clubs. She was fined £7000 with £4436 costs when she was found guilty of seven offences under the Act by Dudley magistrates. An undercover trading standards officer discovered that she had been falsely telling slimmers that they were losing weight.[2]

NON-FATAL OFFENCES AGAINST THE PERSON
Physical offences

Assault and battery This is a statutory offence under Section 39 of the Criminal Justice Act 1988. The *actus reus* of assault is putting someone in fear of immediate force and the *mens rea* is the intention or recklessness in causing the fear. The *actus reus* of battery is the actual infliction of force on a person and the *mens rea* is that the defendant intentionally or recklessly applied force.

Assault occasioning actual bodily harm Section 47 of the Offences Against the Person Act 1861 defines this offence. This *actus reus* is

- an assault
- which causes
- actual bodily harm.

The *mens rea* is the intention or recklessness in doing the deed.

In a recent case the House of Lords decided that the offence could be committed by a person making silent telephone calls which caused psychiatric injury to the victim since this amounted in law to the infliction of bodily harm and an assault.[3] It held that:

An assault was an ingredient of an offence under section 47. An assault might take two forms: the first was battery which involved the unlawful application of force by the defendant upon the victim. The second form was an act causing the victim to apprehend an imminent application of force upon her. It was not reasonable to enlarge the generally accepted legal meaning of what was a battery to include the circumstances of a silent caller who caused psychiatric injury.

The critical question was whether a silent caller might be guilty of an assault. The answer seemed to be 'yes, depending upon the facts'. There was no reason why a telephone caller who said to a woman in a menacing way, 'I will be at your door in a minute or two' might not be guilty of an assault if he caused his victim to apprehend immediate personal violence.

Other offences There are the further offences of malicious wounding and inflicting grievous bodily harm (section 20) of the 1861 Act and wounding and causing grievous bodily harm with intent (section 18).

Protection from Harassment Act 1997

This Act was passed to provide a remedy for those who were victims of stalking. The Act creates or allows:

1. A criminal offence of harassment (section 1) which is defined as a person pursuing a course of conduct which amounts to harassment of another and which he knows or ought to know amounts to harassment of the other (the reasonable person test is applied).

2. A civil wrong whereby a person who fears an actual or future breach of section 1, may claim compensation including damages for anxiety and financial loss.

3. The right to claim an injunction to restrain the defendant from pursuing any conduct which amounts to harassment.

4. The right to apply for a warrant for the arrest of the defendant if the injunction has not been obeyed.

5. An offence of putting people in fear of violence, i.e. where a person by his conduct causes another person to fear on at least two occasions that violence will be used against him.

6. Restraining orders to be made by the court for the purpose of protecting the victim of the offence or any other person from further conduct amounting to harassment or to fear violence.

Certain defences are permitted in the Act including that an individual is preventing or detecting crime.

Therapists and healthcare workers are particularly vulnerable and any therapist who is harassed by a former client should contact the police to obtain their guidance on action which can be taken. If as a result the therapist suffers financial loss or mental or physical harm, compensation may be recoverable in the civil courts.

Malicious Communications Act 1988

This Act makes it an offence for any person to send a letter or other article which conveys:

- a message which is indecent or grossly offensive
- a threat
- information which is false and known or believed by the sender to be false
- any other article which is, in whole or in part, of an indecent or grossly offensive nature.

To constitute the offence there must be the *mens rea* element in that the purpose in sending it is that it could cause distress or anxiety to the recipient or to any other person to whom the offender intends that it or its contents should be communicated. There is no offence if there was a threat which was used to reinforce a demand which the sender believed he had reasonable grounds for making and he believed the use of the threat to be a proper means of reinforcing the demand, e.g. a request for monies due threatening legal proceedings is not an offence.

FATAL OFFENCES AGAINST THE PERSON

Murder

Murder is an offence defined at common law. A conviction for murder results in life imprisonment. The judge has no discretion although as 'life imprisonment' does not mean what it says a minimum sentence can be recommended. Where the offender is under 18 years the verdict is 'at Her Majesty's pleasure', the case being kept under review and the defendant being released when the authorities deem it appropriate.

Manslaughter

Manslaughter is classified as either involuntary or voluntary.

Involuntary This arises from recklessness or gross negligence, or can be constructive manslaughter (e.g. killing in the course of committing an unlawful act).

Voluntary This is where death has occurred as the result of:

- provocation (Homicide Act 1957 section 3)
- diminished responsibility (Homicide Act 1957 section 2)
- killing in pursuance of a suicide pact (Homicide Act 1957 section 4)

Following a manslaughter conviction, the judge has complete discretion to sentence according to the circumstances of the case. At one extreme this could be conditional discharge or at the other a substantial period of imprisonment.

Negligence by a professional

The House of Lords has given a ruling on the directions that a judge gives to a jury in the case of death resulting from negligence by a professional.[4]

Case 1 Negligence in the operating theatre

An anaesthetist was charged with the death of a patient. The facts were that at approximately 11.05 am a disconnection occurred at the endotracheal tube connection. The supply of oxygen to the patient ceased and led to a cardiac arrest at 11.14 am. During that period the defendant failed to notice or remedy the disconnection.

He first became aware that something was amiss when an alarm sounded on the Dinamap machine, which monitored the patient's blood pressure. From the evidence it appeared that some four and a half minutes would have elapsed between the disconnection and the sounding of the alarm.

When the alarm sounded the defendant responded in various ways by checking the equipment and by administering atropine to raise the patient's pulse. But at no stage before the cardiac arrest did he check the integrity of the endotracheal tube connection. The disconnection was not discovered until after resuscitation measures had been commenced.

He accepted at his trial that he had been negligent. The issue was whether his conduct was criminal. He was convicted of involuntary manslaughter but appealed against his conviction. He lost his appeal in the Court of Appeal and then appealed to the House of Lords.

The House of Lords clarified the legal situation. The stages which they suggested should be followed were:

1. The ordinary principles of the law of negligence should be applied to ascertain whether or not the defendant had been in breach of a duty of care towards the victim who had died.

2. If such a breach of duty was established the next question was whether that breach of duty caused the death of the victim.

3. If so, the jury had to go on to consider whether that breach of duty should be characterised as gross negligence and therefore as a crime. That would depend on the seriousness of the breach of duty committed by the defendant in all the circumstances in which the defendant was placed when it occurred.

4. The jury would have to consider whether the extent to which the defendant's conduct departed from the proper standard of care incumbent upon him (involving as it must have done a risk of death to the patient), was such that it should be judged criminal.

The judge would also be required to give the jury a direction on the meaning of gross negligence as had been given in the present case by the Court of Appeal.

The jury might properly find gross negligence on proof of
- indifference to an obvious risk of injury to health or of
- actual foresight of the risk coupled either
  - with a determination nevertheless to run it or
  - with an intention to avoid it but involving such a high degree of negligence in the attempted avoidance as the jury considered justified conviction

or of
- inattention or failure to advert to a serious risk going beyond mere inadvertence in respect of an obvious and important matter which the defendant's duty demanded he should address.

[Bullet points added for clarity]

The House of Lords held that the Court of Appeal had applied the correct test and the defendant's appeal was dismissed.

(An amended test is used in the case of a charge of involuntary death in motor accidents.)

Applying this to the work of a complementary therapist

If a death occurs of a client and it is alleged that the therapist was grossly reckless or grossly negligent in respect of the care of the patient then as well as civil litigation in respect of the death brought by the relatives of the deceased there could also be a prosecution brought by the crown prosecution service.

THE MEDICINES ACT 1968

This Act set up an administrative and licensing system to control the sale and supply of medicines to the public, retail pharmacies and the packing and labelling of medicinal products. It classifies medicines into the categories shown in Box 5.3.

Box 5.3 Classification of medicines under the Medicines Act 1968

1. **Pharmacy only products** These can only be sold or supplied retail by someone conducting a retail pharmacy when the product must be sold for a registered pharmacy by, or under the supervision of, a registered pharmacist.
2. **General Sales List** These are medicinal products which may be sold other than from a retail pharmacy so long as the provisions relating to Section 53 of the Medicines Act are complied with. This means that

- the place of sale must be the premises where the business is carried out
- the premises must be capable of excluding the public
- the medicines must have been made up elsewhere and
- the contents must not have been opened since make up.

3. **Prescription-only list** The medicines are only available on a practitioner's prescription. Schedule I of the Regulations lists the prescription only products and Part II of the schedule lists the prescription-only products which are covered by the Misuse of Drugs Act 1971.

Once a product is defined as a medicinal product by the Medicine Control Agency, then all the provisions of the Act in relation to licensing and marketing apply. Statutory Instruments made under the Medicines Act provide detailed regulations on marketing and other aspects of the Act. Some of the significant ones in the field of complementary therapy are given below.

Marketing authorisation

The Medicines for Human Use (Marketing Authorisations etc.) Regulations 1994 (SI 1994/3144), provide that unless exempt, no medicinal product shall be placed on the market unless a marketing authorisation has been granted by the licensing authority or the European Commission. It is an offence to sell or supply, or to advertise a medicinal product without a licence. (This is further discussed in Chapter 27 on homeopathy.)

Definitions

Article 1 of Council Directive 65/66/EEC defines a medicinal product as:

Any substance or combination of substances presented for treating or preventing disease in human beings or animals. Any substance or combination of substances which may be administered to human beings or animals with a view to making a medical diagnosis or to restoring, correcting or modifying physiological function in human beings or in animals is likewise considered a medicinal product.

Disease includes any injury or ailment or adverse conditions of body or mind. Administered means administered orally, by injection or by introduction into the body in any other way, or by external application, whether by direct contact with the body or not.

Exempt medicinal products

Regulation 1(3) of SI 1994/3144 allows some medicinal products to be supplied by certain individuals without the need for the remedy to undergo the normal marketing authorisation procedures.

Section 12(1) of the Medicines Act 1968 allows persons including aromatherapists to make, sell and supply any herbal remedy in the course of their business in the circumstances described. They may also sell or supply herbal remedies in the same circumstances which have been manufactured for them by the holder of the appropriate manufacturing licence (SI 1971/1450).

Section 12(2) of the Medicines Act 1968 sets out the terms of an additional exemption for herbal remedies prepared in strictly limited ways i.e. crushed, dried or comminuted. Section 132 defines herbal remedy as

a medicinal product consisting of a substance produced by subjecting a plant or plants to drying, crushing or any other process, or of a mixture whose sole ingredient are two or more substances so produced, or of a mixture whose sole ingredients are one or more substances so produced and water or some other inert substance.

Advertising

Regulation 3(1) of the Medicines (Advertising) Regulations SI 1994/1932 provides that no person shall issue an advertisement relating to a relevant medicinal product in respect of which no product licence is in force. Regulation 92 defines advertisement to cover 'every form of advertising whether in a publication or elsewhere'.

In July 1997 the Food Commission, an independent consumer organisation published a report stating that dietary supplements are regulated simply as foodstuffs, while they are often marketed as if they were medicines.[5] The Commission examined labels, leaflets and press releases distributed by manufacturers, importers and retailers of dietary supplements. Out of 314 supplements (which included vitamins, minerals, fish oils, amino acids, enzymes, algae, herbal remedies and slimming aids) a total of 741 health claims were advanced. The report pointed out that any claim that a product can cure, treat or prevent a disease is generally regarded as a medicinal claim and should be made only where the product has a medicines licence. A spokesman for the Medicine Control Agency is quoted as stating that

Claims that a food supplement can prevent, treat or cure a disease are illegal unless the product has a licence proving that it can do what is claimed, and that it is safe to use, but there is a burgeoning market in health foods and alternative medicines where claims fall in a grey area and are difficult to police.[6]

MISUSE OF DRUGS ACT 1971

This Act and subsequent legislation makes provision for the classification of controlled drugs and their possession, supply and manufacture.

The Act makes it a criminal offence to carry on the manufacture, supply and possession of controlled drugs contrary to the regulations. Controlled drugs are divided into three categories shown in Box 5.4.

Box 5.4   Controlled drugs under the Misuse of Drugs Act 1971

Class A includes, amongst others: cocaine, diamorphine, morphine, opium, pethidine and class B substances when prepared for injection.
Class B includes, amongst others: oral amphetamines, barbiturates, cannabis, codeine.
Class C includes, amongst others: most benzodiazepines, meprobamate.

The Misuse of Drugs Regulations 1985 SI 1985/2066 divides controlled drugs into five schedules each specifying the requirements governing activities such as import, export, production, supply, possession, prescribing and record keeping.

Schedule 1 Cannabis, lysergic acid etc. Possession and supply are prohibited except in accordance with Home Office authority.

Schedule 2 diamorphine, morphine, pethidine etc. Regulations control the prescriptions, safe custody and the keeping of registers.

Schedule 3 barbiturates, subject, apart from phenobarbitone, to special prescription requirements.

Schedule 4 benzodiazepines etc. subject to minimum control. Not subject to safe custody and the controlled drug prescriptions requirements do not apply.

Schedule 5 drugs containing only minute strengths of controlled drugs. Exempt from virtually all controlled drug requirements other than retention of invoice for two years.

OFFENCES IN OFFERING/PROVIDING CERTAIN HEALTH SERVICES

Attendance at childbirth

Section 16 of the Nurses, Midwives and Health Visitors Act, 1997 (replacing Section 17 of Nurses, Midwives and Health Visitors Act 1979) is designed to protect women from untrained persons claiming to be able to assist in childbirth.

Box 5.5   Nurses, Midwives and Health Visitors Act 1997, section 16

(1) A person other than a registered midwife or registered medical practitioner shall not attend a woman in childbirth.
(2) Subsection (1) does not apply —
    (a)   where the attention is given in a case of sudden or urgent necessity; or
    (b)   in the case of a person who, while undergoing training with a view to becoming a medical practitioner or to becoming a midwife, attends a woman in childbirth as part of a course of practical instruction in midwifery recognised by the General Medical Council or one of the National Boards.
(3) A person who contravenes subsection (1) shall be liable on summary conviction to a fine not exceeding Level 4 on the standard scale.

Children legislation[7]

The welfare of the child is the paramount consideration for those with responsibilities in caring for the child. Parents could be prosecuted if they fail to obtain assistance from a registered medical practitioner in the event of their child becoming seriously ill. In a recent case parents were convicted, the father imprisoned and the mother given a suspended sentence when they sought homeopathic remedies instead of insulin for their diabetic daughter, who died as a result.[8]

Cancer Act 1939

This Act makes it, amongst other provisions, illegal to place certain advertisements for the treatment of cancer. Section 4 is set out in Box 5.6.

Box 5.6   Cancer Act 1939, section 4(1), (4) and (5)

(1) No person shall take any part in the publication of any advertisement containing an offer to treat any person for cancer, or to prescribe any remedy therefor, or to give any advice in connection with the treatment thereof.
(4) In any proceedings for a contravention of subsection (1) of this section, it shall be a defence for the person charged to prove —
(a) that the advertisement … was published only so far as was reasonably necessary to bring it to the notice of persons of the following classes…
 (i) members of either House of Parliament or of a local authority or of the governing body of a voluntary hospital;
(ii) [repealed]
(iii) registered medical practitioners;
(iv) registered nurses;
 (v) registered pharmacists…
(vi) persons undergoing training with a view to becoming registered medical practitioners, registered nurses or pharmacists;
(b) that the said advertisement was published only in a publication of a technical character intended for circulation mainly amongst persons of the classes mentioned in [(a) above]; or
(c) that the said advertisement was published in such circumstances that he did not know and had no reason to believe that he was taking part in the publication thereof.
(5) Nothing in this section shall apply in respect of any advertisement by a local authority or by the governing body of a voluntary hospital or by any person acting with the sanction of the Minister.

The approval of the Attorney or Solicitor General is necessary before a prosecution can be brought under the Cancer Act 1939. Advertisement is defined in the Act to include 'any notice, circular, label, wrapper or other document, any announcement made orally or by any means of producing or transmitting sounds'.

OTHER ACTS

Fair Trading Act 1973

This Act aims at ensuring competition in the supply of goods. Under the Act powers are given to the Director General of Fair Trading to control monopolies. A monopoly is defined in section 6 as including the situation where one quarter of all the goods of that description which are supplied in the United Kingdom are supplied by one and the same person or company.

Health and Safety at Work etc. Act 1974

Relevant offences under this Act and subsequent Regulations are considered in detail in Chapter 13.

Fraudulent Mediums Act 1951

This is discussed fully in Chapter 20.

Road Traffic Act 1988 (as amended)

Therapists need to be aware of the regulations made under this Act which make it a criminal offence in certain circumstances for a persons to drive when medically unfit to do so.

Situation 2   Unfit for driving

A client visited a homeopath for advice in controlling his diabetes. He had recently had a coma. The therapist gave advice which included the suggestion that he should obtain a referral to the diabetic clinic at the hospital. The client was later involved in a serious accident. The police have asked the therapist for evidence as to what took place at the session.

The therapist would have to co-operate with the police and could not claim any professional immunity from answering questions about the client's knowledge and fitness to drive. If a prosecution was initiated, the prosecution could use the fact that the client knew that he was unfit to drive a car as his diabetes was not under control.

Questions and Exercises

1. Following a psychotherapy session, the therapist is constantly pursued by a client. In what circumstances do you consider that the therapist should take action to draw the attention of the police to what could be regarded as criminal activity?
2. A client is claiming that a therapist has obtained property by deception in offering healing services to cure her cancer. In what circumstances could a prosecution succeed against the therapist?
3. Professions which are state registered have the support of the criminal law in making it an offence to use certain titles. To what extent do you consider that the criminal law should be used to support complementary therapies?

REFERENCES

1. Dyer C 1992 Manufacturers fined for vitamin claims. British Medical Journal 305: 974
2. News item. The Times 23 July 1997
3. R. v. Ireland; R. v. Burstow The Times Law Report 25 July 1997
4. R. v. Adomako House of Lords The Times Law Report 4 July 1994
5. Food supplement claims. The Food Commission, 1997 London
6. Young R Watchdog finds health claims hard to swallow. The Times 21 July 1997 p 9
7. For further information on the law relating to child health care see B Dimond The Legal Aspects of Child Health Care Mosby 1996
8. News report. The Times 6 November 1993

6

Regulation of Therapy

This chapter discusses the extent to which the state is prepared to regulate the groups who practise complementary or alternative medicines and the principles upon which the state does so.

THE BASIC LAWS WHICH APPLY

It is wrong in one sense to state that complementary therapies are not regulated since both the organisations and the members are subject to all those civil and criminal laws which create a framework for every individual and organisation in this country. This legal context is discussed in this book in Chapter 3 on the law of negligence, Chapter 5 on the criminal law, Chapter 13 on health and safety laws, Chapter 15 on laws relating to property and Chapters 9 and 10 on consent, confidentiality and access to health records. In addition the individual chapters on specific therapies give details on laws relevant to those topics. It will be clear from these diverse and extensive provisions, that complementary therapies hardly operate in a legal vacuum. What people mean when they use the word 'unregulated' is that there is an absence of specific state regulation for individual therapies.

Any practitioner can set up in business and offer a service to clients. In the absence of fraud or misrepresentation, no action could be brought to prevent this activity, although of course all the laws relating to health and safety, planning permissions, taxation law and small businesses would have to be complied with. Moreover in the event of any harm occurring the client would have the right to sue the therapist/practitioner for negligence or for breach of contract. There is at the time of writing no Bill of Rights in this country which stipulates certain inalienable rights for each citizen, but citizens can carry on their lawful business unless harm is caused to any person and unless any other laws limiting their activities or requiring them to be conducted in a particular way apply. The Human Rights Bill is before Parliament (see Chapter 2).

The absence of any overall state regulation for complementary/alternative medicine has been considered to raise specific issues for consumers:

- need for choice and information
- safety protection
- redress.[1]

WHY STATE REGISTRATION?

The state has intervened to require registration by specific registration bodies set up in respect of the practice of medicine, dentistry, nursing, midwifery and health visiting. There are specific Acts of Parliament governing each of these professions and in addition under the Professions Supplementary to Medicine Act 1960 certain other health professionals obtained registered status (see below).

Box 6.1   The benefits of state registration

A profession which is state registered has the following advantages:
1. It becomes a criminal offence wrongly to hold oneself out as having that specific title.
2. Minimum standards of competence can be established and enforced.
3. There is an established mechanism for discipline, admission to and removal from the Register.
4. The Register can be published to the general public.
5. The registration authority can issue directions on legal and ethical issues and enforce minimum standards of practice.
6. Pressure groups can work through the Registration body to influence the government over future developments.

There are of course different attitudes over whether state registration is appropriate for some of the complementary therapies. Some may value the state being prepared to intervene to regulate through a system of state registration if this is warranted by the need to protect the public. Other associations may want state registration for their own interests e.g. to protect the standards of their associations, to prevent unauthorised persons practising in that field, and to give them additional status thereby protecting their economic interests. Other groups see state registration as an unwelcome intrusion and feel that their liberty would be unduly restricted through that system.

Baroness Trumpington[2] put forward the official view in 1987 when, as Parliamentary Under Secretary for State, she said

I am firmly of the view that alternative therapists must themselves address the question of standards and qualifications ... Another reason for registration is professional status – a worthy aim, but one that alternative practitioners must convince society they deserve. A problem that prevents the further development and acceptability of alternative therapies is the super-abundance of organisations concerned. To the outsider they all seem to be making similar claims and have common objectives. This can only confuse the public. ... If the organisations representing alternative practitioners are going to get their message across then they need unison and harmony, but not discord.

A cynic might suggest that state regulation of a therapy in terms of registered status is only appropriate when those in power in orthodox medicine are prepared to recognise its validity. Thus the history of the acceptance of osteopathy and chiropractic shows considerable opposition from orthodox medicine to acceptance and state registration. Wardwell[3] describes the battle of osteopathy and chiropractic to obtain acceptance and quotes Morris Fisbein who expressed the view in 1925:

Osteopathy is essentially a method of entering the practice of medicine by the back door. Chiropractic, by contrast, is an attempt to arrive through the cellar. The man at the back door at least makes himself presentable. The one who comes through the cellar is besmirched with dust and grime; he carries a crowbar and he may wear a mask.

CRITERIA

When state registration was considered to be necessary the criteria suggested by the Review body for the Professions Supplementary to Medicine Act 1960 (see below) were based on the need to protect the public. It suggested that protection is required over occupations which involve the elements shown in Box 6.2.

Box 6.2   Criteria for state registration

Occupations which involve either:

- invasive procedures or clinical intervention with the potential for harm; or
- the exercise of judgment by the unsupervised professional which can substantially impact on patient health or welfare;

and where such procedures or judgment are not already regulated by other means (for example through supervision or other legislation).

CPSM 1960 AND ITS PHILOSOPHY

The Council for the Professions Supplementary to Medicine (CPSM) was established under the Professions Supplementary to Medicine Act 1960. It is an independent, self-regulating, statutory body. At present it covers the professions shown in Box 6.3.

> **Box 6.3** Professions covered by the CPSM
>
> - chiropody
> - dietetics
> - medical laboratory science
> - occupational therapy
> - orthoptics
> - physiotherapists
> - radiography.

Discussions are also in hand with art therapists, orthotists, and prosthetists and many other groups seeking registered status.

There is a Board for each of the seven professions under its aegis. The CPSM reports to the Privy Council but there is direct access from the professional Boards to the PC. The CPSM appoints a registrar who runs a secretariat for the CPSM and the Boards, administering the registration scheme and providing support services. The Chairman of the Council is appointed by the Privy Council.

Activities of the CPSM

Under section 1 of the Act the CPSM has the general function of co-ordinating and supervising the activities of the Boards established under the Act and the additional functions assigned to it. These functions are set out in Box 6.4.

> **Box 6.4** Functions of the CPSM
>
> 1. General function of co-ordinating and supervising the activities of the Boards (section 1).
> 2. Making to each Board or inviting the Boards to make to Council, proposals as to the activities to be carried on by the Board.
> 3. Recommending a Board to carry on such activities, or to limit its activities in such manner, as the Council considers appropriate after consultation with the Board on the proposals.
> 4. Concerning itself with matters appearing to it to be of special interest to any two or more of the Boards, and by giving the Boards such advice and assistance as it thinks fit with respect to such matters.
> 5. Exercising its powers under the provisions of the Act in such manner as the CPSM considers most conducive to the satisfactory performance by each Boards of that Board's function under the Act.
> 6. Keeping the registers from each Board and lists deposited open at all reasonable times for inspection by members of the public.

The CPSM acts as the mediator between the Boards and the Privy Council. In its explanatory booklet published in March 1995, it describes itself as having eight primary areas of activity shown in Box 6.5.

Box 6.5 Primary areas of activity of the CPSM

1. NHS purchasers and providers, current changes, private practice and insurance cover
2. Educational changes and relationships
3. Department of Employment, Occupational Standards Council (NVQs)
4. Issues relating to regulation and relationship with educational providers, government departments, disciplinary functions, and statements of conduct
5. Professional bodies
6. European and International dimension
7. Reviewing possible changes to the 1960 Act and the framework for regulations and registration set up under it
8. Internal efficiency of the CPSM

Composition of the council

The Council is constituted in accordance with Part 1 of the First Schedule to the Act. There are 23 members of whom:

- Four are appointed by the Privy Council (one of these must be resident in Scotland and one in Wales).
- One is appointed by the Secretary of State

None of these can be a registered medical practitioner or a member of the stated professions.

- Four persons are appointed jointly by the Secretary of State for Social Services, the Secretary of State for Wales, the Secretary of State for Scotland and the Minister of Health and Local Government.

Two of these only shall be registered medical practitioners and none shall be a member of the stated professions.

- Seven shall be representative members of the Council appointed by each Board.
- Three registered medical practitioners are appointed, one by each of English colleges.
- Three registered medical practitioners are appointed jointly by the Scottish Corporation.
- One registered medical practitioner is appointed by the General Medical Council.

Each Board is entitled to appoint an alternate member for each representative member (Paragraph 1(2)). In addition each Board may appoint two persons to act as additional members of the Council (without right to vote) at any meeting at which the Council is considering a matter appearing to the Council to be of special interest to registered members of the professions for which the Board is established.

Functions of the boards

Each Board has the following functions.

1. To promote the high standards of professional education and professional conduct (section 1(2)).

2. To prepare and maintain a register of the names, addresses and qualifications, and such other particulars as may be prescribed, of all persons who are entitled in accordance with the provisions of the Act to be registered by the Board and who apply in the prescribed manner to be so registered.

3. To cause the register to be printed, published and put on sale to members of the public.

4. To publish corrections to the register.

5. To cause a print of each edition of the register and of each list of corrections to be deposited at the offices of the CPSM.

6. It may approve

- any course of training
- any qualification
- any institution

with a view to registered status being conferred. It may also refuse its approval or withdraw such an approval previously given.

7. It has a duty to keep itself informed of the nature of:

- the instruction given at approved institutions to persons attending approved courses of training; and
- the examinations as the result of which approved qualifications are granted

8. It can appoint persons to visit approved institutions or attend examinations for the purposes under 6 above. The visitor has the duty to report to the Board as to the sufficiency of the instruction given to persons attending approved courses of training at the institutions or the sufficiency of examinations, and as to any other matters relating to the institutions or examinations; but no such visitor shall interfere with the giving of any instruction or the holding of any examination.

When the Board approves a course of training or a qualification:

- the Board sends its recommendations to the Council
- the Council shall send the application and the recommendations together with its own recommendations to the Privy Council
- the Privy Council shall determine whether the approval is to be given or refused.

An opportunity must be given to the applicant by the Privy Council to make representations to it, before approval is refused.

When the Board approves an institution for training the approval does not have to go before the Council or the Privy Council.

The Board can publish statements of 'infamous conduct' and enforce professional discipline (see below). Ultimately it can strike a practitioner from the register.

The Board appoints its own chairman, usually from amongst the profession that the Board represents. Other members of the Board are directly elected from the profession, the Royal Medical Colleges, Universities, employers and other specialist interests. Each Board elects a practising member of the Profession to the CPSM.

Registration machinery

Each Board under the CPSM maintains a register. The NHS require professions supplementary to medicine to have registered status to work in the NHS. The CPSM describes state registration as

guaranteeing a threshold of competence, an acceptance of professional discipline, and duties of care to cover 'omission' as well as 'commission'. It acts as a gateway into the NHS and to the wider 'family' of medical professions.[4]

In the annual report for 1993–4 the CPSM set out a statement about state registration[5] defining more fully what benefits this gives to those registered.

Box 6.6   CPSM statement on state registration

The unique qualities of State Registration.
Only relevant practitioners able to demonstrate current 'State Registration' (as opposed to just 'registration')
- are intentionally defined in a range of statutes as 'health professionals',
- have attended courses and gained qualifications under a system of quality control approved by the Privy Council,
- accept the discipline of the judicial sanction of being 'struck off' for 'infamous conduct',
- are automatically accepted on that basis alone by the General Medical Council and the British Medical Association as being persons to whom it is proper for medical practitioners to delegate treatment,
- have their qualifications statutorily recognised in other European countries under the EC directive on mutual recognition of higher education diplomas,
- are automatically deemed in statutes governing local authorities to be of such probity as not to require (medical) inspection of their professional activities,
- are recognised by the great majority of private health care and medical insurance providers as meeting the highest standards in their profession (and state registration is a requirement for all but a handful of these providers), and
- if Chiropodists, are legally able to administer local anaesthetics (and perform surgery on the foot) and to be exempted from relevant prescription-only drugs regulations.

State registration can thus be seen as a universal standard and a kitemark of excellence. It is a specific offence to make a false claim to state registration.

THE 1996 REVIEW AND RECOMMENDATIONS

A review of the Professions Supplementary to Medicine Act 1960 has recently been undertaken by JM Consulting Ltd under a steering group chaired by Professor Sheila McLean. Following a consultation document issued in October 1995, a report was published in July 1996.[6]

The report described the present weaknesses of the Professions Supplementary to Medicine Act, identifying two broad types, the weaknesses in the powers provided by the 1960 Act and those in the statutory bodies and working arrangements. It explored the developments which had taken place since 1960 including:

- the development of primary care
- the internal market

- the use of multi-disciplinary teams and the possibility of non state registered professionals being employed in the NHS by GPs
- the growth of private sector provision
- the changes which have taken place within the professions such as the development of strong professional associations with regulations for discipline
- the inappropriateness of the term 'Professions Supplementary to Medicine'.

  Other changes include:

- the new professions which have sought state registered status
- developments within higher education and degree status for many professions and education provision being made outside the NHS
- changing attitudes in society and public expectations.

Its recommendations cover the following areas:

- basic recommendations
- the establishment of a Council for Health Professions (CHP)
- the establishment of Statutory Committees and a Panel of Professional Advisers
- protection of title.

Basic recommendations

Basic recommendations of the review body on the 1960 Act are as follows:

1. A new statutory body should be established with new powers.
2. Legislation should allow for the growth in the number of professions.
3. The purpose of the new legislation should be the protection of the public.
4. Professions to be covered should be based on the potential for harm arising from either invasive procedures or the application of unsupervised judgment by the professional which can substantially impact on patient/client health or welfare.
5. The seven existing professions under the CPSM should be included plus arts therapy, prosthetics and orthotics.
6. Other professional groups may be eligible.
7. Protection of common title for all of the regulated professions should be established.
8. The new statutory body should have more effective and flexible powers.
9. The government, through the Secretary of State or Privy Council should continue to provide oversight and the ultimate court of appeal, but with reduced involvement in policy and administrative matters.
10. The normal costs of the regulatory body should be funded from registration fees.

Recommendations on the council

The recommendations of the review body on the Council are:

1. A new enlarged Council for Health Professions (CHP) should be established,

with stronger powers to decide on matters currently referred to the Privy Council and with broader membership.

2. The overall function of the CHP should be 'to provide protection to the public by specifying and monitoring standards of education, training and conduct for health professions'.

3. The Council should be a policy-making and supervisory body rather than an executive one.

4. There should be three main types of duty for the CHP:

- matters which it could determine itself
- matters needing Government approval
- major matters which would eventually require placing before Parliament for affirmative resolution.

5. Membership of the Council should be:

- one third lay members (i.e. not registered professionals)
- each professional group to be represented equally
- professional representatives to be elected by registrants
- other interests to be represented: i.e. medical, other health professions, consumer
- nominations by Secretary of State or Privy Council.

6. The government should appoint the initial Council, following these principles, but in future the Council should be allowed to recommend changes to adapt to future circumstances.

Recommendations on statutory committees

The recommendations body on statutory committees are that the Council should delegate much of its work to statutory committees:

1. Preliminary Proceedings Committee – to investigate and deal with all initial complaints or other professional performance matters.

2. Professional Conduct Committee – to define and enforce standards of conduct, acting as a judicial committee when cases are heard.

3. Health Committee – to deal with matters of conduct possibly originating from health causes.

4. Education Committee – dealing with

- pre-registration qualifications
- continuing professional development (CPD)
- registration criteria including for overseas and European Economic Area applicants.

5. A Panel of Professional Advisers should be appointed by Council to provide the resources and the expertise to carry out much of the detailed work in education and other areas. Members of the Panel would be nominated by professional bodies and would provide:

- members of working parties
- members of Committees
- members of course validation panels
- members of the Education Committee's working committees
- a source of consultation on specific issues.

The Council could set up other non-statutory committees.
  The Government's role would be:

- to establish the initial Council
- to appoint specific members to the Council on a continuing basis to approve minor matters such as the rules and procedures of the Council
- to receive and consider applications for major changes such as the admission of the new professions and to submit these to Parliament
- to act as a final appeal forum when appropriate.

Protection of title

The report recommends that all professions regulated under the CHP would have a protected title. This would be agreed by affirmative resolution of Parliament. The Council would promote and publicise the titles and their significance to the public and employers, and would also have powers to monitor compliance with the protected title regime and to request court action against non state registered practitioners using protected titles or otherwise holding themselves out to be state registered.

Comment on the recommendations

Perhaps the most controversial of the suggestions is the recommendation that the existing statutory Boards should cease to exist and the CHP should be the umbrella organisation, emphasising the shared approach of all the professions. The report looks at the opposition to this proposal which is based on a perceived loss of professional autonomy and emphasises the lack of commonality across the professions. The report concluded

It is illogical to welcome the thought of fifteen or twenty autonomous professional boards, each with its own sub-structure of education, discipline, investigation and liaison committees. This cannot be efficient or effective.

Legislation is now awaited following this report and its future depends as much on the willingness of the new Labour Government to continue with these proposals as on the overall support that the proposals receive from the existing professions covered by the CPSM.

FUTURE CHANGES AND COMPLEMENTARY THERAPIES

The review of the Professions Supplementary to Medicine Act 1960 considered the place of state registration for complementary medicines.

The report emphasised the importance of creating a flexible structure which can adapt to the changes ahead including the requests of new professions to be included under the umbrella of the CHP. It recommends that the following criteria should be used to decide whether an occupational group should be eligible for regulation.

Box 6.7   Criteria for state regulation

Such professions:
- cover a discrete area of activity (not all of which need be exclusively theirs) displaying some homogeneity
- apply a defined body of knowledge and practice based on evidence of efficacy (a good test of efficacy for many groups will be acceptance on the part of the medical profession)
- have an established professional body (which accounts for a significant proportion of the practitioners in that occupational group)
- already (through this body) operate a voluntary register (with defined routes of entry into the profession and entry qualifications which are independently assessed)
- operate to a defined code of practice and ethical standards with disciplinary procedures[7]

THE OSTEOPATHS ACT AND CHIROPRACTORS ACT

In 1993 and 1994 respectively legislation setting up statutory registration for osteopaths and chiropractors was passed based very much on the model of the Medical Act 1983. The legislation at the time of writing is not fully implemented. Each Act is considered in detail in the relevant chapters in Section 2.

These two professions were not included in the umbrella organisation of the new Council for Health Professions which the review body recommended should be established since, as a result of the timing, they obtained their own separate legislation and regulations rather than being brought under the umbrella of the Professions Supplementary to Medicine.

NHS AND PROFESSIONAL SUPPORT AND CONTROL

Many professional associations of health professionals working in the NHS have provided advice and guidance for members who, whilst state registered in a traditional field, seek also to become skilled in a complementary therapy. Examples will be taken from the Royal College of Nursing (RCN) and the British Medical Association (BMA). In addition the state registration bodies have considered the role of their registered practitioners in relation to complementary therapies. The advice of the UKCC and the GMC will be considered and the role of the Royal Pharmaceutical Society of Great Britain explored.

The Royal College of Nursing

The RCN set up in 1991 a specialist interest group in complementary therapies. Now known as the Complementary Therapies in Nursing Forum, its aim is to promote research, standard setting and the overall advancement and development of this area of nursing practice. It set out in 1994 a revised statement of beliefs. These are summarised in Box 6.8 below. It has also published an extremely useful consumer checklist in relation to complementary therapies.[8] This gives advice to the consumer on the following areas:

- Why choose a complementary therapy
- How to choose a complementary therapy
- Questions to ask after the choice has been made.

The RCN Forum also issues position statements such as that on homeopathic preparations and herbal substances used by nurses. It has also prepared a guide to the levels of training available in complementary therapy courses which nurses may wish to undertake. The guide only includes courses with university accreditation and analyses them at five levels: certificate, diploma, degree, masters degree and doctorate.

It is clear from the growth of membership of the Forum and the popularity of the annual conference that there is considerable interest by practitioners registered with the UKCC in the value of complementary therapy in conjunction with their nursing practice and the RCN is at the forefront in providing advice for its members.

In its position statement on homeopathic preparations and herbal substances used by nurses, the RCN quotes from the UKCC guidance (see Box 6.9 and Box 27.1) and states that the RCN Indemnity Insurance scheme covers RCN members for all aspects of their nursing practice provided that:

1. They have undergone some form of training or preparation for the activities they undertake.
2. They are competent to undertake these activities.
3. They undertake such activities with the knowledge and approval of their employer.

Box 6.8 RCN Complementary Therapies in Nursing Forum statement of beliefs

1. Nurses using complementary therapies should follow the UKCC requirements on personal and professional responsibilities.
2. All patients and clients have the right to be offered and receive complementary therapies either exclusively or as part of orthodox nursing practice.
3. All patients have the right to expect that their religious, cultural and spiritual beliefs will be observed.
4. All complementary therapies available to patients must have the support of the collaborative care team.
5. A nurse who is appropriately qualified to carry out a complementary therapy must agree and work to locally agreed protocols for practice and standards of care.
6. The patient/client and nurse should determine the suitability of any proposed therapy. Informed consent should be obtained and records kept with the care record of the patient/client.
7. Where possible research based complementary therapy practices should be used.
8. Nurses should develop their self awareness and interpersonal skills.
9. Nurses using complementary therapies should be prepared to instruct carers and clients/patients.
10. Nurses have a responsibility to evaluate the outcomes of therapy.
11. There should be an annual clinical audit of nurses working in the field.

The British Medical Association

The BMA undertook research into the status and present position of complementary medicine the report of which was published in 1993,[9] but it has not since then undertaken any further work. Its remit does not cover giving advice to doctors on how they practice, nor does the BMA become involved in litigation between doctor and patient.

The UKCC

The UK Central Council for Nursing, Midwifery and Health Visiting has no responsibility for the standards of educational courses which are outside nursing, midwifery and health visiting and therefore has no direct impact upon courses in complementary therapies. However it sets out its principles in relation to a registered practitioner practising in complementary therapies in paragraphs 8 to 11 of the *Scope of Professional Practice*, which is concerned with developing practice. Other guidance is given in its advisory paper *Standards for the Administration of Medicines* (see Box 6.9) and in the *Midwives' Rules* (see Box 6.10) and the *Midwife's Code of Practice*.

From these principles it can be seen that the UKCC regards it as the responsibility of the individual practitioner to determine her competency to practice within a complementary therapy. The UKCC also requires a registered practitioner to work with colleagues in the health care team in the use of complementary therapies as in orthodox medicine. It recognised that employers may establish local protocols to provide a framework for the use of complementary therapies. It also advises its practitioners to check on the insurance cover which is available.

Box 6.9   UKCC Advice in standards for the administration of medicines[10]

Paragraph 39: Some registered nurses midwives and health visitors, having first undertaken successfully a training in complementary or alternative therapy which involves the use of substances such as essential oils, apply their specialist knowledge and skill in their practice. It is essential that practice in these respects, as in all others, is based upon sound principles, available knowledge and skill. The importance of consent to the use of such treatment must be recognised. So, too, must the practitioner's personal accountability for her or his professional practice.
  (See also Chapter 27 and UKCC advice on homeopathic medicines.)

Box 6.10   Midwives rules[11]

Rule 41 (3) Unless special exemption is given by the Council to enable a particular hospital, or other institution, to investigate new methods, a practising midwife must not administer any form of pain relief by the use of any type of apparatus or by any other means, which has not been approved by the Council other than on the instructions of a registered medical practitioner.

See also Chapter 27 and the UKCC advice to midwives in the Midwife's Code of Conduct on homeopathy.

The General Medical Council

Like the UKCC, the registration body for doctors is not directly concerned with the use of complementary therapies. However its general guidance set out in its booklet *Good Medical Practice*[12] covers the whole of the doctor's work and therefore indirectly relates to a situation where the registered practitioner is using or referring a patient to complementary therapies.

Referral

Paragraph 28 in relation to the delegation of care to non-medical staff and students would cover referral of patient by a registered medical practitioner to a complementary therapist and states:

You may delegate medical care to nurses and other health care staff who are not registered medical practitioners if you believe it is best for the patient. But you must be sure that the person to whom you delegate is competent to undertake the procedure or therapy involved. When delegating care or treatment, you must always pass on enough information about the patient and the treatment needed. You will still be responsible for managing the patient's care.

Paragraph 29 warns that

You must not enable anyone who is not registered with the GMC to carry out tasks that require the knowledge and skills of a doctor.

Both paragraphs 28 and 29 raise some legal concerns. The final sentence of paragraph 28 would suggest that the doctor becomes responsible for any harm caused by the complementary therapist to the patient, thus implying a vicarious liability on the doctor's part. This would not be so, however, unless doctors actually employ a complementary therapist. If they are simply purchasing services on behalf of a patient, then such complementary therapists would be liable in their own right to the patient. If, of course, the doctor has been negligent in a referral (chosen the wrong therapy for the patient's condition, chosen a person known to be incompetent, or given the therapist wrong or inaccurate or incomplete information about the patient) then the doctor would be directly liable in his or her own right for any harm which befalls the patient as the result of this negligence.

Paragraph 29 gives rise to issues in relation to a judgment on the skills necessary to carry out complementary therapies and when a medical training is an essential prerequisite. This judgment is not easy to make unless the referring doctor has a good understanding of the individual therapy to which the patient is being referred.

Doctors using complementary therapy skills

The GMC expects registered medical practitioners to abide by its guidance in whatever role they are caring for patients. Thus in the *Good Medical Practice* guidelines paragraph 1 states:

Patients are entitled to good standards of practice and care from their doctors. Essential elements of this are professional competence, good relationships with patients and colleagues and observance of professional ethical obligations.

This principle would apply to both the practice of conventional and complementary medicine.

In July 1992 the professional conduct committee of the GMC heard five charges of professional misconduct brought against Dr Keith Mumby which arose in connection with his practice of clinical ecology. He was found guilty of two of the charges, touting for publicity and failing to give a patient adequate medical attention.

The policy of the GMC has been criticised by Dr Kay who appeared as an expert witness in the case on the grounds that the GMC failed to consider the wider issue of the use of treatments that are not scientifically validated.[13] Dr Kay states that

The basic concepts of clinical ecology are unproved. Clinical ecologists therefore attempt to diagnose and treat a disease [total allergy syndrome] which conventional doctors believe does not exist ... The GMC must face the issue of alternative allergy practice, particularly when a diagnosis is given of an illness which conventional doctors believe does not exist and when potentially dangerous dubious substances are injected.

Dr Kay also quotes the GMC charging Dr James Sharp in 1989 over his adoptive immuno-therapy treatment with advising and treating patients with AIDS, AIDS related complex and HIV infections without sufficient knowledge, training or experience to treat the conditions competently and offering the treatment without proper clinical trials and despite inadequate independent scientific evidence to support it.

He recommends that the GMC should review its policy on advertising to prevent outrageous advertisements while at the same time permitting the public's access to proved specialist services.

Dr Kay raises a fundamental principle about the role of the state registration bodies when their registered practitioners take part in or refer patients to therapies which have not been scientifically validated. Given the difficulties of establishing, according to conventional methods of scientific validation (see in particular homeopathic medicine), the benefits of many of the therapies discussed in this book, is it right to give to a registration body the power to prevent its registered practitioners practising in these alternative fields? The same principles could of course apply to the UKCC and the CPSM and their registered practitioners.

It is relevant to note that several organisations for complementary therapies have been set up where the membership is restricted to those already registered as medical practitioners or dentists such as the British Medical Acupuncture Society and the Faculty of Homeopathy.

Royal Pharmaceutical Society of Great Britain

This organisation is responsible for the admission, regulation and monitoring of registered pharmacists. It was criticised recently by Dr Charles Shepherd Medical Adviser to the M.E. Association[14] in a documentary on BBC2 which investigated

Signalysis Laboratories in Gloucester run by non-medical practitioners, which purported to diagnose and prescribe treatments from heating urine and blood samples. The business described itself as preparing products under the supervision of a registered pharmacist on premises registered with the Royal Pharmaceutical Society of Great Britain. Dr Shepherd said that the Royal Society had been complacent and should be more active in protecting the public. Disciplinary hearings have been held by the Royal Society and at the time of writing the outcome is still awaited.

Medical protection organisations

To what extent do the main providers of protection for doctors and dentists provide the cover for members who practise in complementary therapies?

The Medical Defence Union

The MDU only provides cover for registered medical and dental practitioners. It does not have members who are practising in the field of complementary therapies who are not medically qualified.

The Board of Management has the power to decide not to assist a member in a particular circumstance and is not bound by a contractual arrangement as would be the case with an insurance policy. In practice, however, this is hardly ever exercised and discretion can of course act in favour of the member. Having said that, the Board of Management would expect that any member undertaking a particular procedure or providing a specific therapy would have the necessary training, skill and experience, equipment and assistance safely to provide a service to patients.[15]

The MDU asks members to tell it about their areas of clinical activity, but admits that sometimes it only hears of their practice when a claim or complaint arises. It states:

We do not restrict clinical activity at present, but this is a subject under review, and we already charge an additional subscription, for example, to GP members who are undertaking cosmetic surgery – an area which gives rise to a disproportionate number of claims and complaints.

The MDU provides no written guidance about alternative medicine but would respond to individual questions by members.

The Medical Protection Society

Like the MDU the MPS only accepts into its membership practitioners who have a medical or dental qualification. Therefore all its members who practise in homeopathy or alternative medicine are also medically trained and registered.

In terms of the standard of care which members practising in complementary therapies should follow, the MPS encourages its members to adopt practices which command the support of a respectable and responsible body of professional opinion i.e. the Bolam test.

Provided the member can command Bolam type support we would be prepared to defend his acts and omissions. If a member could not obtain expert opinion support then the

Society is likely to have to settle the claim (always assuming that the member was in benefit at the time of the incident giving rise to the matter).[16]

The MPS has dealt with claims in relation to alternative or complementary medicine. The Secretary and Medical Director cited such cases as:

- pneumothorax following the insertion of acupuncture needles
- adverse skin reactions following homeopathic treatments
- omissions of treatment for certain conditions (e.g. underlying breast lumps, bowel neoplasms, etc.) for which inappropriate remedies were given and the patient was inadequately investigated and treated.

The MPS is not an academic institute or clinical body. It would therefore expect members to receive advice about clinical management from their universities, postgraduate institutions, Royal Colleges etc. Its guidance is purely of a medico-legal kind and it does not have anything specific in relation to complementary therapies. The Medical Director stated:

We do try to ensure that our members have a clear understanding of the responsible boundaries of clinical practice as mapped out by the Bolam test.

Conclusions

From the responses from both MDU and MPS it is clear that there is no tight distinction between providing protection for orthodox medicine and for complementary therapies. Both associations, however, require members to be registered medical or dental practitioners. Nevertheless this does not prevent claims being made in respect of activities in the field of complementary therapies. Both associations admit that claims are being settled in respect of harm arising from the practice of complementary therapies by their members.

REGULATION THROUGH LOCAL AUTHORITIES

The local authority is the enforcement agency for several Acts of Parliament which relate to the practice of complementary therapies. The legislation is considered in detail in the relevant chapters including Chapter 13 on health and safety.

The trading standards department

The trading standards department of a local authority has enforcement powers under the Trade Descriptions Act 1968, the Weights and Measures Act 1985, Part II and Part III of the Consumer Protection Act 1987 and the Consumer Credit Act 1974. It will follow up any complaint about a practitioner in complementary therapy offering services to the public if there appears to be a breach of the law, for example it will pursue a case where a practitioner has fraudulently claimed qualifications to which he or she was not entitled. If, however, the client is complaining that the therapy did not appear to be effective, then the department would advise the client to refer that complaint to the appropriate association for that therapy.

The environmental protection department

The environmental protection department is the enforcement agency in relation to the Health and Safety at Work etc. Act 1974 for those premises which come under the jurisdiction of the local authority. Where a licence is required (see below) it will visit the premises and prepare a report for the licensing department. Owners of offices, shops and railway premises are required to register with the local authority and the environmental health department is able to inspect the premises. The frequency of their inspection visits will depend upon their assessment of risks involved. Thus premises used for electrolysis or ear piercing or acupuncture would be visited relatively frequently because of the greater risk of infection than with a therapy which was not invasive. The environmental health offices also act as the enforcement agency of the COSHH regulations (see Chapter 13) in the relevant premises. Where a therapist is working from home, then the Health and Safety Executive would be the enforcement agency for the provisions of the Health and Safety at Work etc. Act 1974.

Licensing function of the local authority

Certain therapies are required to obtain a licence from the local authority to practise. These include acupuncture (see Chapter 16) and services such as ear piercing and tattooing. Licences are also required for public entertainment (see Chapter 28 and licenses for hypnosis).

REGULATION THROUGH THE CHARITY COMMISSIONERS

Many organisations involved in complementary therapies are registered as charities. They are thus subject to the requirements of the law as set out in the 1960 and 1992 Charities Acts and come under the control of the Charity Commissioners. Guidance is available from the Charity Commissioners (see bibliography). There are currently over 150 000 organisations which are registered charities. The Commissioners encourage any organisation considering registering as a charity to consider linking up with an existing registered charity, to take advantage of size and save on administrative costs. The register is available for inspection.

Registration with the Commission is possible if

- the organisation carries out charitable purposes
- all or a majority of the charity trustees are normally resident in England and Wales
- all or most of the assets are held in England and Wales
- the organisation, being a company, is incorporated in England or Wales.

Charitable purposes include:

- the relief of the elderly, vulnerable or hardship
- the advancement of education
- the advancement of religion
- other charitable purposes for the benefit of the community.

The organisation must satisfy at least one of these purposes and in addition be established for the public benefit.

Charities which do not hold capital, or have less than £1000 income, or do not have the use or occupation of rateable land in this country are exempt from registration. Others are exempt by specific regulation. These include some special schools and some charities for the advancement of religion. Organisations registered under the Friendly Societies Act 1974 are also exempt.

The advantages of being registered as a charity include benefits in relation to exemption from income and corporation tax and VAT, lower business rate, and assistance from the Commissioners. In addition fundraising is facilitated by being a registered charity. An example of a conflict fought by executors of a will over whether the bequest was a charitable one is discussed in Chapter 25 on healing.[17]

Any charity will have a governing document. This states the information shown in Box 6.11.

Box 6.11   Governing document of charity

This will state:
- objects of the charity
- powers of the charity
- trustees of the charity
- administrative provisions (voting, meetings, financial arrangements etc.)
- provisions for dissolution of the charity.

The drawbacks (or statutory obligations of being a registered charity) relate to the control over the name of the organisation and the accounts which have to be submitted to the Commissioners. The nature of the accounts and the type of audit depends upon the size of charity. Charities with gross expenditure over £100 000 per year must submit the full annual accounts and an annual report and have a full audit once a year. The accounts are to be made public. In contrast a charity with less than £1000 income which has voluntarily registered as a charity, only has to submit simplified accounts, with an independent examination rather than an audit.

Criminal sanctions against those who fail to comply with the requirements were introduced by the 1992 Act. There are also strict regulations relating to the role of the trustees on any charity. However regulation is more in respect of the fiduciary duties of trustees, not to make an inappropriate profit from their position and to ensure that the charity's monies are well spent, rather than enforcing a suitable code of behaviour and ethics in respect of relations with patients and potential patients.

Case 1   Appeal to the charity commissioners[18]

A complaint was made to the Charity Commissioners by a group of breast cancer patients who challenged a scientific study in which they were subjects. The study was funded by the Cancer Research Campaign and the Imperial Cancer Research Fund and the results, which were widely publicised, appeared to show that women treated at an alternative therapy clinic in Bristol were twice as likely to die of the disease as those treated with conventional medicine. Subsequently the study was found to be flawed, allowance not being made for the fact that more seriously ill patients were being treated at the clinic.

An investigation by the Charity Commissioners criticised the failure of the charities to control the allocation of funds to research and for allowing research to be published under their name without ensuring its soundness.

SELF-REGULATION

Self-Regulation is like putting Dracula in charge of the Blood Bank.[19]

These words were spoken by Robert Packman on the BBC when commenting upon the reliance on self-regulation by the London Stock Exchange in comparison with that in the USA where there was greater state control. However the words could apply to any area of customer service where similar organisations establish a body regulating professional conduct between members. Thus estate agents, builders, travel agencies and operators, care agencies providing personal services in individual homes, to name but a few of the wide variety of organisations, all have an umbrella organisation which sets standards and codes of practice for members.

The function of the umbrella organisation is usually two-fold. On the one hand it provides some measure of protection for the disgruntled consumer, possibly through establishing a Code of Conduct for all its members and a complaints procedure, and rarely as a means of obtaining compensation for harm; and on the other hand it provides some protection for the honest, conscientious supplier of services – an accreditation, so that potential customers will know that, in using services of a member of the organisation they can be assured of a provider who follows standards and is trustworthy (thus implicitly deprecating those who are not members of the organisation and warning the public against quacks).

Where it works well the system is a good one; it is, after all, in the interests of all that high standards should be maintained. However when it fails the public is left unprotected. An example of a situation where self-regulation has been considered by the government to be unsatisfactory and has not prevented rogue firms exploiting the public, and has thus led to state intervention, is that of private security firms. The government announced in July 1997 its intention of introducing new legislation to control the activities and standards of such firms. The announcement was welcomed by the British Security Industries Association which had complained that these rogue firms were tarnishing the reputation of the industry. Here the umbrella organisation was being let down by some of its members. In other cases the organisation itself is at fault.

An example of the meaninglessness of some lists of members of some associations is vividly illustrated by a letter sent to the financial advice column in the *Sunday Times* run by Roger Anderson. On 18 May 1997 he printed a letter as follows:

Case 2   Meaningless 'qualifications'

I paid £15 to Empathy International for introductory literature on how to practise hypnotherapy. I did not like what I saw and chose not to pay for the full course. Although I received the guaranteed refund, Empathy International has now included me in a list of associate members, with the letters Assc MEACH after my name, plus my address and telephone number.

Roger Anderson's reply pointed out that the form that the correspondent had signed included an agreement that he would be put on the list so that other members could contact him 'on matters hypnotherapeutic'. He also commented that the letters 'Assc MEACH' could mean that the 'therapist' has had no training whatsoever.

The lessons from the correspondent's experience are that members of the public should be wary, both of signing forms to accept offers when they could be agreeing to commitments they do not appreciate or understand and also of making use of the services of therapists without checking the actual meaning of credentials which they put forward.

In practice many therapists and their organisations have shown clear commitment to high standards and ethical practice and the chapters in Section 2 of this book give examples of some of the main organisations which provide high standards of self-regulation for their members.

Central organisations

In addition there are some central organisations covering several different therapies which are dedicated to the maintenance of high standards of practice.

British Complementary Medicine Association

The BCMA was formed in 1990. Fifty different organisations come under its rules and they have a total of over 25 000 individual members representing over 30 different therapies. It has produced a Code of Conduct[20] which the members of the organisations affiliated with it are required to observe and to which such organisations attach, as an appendix, provisions relevant to their therapy. This Code covers:

- An introduction
- The Code of Conduct
- Disciplinary and complaints procedures
- Explanatory notes on the law and ethics.

In the Code of Conduct the BCMA recognises the necessity of its members working alongside orthodox medicine and the importance of their patients receiving medical advice.

To this end new patients/clients must be asked what medical advice they have received. If they have not seen a doctor, they must be advised to do so.

The BCMA is a non-profit making body with an elected unpaid committee.

The Institute of Complementary Medicine

The Institute of Complementary Medicine was formed in 1982 as an educational charity supporting research and development of all forms of complementary medicine education, training and national registration. It established a register of practitioners in the various fields. In 1989 it set up the British Council for Complementary Medicine with the intention of this organisation taking over the British Register of Complementary Therapists within a few years. The Divisions on the Register include:

- Aromatherapy
- Chinese medicine
- Chromotherapy
- Counselling
- Energy medicine
- Healing/counselling
- Homeopathy
- Hypnotherapy
- Indian medicine
- Japanese medicine
- Massage
- Nutrition
- Osteopathy
- Reflexology
- Remedial massage and
- a general division.

The ICM sees 'complementary' as 'complementing what the body, mind or spirit requires', it does not mean 'to complement another service or treatment'. Its mission statement is shown in Box 6.12.

With 423 courses and organisations affiliated to the ICM, it considers that it thus represents 80% of the field out of an estimated 60–70 000 practitioners. It is concerned with standards and methods of practice and education and would like to see complementary medicine brought under state regulation. It requires persons on the British Register to have adequate insurance cover but does not arrange this itself. Affiliated organisations are required to follow its Code of Ethics and Practice, which is regularly updated. It has devised protocols for research designed to bridge the gap between the individual holistic nature of the therapies and the demands for randomly controlled trials. Professional associations are encouraged to use the ICM's Code of Ethics and Practice for members as the basis on which to build their individual requirements. Each Division of the British Register is autonomous and there is provision for the introduction of variations and additions to the requirements for admission to any Division from time to time.

Box 6.12 Mission statement of ICM

The Institute is the focal point of learning and healing for those concerned with the future of humanity, the future of health care and the way in which people are educated in personal development.

It is a meeting point for those wishing to share in the deeper understanding of the philosophies of life and living.

Complementary medicine is holism in practice.

The Council for Complementary and Alternative Medicine

This was established to provide a forum for communication and cooperation between the professional organisations for the complementary therapies of acupuncture, herbal medicine, homeopathy, naturopathy and osteopathy. It is not an accreditation body.

The Federation of Holistic Therapists

There are other umbrella organisations which cover a wide variety of therapies.
The Federation of Holistic Therapists represents the following:

- International Federation of Health and Beauty Therapists (which covers the Society of Health and Beauty Therapists, the Association of Therapy Teachers and the Health and Beauty Employers Federation)
- The International Council of Holistic Therapists
- The International Council of Health, Fitness and Sports Therapists (which covers the Finnish Sauna Society and the Institute of Massage and Movement)
- The Federation of Professional Sugaring

All members of the Federation of Holistic Therapists must abide by the Code of Ethics and subsidiary ethical rules. A list of the qualifications it recognises for membership of the Federation is given and this includes over 90 different qualifications including City and Guilds and NVQs. It notes that whilst membership at associate or fellowship level is normally restricted to those who have obtained one of the listed qualifications, a small number of candidates have been allowed into membership without the necessity of taking such examinations. This is primarily for those possessing an alternative therapy qualification and this will be investigated on payment of a small fee.

The declaration of those applying to join the Federation of Holistic Therapists is shown in Box 6.13.

Box 6.13   Federation of Holistic Therapists' declaration

I solemnly declare that I will observe all the conditions of the FHT constitution together with By-Laws, ethical and Other rules and Regulations thereof and I will conduct myself honourably in the practice of my profession and maintain the dignity and welfare of the Federation to the utmost of my power...

The Federation of Holistic Therapists provides insurance cover for its members. This requires information on the qualifications of the individual, the field in which they practice, the treatments which are performed, and specific cover which is required e.g. product, public and treatment liability for £2 million, student placement cover, employer's liability cover etc.

A Code of Practice for Hygiene in Salons and Clinics and also bye-laws, a Code of Ethics and subsidiary ethical rules must be followed. Specific therapies are excluded under the subsidiary ethical rules unless specific qualifications in these fields are obtained. Therapies excluded are: physiotherapy, chiropody, cutting of skin, acupuncture, anaesthetics, ultra-violet radiation, lasers, skin peeling, hair removal on the body, varicose veins, moles, warts, veins and capillaries, and the use of ozone and ultrasonic devices. In addition treatments of the opposite sex are considered undesirable except in an emergency and guidelines are put forward.

REGULATION THROUGH INSURANCE COMPANIES

In Chapter 4 the law relating to contracts of insurance is considered. It was noted that insurance companies are laying down specific requirements for providing cover. These requirements could be seen as another mechanism regulating the offer of complementary therapies to the public and may prove significant in ensuring that individual practitioners are members of a recognised and accredited organisation. The importance of the insurance industry in the protection of the public should not be ignored. Of note, too, is the extent to which certain requirements are being laid down in relation to, for example, the need for a therapist to work in conjunction with a doctor and the exclusion of certain activities such as diagnosis from cover.

THE FUTURE

There will be many groups/associations etc. of complementary medicine practitioners who will feel frustrated and excluded by the recommendations of the review of the 1960 Act. Many seek state registration as a protection of their practice – to ensure that unqualified persons do not practise creating a risk to the public. However through self-regulation they can to a considerable extent secure the advantages which state registration can bring, providing that they educate the general public in understanding the significance of membership of the organisations which provide this self-regulation. It may be that once the recommendations of the review body on the CPSM are implemented many more therapies will be brought under the umbrella of the new Council for Health Professions. Although it seems unlikely now that other therapies will secure their own legislation comparable to that of the osteopaths and the chiropractors.

The influence of insurance companies, existing registration bodies and professional associations of state registered practitioners who also work in the field of complementary therapies should not be underestimated in identifying the forces of control which exist.

At present practitioners are awaiting the European Commission's response to the Lannoye Report on the future of complementary medicine in Europe. This and the UK government's response will be crucial in determining the format and nature of the regulation of complementary therapy practitioners in the 21st century.

In the meantime the NHS Confederation has called for complementary medicine to be more tightly regulated.[21] The Report stated that the GPs and trusts were finding it difficult to make informed choices about complementary medicine because of the bewildering range of professional organisations and training courses. The Confederation seeks a government review of complementary medicine's effectiveness and training and regulation procedures. The Report surveyed 651 health professionals and alternative practitioners in Leicestershire found that complementary medicine was used at a low but significant level within the NHS. More than a third of midwives said that they used complementary techniques, mostly aromatherapy and 28% of GPs referred patients to alternative practitioners. At the time of writing Government response to the recommendations in the Report is awaited.

Questions and Exercises

1. Should you regulate a religion? If so, how do you regulate a religion?
2. There is a strong hostile move against regulation (see Chapter 35 on psychotherapies); what do you see as the advantages to a therapy of being neither state nor self-regulated?
3. It has been argued by Julia Stone and Joan Matthews that state regulation of some complementary therapies is inappropriate and the medical model is inapplicable to many therapies. What alternative do you consider is appropriate?

REFERENCES

1. Flynn D 1993 Regulation of non-conventional medicine. Consumer Policy Review 3(4): 225–31
2. Trumpington 1987 Alternative medicines and therapies and the DHSS. Journal of the Royal Society of Medicine 80: 336–8
3. Wardwell WI 1994 Alternative medicine in the United States. Social Science & Medicine. 38(8): 1061–8
4. CPSM 1995 Who we are and what we do. CPSM, London
5. CPSM Annual Report 1993–4. p 14. CPSM, London
6. The regulation of health professions: Report of a review of the professions supplementary to Medicine Act (1960) with recommendations for new legislation, conducted and published by JM Consulting Ltd July 1996
7. Taken from Lord Benson's speech in the House of Lords debate July 1992
8. RCN 1993 Complementary therapies: a consumer checklist. Scutari Press, London
9. British Medical Association 1993 Complementary Medicine: New approaches to good practice. OUP/BMA, Oxford
10. UKCC 1992 Standards for the administration of medicines. UKCC, London
11. UKCC 1993 Midwives rules. UKCC, London
12. General Medical Council Good medical practice. GMC, London
13. Kay AB 1993 Alternative allergy and the General Medical Council. British Medical Journal 306: 122–4
14. Home Ground BBC2 (Documentary on Complementary Medicine) 15 July 1997
15. Personal communication to the author
16. Personal communication to the author from the Secretary and Medical Director of the MPS. 9 May 1997
17. Funnel and another v. Stewart and others The Times Law Report 9 December 1995
18. Hunt E Independent 7 January 1994 p 5
19. Packman R News item BBC1 24 October 1996
20. BCMA Code of Conduct. BCMA, Leicester
21. NHS Confederation 1997. Complementary Medicine in the NHS. Brimingham NHS Confederation

7

Employment law

The complementary therapist may be an independent self-employed practitioner and/or an employee working within a health care setting such as an NHS trust or General Practice. If a self-employed person, the therapist may employ other persons to carry out certain activities. This chapter therefore covers employment law from these different perspectives. In particular the topics shown in the box above will be covered. Reference should be made to Chapter 4 on contract law, setting out the basic principles of law covering contracts including contracts of employment. Reference should also be made to Chapter 13 on health and safety laws which includes comment on the employer's obligations in relation to health and safety.

THE EMPLOYMENT CONTRACT

Distinguished from other contracts

A contract of employment relates to a situation when one individual or organisation, 'the employer', contracts with an individual, 'the employee', to provide remuneration in consideration of the other acting as an employee and rendering services in that capacity. It is known as a 'contract of service'. Once the contract is agreed the existence of the employment relationship means that the employer is held in law vicariously liable for negligence and other civil wrongs of the employee, if they occurred in the course of the employment (see Chapter 3 on negligence where the concept of vicarious liability is further explained). As a consequence of the employment relationship other duties for both the employer and the employee arise resulting from statutory and common law provision (see statutory and implied terms below).

A contract of service is the employment contract and must be distinguished from a 'contract for services'. The latter is the hiring of an individual or organisation to provide services (often on a short term basis) where a contract of employment is not created. A contract for services does not give rise to the vicarious liability of the hirer for the wrongful acts of the individual or organisation whose services have been used. Although the hirer may, of course, be directly liable if he has used a firm knowing that they were incompetent and likely to cause harm, or if he gave them negligent instructions as a result of which harm has occurred.

The situation shown in the following box illustrates the difference.

Situation 1 Contract of service and contract for services

A. An acupuncturist employed a receptionist who was zealous in protecting the interests of her employer. On one occasion she was concerned that a client was drunk and disorderly and attempted to remove him from the waiting area. In so doing she broke the client's arm. It was subsequently established that the client was suffering from a stroke and the receptionist had acted in an inappropriate and excessive manner. The client has indicated that he will be seeking compensation.
B. An acupuncturist asked a window cleaner to clean the windows of his consulting rooms both inside and outside. The window cleaner was suspicious about a person who entered the premises and assaulted him whilst removing him from the room. It was subsequently established that the person thought to be trespassing was a prospective client.

In situation A, if it can be shown that the receptionist was acting in the course of employment and in the interests of her employer although her actions were excessive, her employer would be held vicariously liable for her actions and therefore would have to pay compensation to the client. In situation B however the window cleaner is not an employee and the acupuncturist does not therefore become vicariously liable for the harm which he has caused to the prospective client. Only if it can be shown that the acupuncturist is directly liable, e.g. in hiring a person who was clearly unsuitable to do that activity, could the acupuncturist be held liable.

Therapists should have a clear understanding of whether the services of a person working for them are used under a contract of service or a contract for services, because of the different duties which can arise. National insurance and income tax may also be payable in respect of an employee.

Sources of terms

A contract is an abstract concept: it relates to a relationship recognised in law between two persons or parties. It may be contained in writing but in fact the law only requires a contract to be evidenced in writing in very few situations (such as a contract for the sale of land). A contract comes into being once there has been an acceptance of an offer, where consideration will be provided and there is an intention to create legal relations (see Chapter 4).

The terms of a contract of employment derive from a variety of sources as can be seen from Box 7.1.

Box 7.1   Sources of a contract of employment

- Express terms agreed between the parties
- Terms implied by law
- Terms required by statutory provision
- Terms which result from collective bargaining

Express terms

Express terms will be agreed between the parties, perhaps at the interview, or will be set out in the information which preceded any application. An appointment letter may also include the terms on which the offer of the post is based. They may include: the title of the post, the starting date, the hours and salary, holidays, pension schemes etc.

Implied terms

Implied terms which the law expects the parties to recognise are shown in Box 7.2.

Box 7.2   Terms implied by law into a contract of employment

Terms implied as binding on the employee:
- the employee will obey the reasonable instructions of the employer
- the employee will act with reasonable care and skill
- the employee will be loyal to the employer
- the employee will respect any duty of confidentiality

Terms implied as binding on the employer:
- the employer will take reasonable care of the health, safety and welfare of the employee
- the employer will pay the employee
- the employer will act reasonably to the employee

Failure to observe the implied terms could lead to an action by either side for breach of contract.

STATUTORY RIGHTS IN EMPLOYMENT

Many rights are now given to an employee by Act of Parliament. These are known as statutory rights and are shown in Box 7.3. They have been consolidated in the Employment Rights Act 1996. The parties may agree more generous terms than those given by Act of Parliament but cannot agree to worse, unless there are specific opting out provisions (e.g. in a fixed term contract the parties may agree that failure to renew the contract after the fixed term will not count as a dismissal and so will not give rise to an unfair dismissal claim).

Box 7.3 Statutory rights

- right not to be unfairly dismissed
- right to receive a written statement of the employment particulars
- right to an itemised pay statement
- right not to suffer unauthorised deductions from wages
- right not to suffer detriment in health and safety cases
- right to have time off for certain public duties and in a redundancy situation
- right to have time off for ante-natal care and other maternity rights
- right to have time off for employee representation
- right to remuneration on suspension for medical grounds
- right to minimum period of notice
- right to a written statement of reasons for dismissal
- right to receive redundancy payments

The rights shown in Box 7.3 sometimes require a minimum period of service in order that the employee can claim eligibility; others, such as the right not to be dismissed in health and safety cases (Section 100 Employment Rights Act 1996) do not require any minimum length of continuous service but can be enforced by the employee as soon as the contract commences. Some rights only exist if the employer has more than a specific number of employees; others exist whatever the size of the employer's organisation. Further information on the rights of the employee can be obtained from the offices of the Department for Education and Employment.

TERMINATION OF CONTRACT

A contract of employment can be ended in the ways shown in Box 7.4.

Box 7.4 Termination of contract of employment

1. By notice
2. By performance
3. By breach
4. By frustration

Notice

Either side can end a contract of employment, but there will be a minimum notice required: either one that has been agreed by the parties or one that is set by Act of Parliament, or one that is deemed to be reasonable. The Employment Rights Act 1996 Part IX sets out the statutory periods of notice which are shown in Box 7.5.

Box 7.5 Statutory notice periods to be given by employer

- not less than one week notice if less than two years continuous service
- not less than one week notice for every year of service between two and twelve years continuous service
- not less than twelve weeks notice if more than twelve years continuous service

---

The notice required to be given by an employee is not less than one week for an employee who has been continuously employed for more than one month. Either party can waive the right to notice by agreeing payment in lieu of notice and can also treat the contract as ended without notice by reason of the conduct of the other party (i.e. contract ended by breach see below).

Performance

A fixed term of contract of employment will end when that term comes to an end i.e. the contract has been performed. However for the purposes of the law on unfair dismissal, ending a fixed term contract without continuing it equates with a dismissal and so failure to renew the fixed term could give rise to an action for unfair dismissal. However it is possible for the parties to agree before the contract begins that the right to apply to an industrial tribunal when the contract is not renewed is excluded.

Breach

Where either party in a contract of employment is in fundamental breach of its terms, this gives a right to the innocent party to regard the contract as ended by the breach of contract on the part of the other. The right of the employer to end the contract in this way is subject to the employee's right to bring an action for unfair dismissal before an industrial tribunal (see below).

Frustration

An event not envisaged when the contract was made which makes the contract radically different from what was envisaged can bring a contract of employment to an end. This is by operation of law, i.e. without the necessity of any notice to be given. Thus where an employee is sentenced to prison for a significant time the contract of employment will be frustrated by operation of law and will end automatically without notice.

UNFAIR DISMISSAL

If an employer gives the length of notice required by the contract of employment to terminate a contract that is not a breach of contract. However it could be extremely unfair on a person who has worked loyally and conscientiously for several years when there appears to be no justification for ending the contract. The concept of an unfair dismissal was therefore introduced into our law by statute. This law requires the employer to have a reason recognised by statute as the basis of the dismissal and to act reasonably when using that reason to justify the dismissal.

A recognised reason

Reasons which can be used as the ground for dismissal are shown in Box 7.6.

Box 7.6 Reasons recognised by statute as grounds for dismissal

- capability or qualifications
- conduct
- redundancy
- legal impossibility

Acting reasonably

Even where the dismissal was for a recognised reason the tribunal must decide if the employer acted reasonably or unreasonably in treating that reason as sufficient for dismissing the employee. In determining the issues the tribunal would have regard to all the circumstances including the size and administrative resources of the employer's undertaking. Other factors which are considered are:

- the extent to which the employer followed any Code of Practice for handling disciplinary matters,
- whether there was a fair investigation,
- whether the dismissal was consistent with how other employees were treated, and
- if the employer heard the employee's views.

The tribunal is required to determine the issue in accordance with equity and the substantial merits of each case.

The following is a situation where an NHS employee also wished to practise complementary therapy and in the circumstances his dismissal was held to be fair.

Case 1 A second job in the lunch hour

One of the conditions on which an occupational therapist was employed was that he would obtain permission to engage in any outside work and he would only see private clients in the evenings and at the weekend. In 1990 he was seen by an area manager seeing a private client during the normal working week. He was given a strong warning that when he saw his private clients for alternative therapy this was to be outside his normal working hours. In 1993 there was again evidence that he was seeing a patient in ordinary working hours, and that he was calling up a private client during his working time.

A disciplinary hearing was held and he was found guilty of gross misconduct in two respects: firstly in seeing a private patient during working hours, and secondly in ignoring the very clear and emphatic warning which he had been given. He was summarily dismissed for gross misconduct.

He failed in his application to the Industrial Tribunal which found the dismissal to have been fair and he also failed in his appeal to the Employment Appeal Tribunal. His defence that he was doing no more than taking an early lunch was rejected on the grounds that lunch hours are for lunch and not for seeing private patients. It was also alleged on his behalf that the management were aware that he was seeing private clients during the day and that the flexibility which he was permitted in the ordering of his work and the taking of his lunch break, enabled him to see private clients. The Employment Appeal Tribunal was satisfied that the employers had conducted a reasonable and fair enquiry into what had happened and that the decision of the Industrial Tribunal was beyond any sensible criticism.

It is therefore essential for any health professional, if an employee, to obtain the consent of the employer if he or she intends to practise privately during working hours.

EMPLOYMENT GUIDELINES

West Yorkshire Health Authority has issued guidelines aimed at assisting Health Authorities and Trusts to employ suitable qualified complementary therapists.[2] It covers three areas:

- Professional status
- Insurance
- Qualifications.

Employers following these guidelines should be able to set clear protocols to ensure patient safety.

LOCAL BARGAINING

Self-employed therapists who employ staff

Therapists who employ their own staff have complete freedom to agree the level of remuneration. Obviously however the local rates of pay for comparable work would be taken into account to ensure a good standard of applicant. Rises can be agreed with the employee and may include a regular rise reflecting any inflationary element.

Therapists employed within the NHS

Therapists who work in the NHS will have found that the Whitley Council terms and conditions of service are gradually being used less and less by employers in the NHS as local collective bargaining replaces the nationally determined standards. At present for certain categories of staff, such as nurses and doctors, the government sets a nationally fixed minimum level of increase in the light of the recommendations of the Review Bodies and then permits health authorities and trusts to agree further increases within an overall limit. Other terms and conditions such as shifts and holidays are being agreed locally.

Independent therapists providing services to NHS organisations

Some therapists may offer services to health service bodies on a contract for services basis. Thus an aromatherapist may agree with a GP fundholding practice that she will undertake three sessions a week in the practice premises, but may provide those services not as an employee but as an independent contractor on a contract for services. The method and amount of payment due under that contract would be agreed between them. In these circumstances the nature of the contract can be agreed between GPs and therapist and would be subject to the Supply of Goods and Services Act (see Chapter 4). If the therapist is negligent and harms a client, the GP would not be vicariously liable, unless he or she had been negligent in giving information to or in selecting the therapist and was directly at fault.

RIGHTS OF THE PREGNANT EMPLOYEE

The Employment Rights Act 1996 consolidates the statutory rights of the pregnant employee and rights in the event of maternity. These are summarised in booklets available from the Department for Education and Employment. The main rights are shown in Box 7.7.

Box 7.7 Statutory rights in maternity

- Time off work for antenatal care
- Right not to be dismissed on grounds of pregnancy
- Right to return after childbirth
- Right to maternity leave
- Right to receive payment during maternity leave

Maternity provision is very complicated and to ensure that she gets her full entitlement an employee must be certain to give the right notice at the right time. An employee in such a position should obtain current government guidance from a Citizens' Advice Bureau or the Department for Education and Employment.

RIGHTS IN RELATION TO SICKNESS

Employees are entitled to receive statutory sick pay from their employer when they are sick. Those who are not in work or are self-employed may be able to claim state benefits instead. These include: sickness benefit, invalidity benefit, and severe disablement allowance.

Statutory sick pay is payable for up to 28 weeks incapacity – spells separated by a period of not more than eight weeks count as one.

The statutory pay scheme applies to those who have a minimum level of service. Employers used to be able to recover some of the cost of paying out the benefits but this is no longer the case. Many employers will, nevertheless, agree more generous terms with their employees who will then receive superior sickness benefits under their contracts of employment: in the NHS most employees with the necessary continuous service have, under Whitley Council conditions, had six months full pay and six months half pay to cover sickness. However a therapist who provides services to the NHS as an independent practitioner, i.e. not an employee, would have no entitlement to sick pay from the NHS organisation and should consider getting separate insurance cover to top up any state benefits.

PROTECTION AGAINST DISCRIMINATION: RACE, SEX AND DISABILITY

The main legislation protecting persons against discrimination on grounds of race or sex are the Race Relations Act 1976 and the Sex Discrimination Act 1975 and subsequent amendments. The Equal Pay Act 1970 implies an equality clause into any employment contract, that a woman employed on like work to a man is entitled to have similar terms and conditions.

The basic principles under the race and sex discrimination laws apply both within and outside the employment field.

Race discrimination

Principles of protection against race discrimination

Basic principle Discrimination on grounds of colour, race, nationality or ethnic or national origins is unlawful.

Direct discrimination This occurs where one person treats another less favourably on racial grounds than he would treat a person of another race.

Indirect discrimination This exists when an employer applies a requirement or condition which, although applicable to all people, is such that a proportion of people of one race who can comply with it is smaller than the proportion in another, or where the employer cannot show that the requirement is justifiable on other than racial grounds and it is to the detriment of the complainant because she cannot comply with it.

It is also unlawful to victimise or segregate on grounds of race.

Exempt areas Genuine occupational grounds can exist e.g. the essential nature of the job requires a particular physique and authenticity (e.g. the Moor in Othello). There are also grounds of national security and special rules for charitable trusts.

Other provisions It does not apply to immigration rules, or civil service regulations.

Enforcement This is through an application to an industrial tribunal. Assistance can be provided by the Commission on Racial Equality which has a statutory duty to work towards the elimination of discrimination, to promote equality of opportunities and to keep the Race Relations Act under review. The Commission can itself take action in relation to advertisements which indicate an intention to discriminate. It has the power to seek an injunction to prevent discrimination on racial grounds.

Sex discrimination

Principles of protection from sex discrimination

Basic principle To treat a person less favourably on the grounds of sex than a person of the other sex would be treated is unlawful. It is also unlawful for an employer to discriminate against a person on grounds of marital status.

Indirect discrimination This occurs where an employer applies a requirement or condition which, even though it applies equally to all persons, is such that a proportion of people of one sex who can comply with it is considerably smaller than the proportion in the other; where the employer cannot show justification on other than sexual grounds and is to the detriment of the complainant. It is also unlawful to victimise or segregate on grounds of sex.

Exempt areas Sex can be a genuine occupational qualification, i.e. the essential nature of the job requires a person of a different sex (e.g. authenticity, decency and privacy, personal services, work abroad which can only be done by a man) or the job is one of two held by a married couple. Other exemptions are:

- national security
- work in private households
- charitable trusts
- ministers of religion
- sports and sports facilities
- police and police cadets (in respect of certain terms only).

Enforcement This is through an application to the industrial tribunal. Like the CRE the Equal Opportunities Commission has a duty to work towards the elimination of discrimination and promoting the equality of opportunities. It keeps under review the Sex Discrimination Act and can bring action itself in the event of advertising which indicates an intention to discriminate unlawfully. It can also bring an action for an injunction to prevent a person acting in discriminatory fashion.

Case 2 Work of equal value[3]

A test case on the Equal Pay Act 1970 was brought by speech therapists who claimed that they were employed on work of equal value with male principal grade pharmacists and clinical psychologists employed in the NHS whose salaries exceeded theirs by about 60%. Part of the argument circulated around the nature of speech therapy and what was the relevant profession to it in comparative terms. The employers pointed out that speech therapists had been considered in the past to be a profession auxiliary to medicine, and were therefore grouped with almoners, chiropodists, dieticians, medical laboratories technicians, occupational therapists, physiotherapists and radiographers. In contrast clinical psychologists had been treated as comparable to scientists such as physicists and biologists.

The Court of Appeal referred the case to the European Court of Justice.[4] This decided that the fact that the differences in pay were mainly arrived at through collective bargaining was not sufficient objective justification for the difference in pay between the two jobs. It was for the national court to determine whether and to what extent the shortage of candidates for a job and the need to attract them by higher pay constituted an objectively justified economic ground for the difference in pay between the jobs in question. In applying the European ruling it was held that the speech therapists had been unfairly treated.

Disability discrimination

The Disability Discrimination Act was passed in 1995 and will, when fully implemented, give the disabled person certain rights in relation to employment, pensions and insurance, the provision of goods and services, access to premises, education and public transport. The main provisions of the Act are set out below in Box 7.8.

Box 7.8   Disability Discrimination Act 1995

1. Definitions of disability and disabled person
2. Employment: discrimination by employers, enforcement provisions, discrimination by other persons, occupational pension schemes and insurance services
3. Discrimination in other areas: goods, facilities and services, premises, enforcement
4. Education
5. Public transport: taxis, public services vehicles, rail vehicles
6. National Disability Council
7. Supplemental: Codes of Practice, victimisation, help
8. Miscellaneous

The Disability Discrimination Act 1995 defines a person as having a disability if

he has a physical or mental impairment which has a substantial and long-term adverse effect on his ability to carry out normal day-to day duties.

Guidance may be issued by the Secretary of State about the matters which must be taken into account in the application of this definition.

Part II, which covers discrimination in employment, makes it unlawful for an employer to discriminate (i.e. unjustifiably treat the disabled person less favourably) against a disabled person in arrangements for recruitment, and also in the terms of employment which are offered including opportunities for promotion and training and other benefits. The disabled employee is also protected against dismissal or other detriment. Regulations will be made to cover these provisions and also to define further the duties of the employer in relation to physical arrangements.

Small businesses are exempt from these provisions if the employer has fewer than 20 employees. The disabled person has the right to apply to an Industrial Tribunal over any discrimination. There are also provisions covering discrimination of contract workers and discrimination by trade union organisations. Discrimination by occupational pension schemes and insurance services is also made illegal.

Part III covers discrimination in the provision of goods, facilities and services. It will be unlawful for a provider of services to discriminate against a disabled person by refusing to provide him with services, or in relation to the standard or terms of the service. There will be a duty on service providers to take such steps as are reasonable to make alterations to buildings, or to the approach or access, and to provide auxiliary aids, such as audio tapes or sign language. Regulations will be passed to determine what is reasonable and also on the implementation of this duty.

In the provisions relating to discrimination in education, it will be a requirement for the annual report of each county, voluntary or grant-maintained school to include information on the arrangements for the admission of disabled pupils, the steps taken to prevent disabled pupils from being treated less favourably than other pupils and the facilities provided to assist access to the school by disabled pupils. Similar requirements are made in relation to further and higher education.

Taxi accessibility regulations are to be made to ensure that disabled persons and persons in wheelchairs can get into and out of taxis safely and also be carried in safety and in reasonable comfort. Taxi drivers will also have a duty to carry the guide dogs and hearing dogs of passengers without making an additional charge. Regulations may also be made relating to public service vehicles and the access and carriage of disabled persons and wheelchairs.

Part VI establishes the National Disability Council. This Council will, following consultation, advise the Secretary of State on relevant matters as requested, and prepare Codes of Practice. Unlike the Equal Opportunity Commission it will not have the power to take cases to an industrial tribunal.

In theory the framework is in place for a major revolution to take place in the lives of disabled persons. However in practice the value of the Act will depend on the more detailed guidance and regulations still to be passed and the extent to which the government of the day places its weight behind the legislation. Much too will depend upon the new National Disability Council in advising the government and in highlighting unjustified discrimination.

REHABILITATION OF OFFENDERS ACT 1974

The aim of this Act is to prevent discrimination against those who have had criminal convictions. It works by regarding certain offences as 'spent' after a certain length of time. This means that the person does not have to disclose the offence and to dismiss an employee on grounds that she failed to disclose a spent offence is automatically unfair. However the Act does not apply to serious crimes and many occupations are excluded from its effect including health service employment.[5]

TRADE UNIONS

The protection and immunities which trade unions and their members enjoyed in the 1970s and 1980s have been eroded until they have very few rights in relation to protection as a result of industrial action. Industrial action itself is defined in narrow terms if it is to be construed as 'lawful'. Rules are laid down in relation to the holding of elections, and secret ballots are needed before a strike can commence.[6] Secondary industrial action is prohibited so that trade unions are not immune from liability for the effects of any secondary action.

The individual citizen has been given a right to prevent disruption to his supply of any goods or services because of unlawful industrial action. If he can show that he has been or will be deprived of goods or services and that the industrial action is unlawful then he can apply to the court for an order to restrain the action.

The establishment of a Commission for protection against unlawful industrial action enables legal advice and representation to be paid for, though the Commission will not itself bring proceedings on behalf of an individual. Unlawful industrial action includes the following:

- industrial action which constitutes a tort
- industrial action which is not supported by ballot
- where proper notice is not given
- if it is not in furtherance of a trade dispute
- if it is secondary action
- if it promotes a closed shop
- if it is to support an employee dismissed whilst taking part in unofficial industrial action
- unlawful picketing.

The law relating to trade union constitution, membership, elections, funds, accounts and other forms of control was consolidated in the Trade Union and Labour Relations (Consolidation) Act 1992. An employee's right to join an independent trade union and to take part in its lawful activities is protected so that dismissal in relation to such activities is automatically unfair without any continuous service requirement. The office of Commissioner for the Rights of Trade Union Members was established following the Employment Act 1988. His task is to assist trade union members who have complaints against their trade union. He can also give assistance in relation to the right to a ballot before industrial action, the right to inspect a union's accounting records and in relation to complaints about trade union elections and the register of members. Since the Employment Act 1990 the Commissioner has the power to assist in proceedings arising from alleged breaches of the union rules such as appointment to office, disciplinary proceedings and authorisation of industrial action.

WHISTLE BLOWING

This is the term which refers to a person (usually an employee) who draws attention to concerns which have health and safety implications. Because of a fear that such persons, many of whom have a professional duty to draw attention to dangers and hazards, would be victimised as a result of their actions, the Department of Health issued a circular recommending that each trust and authority should set up a procedure whereby an individual employee could draw these concerns to the management internally without being victimised and thus not needing to bring in the media or other external bodies. In February 1996[7] the Public Interest Disclosure Bill was introduced by Don Touhig MP into the House of Commons. With cross party support, the Bill was designed to give legal protection to employees who 'blow the whistle' on crime or malpractice at work. It would have protected such persons from being sacked, denied promotion or being subjected to discrimination if they revealed malpractice in the public interest. The protection would only apply if they first raised the matter privately with their employers and were ignored. The whistle blower would be able to obtain an injunction to prevent threats of reprisals and, where appropriate, claim compensation through the courts for loss or earnings, distress and damage to reputation. The proposed Bill was not enacted. However employees do have some statutory protection if they bring matters of health and safety to the attention of the employer (see Chapter 13 on health and safety).

Therapists who are themselves employers should ensure that they are receptive to any concerns raised by their employees.

GRIEVANCE PROCEDURES

As stated above the Department of Health has recommended establishing a procedure to ensure that an employee can raise any concerns, without being victimised, to the awareness of senior management. It is likely that, as part of the initiative in local collective bargaining, individual employers will establish grievance procedures which will enable individual employees to appeal about pay, promotion or other terms of service which cause concern.

Questions and Exercises

1. A therapist agrees to work in a GP practice undertaking four sessions per week. She is not clear whether she would be regarded as an employee or a self-employed person. How can she tell and what are the differences between the two forms of contract?
2. A therapist sets up a practice in a community health centre with other complementary therapists. They agree that they will employ a receptionist to be shared by them all. What rights does the receptionist have and who would be regarded as her employer?
3. Draw up a leaflet setting out the basic rights of any employee whom you may employ.
4. Referring back to Chapter 4 analyse the legal stages which are followed in creating a contract of employment.

REFERENCES

1. Watling *v.* Gloucestershire County Council Employment Tribunal 23 November 1994, Lexis transcript; EAT/868/94, 17 March 1995
2. News item 1996 Medical Law Monitor Jan/Feb: 6–8
3. Enderby *v.* Frenchay Health Authority and the Secretary of State for Health [1991] IRLR 44
4. Enderby *v.* Frenchay Health Authority and Health Secretary (C–127/92) October 1993 ECJ Current Law 1994 4813; [1993] IRLR 591
5. Rehabilitation of Offenders Act 1974 (Exceptions) Order 1975 SI 1975/1023
6. Dimond BC 1997 Strikes, nurse and the law in the UK. Nursing Ethics 4(4): 269–76
7. Landale J Bid to protect whistleblowers. The Times 14 February 1996, p 2

8

The organisational framework: public and private

As the increase in interest in complementary therapies has developed so there are greater opportunities for practitioners to undertake work within the NHS or for registered homes or private medical organisations rather than simply on a person to person basis. In addition there is a growing demand for complementary therapies to be available on the NHS. A report by *Which?*[1] quoted a MORI survey in 1989 where three out of four respondents believed that alternative medicine should be available on the NHS.[1] The aim of this chapter is to explain how the present structure of the National Health Service and local government operates in order to make it clear what role is played by each as purchasers and providers of care.

THE NHS FRAMEWORK

Founding principles

The National Health Service established on 7 July 1948 under the National Health Service Act 1946 has undergone many organisational changes since that time but two principles have survived almost intact: one is that treatment is available free at the point of delivery of health care, unless there are specific statutory provisions to the contrary (e.g. prescription charges) and the other is that treatment should be available on the basis of equality to those in need. The latter principle was almost lost with the two tier system of access to secondary care as a result of GP fundholding, but the Secretary of State for Health in an announcement on 16 July 1997 made it clear that reforms were to take place to prevent GP fundholding patients having priority and that a common waiting list would be kept for patients who would receive treatment on the basis of need.

The statutory duty upon the Secretary of State is set out in the National Health Service Act 1977 (reenacting the provisions with amendments of the National Health Service Act 1946) and is shown in Box 8.1.

Box 8.1 The National Health Service Act 1977, section 1

(1) It is the Secretary of State's duty to continue the promotion in England and Wales of a comprehensive health service designed to secure improvement —
    (a) in the physical and mental health of the people of those countries, and
    (b) in the prevention, diagnosis and treatment of illness,

and for the purpose to provide or secure the effective provision of services in accordance with this Act.

Section 2 details the Secretary of State's powers and these include the power:

(a) to provide such services as he considers appropriate for the purpose of discharging any duty imposed upon him by this Act; and
(b) to do any other thing whatsoever which is calculated to facilitate, or is conducive or incidental to, the discharge of such a duty.

None of these provisions exclude the possibility of complementary therapies being provided within the NHS in the exercise of the Secretary of State's statutory duties, provided that they can be seen as coming within the definition of health. Section 3 is shown in Box 8.2 and it can be seen that many of these duties could include the provision of complementary therapies for both diagnosis, treatment and prevention of ill-health.

Box 8.2 National Health Service Act 1977, section 3

It is the Secretary of State's duty to provide throughout England and Wales, *to such extent as he considers necessary to meet all reasonable requirements* [author's emphasis] —
(a) hospital accommodation;
(b) other accommodation for the purpose of any service provided under this Act;
(c) medical, dental, nursing and ambulance services;
(d) such other facilities for the care of expectant and nursing mothers and young children as he considers are appropriate as part of the health service;
(e) such facilities for the prevention of illness, the care of persons suffering from illness and the after-care of persons who have suffered from illness as he considers are appropriate as part of the health service;
(f) such other services as are required for the diagnosis and treatment of illness.

The 1990 Act

In 1991 a radical reorganisation took place of the organisation of the National Health Service. The National Health Service and Community Care Act 1990 introduced into the NHS what has since become known as 'the internal market'. Health authorities have the responsibility of purchasing health services for the persons in their catchment area. Hospitals and community health services are grouped under NHS trusts which are the providers of health care, but can also be the purchasers. Contracts known as 'NHS agreements' are drawn up between health authorities and trusts for the provision of services. Under Section 4 of the Act these can not be legally enforced through the courts, but an adjudication system has been set up under the aegis of the Secretary of State.

Both health authorities and NHS trusts are statutory authorities, which can sue and be sued in their own name, and with chairmen and non-executive directors appointed by the Secretary of State.

The 1990 Act also enables GP practices to apply for fundholding status, so that they become the purchasers of secondary health care for patients on their list with funds allocated to them by the health authorities.

Potential purchasers within the NHS

As mentioned above, the basic principles upon which the NHS is founded do not preclude the use of complementary therapies. Under the 1990 reorganisation there are two potential routes through which such health care can be purchased on behalf of NHS patients.

NHS trusts as providers and purchasers

When NHS trusts were set up they transferred into their employment the staff who had previously worked for the unit directly managed by the health authority. These staff were able in law to retain the terms and conditions of service under which they were then working. However new appointments and promotions have often been made on the basis of new conditions of service set by the trusts which have also frequently agreed new conditions with their transferred staff. Increasingly trusts are laying down protocols and procedures for their staff and these can include instructions about the use of complementary therapies. (The requirement of an employee to obey the reasonable instructions of the employer is covered in Chapter 7 on employment law.)

The NHS trust has a duty to provide a service in accordance with any agreement with a health authority or with a GP fundholder. This may involve the trust in purchasing services on a sub-contracted basis.

GPs as purchasers and providers

GPs are independent contractors and have an agreement with a health authority (before April 1996 a Family Health Services Authority) to provide services for the patients on their list in accordance with the terms of service laid down by statutory instrument. In the fulfilment of their duties they may employ a considerable number of personnel depending on the size of the practice. These include receptionists, practice nurses and specialist nurses, and could also include practitioners in complementary therapies such as counsellors or aromatherapists. These persons would usually be employed by the partnership of doctors and the GPs would therefore be vicariously liable for any harm the therapists cause by negligence in the course of their employment.

Those GP practices which have obtained fundholding status provide all the primary care which non-fundholders must provide, but also have the responsibility of purchasing secondary care for their patients. They are not restricted in how they meet this purchasing commitment and could purchase services from the private sector and from complementary therapists.

It is a question of fact as to whether there is a contract of employment between the GP practice and the complementary therapist or whether there is a contract for services, in which case the therapist would remain personally accountable for the care provided and the GPs would not be vicariously liable (see Chapters 3 and 7).

NHS agreements

There is a distinction between contracts with health service body and contracts with non-health service bodies.

Under the NHS and Community Care Act 1990 agreements between health service bodies are not legally enforceable contracts.

Box 8.3   The NHS and Community Care Act 1990, section 4(3)

Whether or not an arrangement which constitutes an NHS contract would, apart from this subsection, be a contract in law, it shall not be regarded for any purpose as giving rise to contractual rights and liabilities, but if any dispute arises with respect to such an arrangement, either party may refer the matter to the Secretary of State for determination under the following provisions.

Thus a dispute between a GP fundholder and an NHS trust over an NHS agreement could not be taken to court to be resolved. However a dispute between a GP fundholding practice and an individual consultant or a practitioner of complementary therapies could result in an action in court. This is because the latter are not defined as health service bodies. It would be different if the consultant was acting as the employee of an NHS trust or the therapist was an employee of a health service body and was providing services to the GP practice in that respect.

The NHS and complementary therapies

There is considerable evidence that complementary therapies are a growth industry. In addition there is clear evidence, quoted in Chapter 1, of a wider availability of complementary therapies through the NHS. All the signs are that this interest and the access through the NHS will continue to grow.

In addition there is evidence of doctors both in general practice and in hospitals carrying out research to compare the effectiveness of complementary therapies with orthodox treatments. The creation of a Chair in Complementary Medicine at Exeter University, for example, will encourage the development of research into and acceptance of the place of complementary therapies in our health care.

No patient has an absolute right to access health care through the NHS. The courts have usually refused to support claims by patients who have sued health authorities for breach of the statutory duty when health care that they hoped for has not been provided. This is subject to the exception that every patient is entitled to be on a GP list and accident and emergency services are available to meet urgent health needs. There is therefore no clear legal right for a patient to insist on being referred to a specific therapy under the NHS. Whether a patient can obtain a specific therapy (such as aromatherapy, acupuncture or healing) through the NHS depends upon the views of the particular general practitioner.

GPs will clearly be influenced by research findings on the clinical effectiveness of each complementary therapy. If these support the value of individual therapies, then we can expect referrals of patients to complementary therapies within the NHS to increase. Indeed, if the research findings show superiority of the complementary therapy over orthodox medicine it could be argued that a GP who failed to refer a patient to the most effective treatment was acting contrary to the Bolam Test, i.e. was not following the reasonable standard of a competent general practitioner (see Chapter 3). Realistically, however, it will probably take a considerable time before referral to a complementary therapy is regarded as the reasonable standard of care. Nevertheless it may be that referral to an osteopath or chiropractor for certain conditions should become part of basic orthodox medical practice. The implications of this development for GPs, consultants and other health professionals are that they must be prepared to learn the strengths and weaknesses of individual complementary therapies so that they can know when a particular patient would benefit.

THE PLACE OF LOCAL AUTHORITIES

Residential and nursing home care

One of the major changes brought about by the NHS and Community Care Act 1990 was that the social services departments of local authorities became the purchasers of residential and nursing home care, instead of the Department of Social Security. The changes came into force on 1 April 1993. (Those who were entitled to social security provision in respect of their nursing home or residential home places before that time had preserved rights, which means they continue to be entitled to obtain resources from social security as long as they remain in that accommodation.)

From April 1993 local authorities have had the responsibility of carrying out an assessment on individuals who appear to be in need of community care services. Where it appears that housing or health services may be required, then they can ask the housing authority or the relevant health authority to join social services in the assessment. If the assessment reveals that an individual requires residential or nursing home care then, unless it is considered to be an NHS duty to provide the care, the local authority is the purchaser of the accommodation. It will, with the involvement of the client and any carer, decide on the accommodation to be purchased and the client will contribute to the fees on a means tested basis.

Each year the local authority has a duty, in conjunction with health authorities and the voluntary sector, to prepare, or revise and publish a plan for the provision of community care services for its catchment area.

The Registered Homes Act 1984

The local authority may be the purchaser of individual places in a residential or nursing home, but it also has a second role as the registration authority for residential care accommodation. The health authority is the registration authority for nursing homes.

The Registered Homes Act 1984 places duties on the local authority in respect of residential care homes, and on health authorities in respect of nursing and mental nursing homes, to register and inspect the accommodation.[2] The authorities can refuse to register or cancel any registration if there has been a failure to comply with the registration requirements. There are also powers to act in an urgent situation. Owners and managers can appeal to the Registered Homes Appeals Tribunal. Regulations laid down under the 1984 Act specify particular requirements relating to the conduct of residential care homes which must be met by the owners including:

- record keeping
- procedures relating to residents' monies
- the facilities and services to be provided in such homes
- the number and qualifications of staff to be employed in such homes
- the number of suitably qualified and competent staff to be on duty in such homes
- the notices which must be given to the registration authority about specific events
- the information to be provided by the applicant for registration.

The court has held[3] that in its capacity as purchaser the local authority can require higher standards than are laid down as part of the registration provisions.

Application to complementary therapies

Many residential and nursing homes are now enabling residents to obtain complementary therapies as part of their care. Those therapists who provide services to these homes should be aware of the contractual nature of their service: whether they are employed on a part time basis for a few sessions a week, in which case the owners of the home will be their employers and will consequently be vicariously liable for their work; or whether they are self-employed contractors entering the home as independent practitioners, personally responsible for their work.

Therapists providing services in these homes should ensure that, where appropriate, they identify and make contact with the resident's doctor to ensure that there are no contraindications to the treatment they are giving.

If therapists become aware that conditions in the home are unacceptable, and that the managers or home owners appear to be indifferent to any criticism, they can make a complaint through the procedures set up under the 1990 Act (see Chapter 12). If this fails, they can bring to the registration authority's attention any concerns they have about the home.

THE VOLUNTARY SECTOR

There are statutory requirements on both health and local authorities to involve the voluntary sector in the provision of care. Thus there must be involvement from the voluntary sector on the joint consultative committee, the statutory body which links health and local authority planning, and on the provision for aftercare for certain patients detained under the Mental Health Act 1983. Many therapists who are members of voluntary organisations may have an opportunity to contribute to the planning of health and social care at both organisational and individual level.

In addition some therapists provide services free of charge for individuals, whether at home, in residential accommodation or in hospitals. They should be aware that regardless of whether they are paid or not they still have legal responsibility for the care they provide (see Chapter 3).

THE PRIVATE HEALTH CARE SECTOR

To what extent do plans for private health care provision include access to complementary therapies as part of the cover provided? The answers from various private health groups to this question is given below.

PPP Health Care Group

Access to certain complementary therapies is provided for subscribers. Those therapies include osteopathy, chiropractic and acupuncture. Practitioners in these areas are individually recognised as being eligible for benefit of outpatient treatment of subscribers, provided those subscribers have been referred by a general practitioner.

The criteria for recognition are as follows:

Osteopathy

1. Completion of the four year full-time course at one of the three colleges recognised by the General Council and Register of Osteopaths.
2. The DO. qualification.
3. Acceptance by the Register – MRO.
4. Lay practitioners to be in full-time osteopathic practice for five years.
5. Medical practitioners to be in full-time osteopathic practice for five years.
6. Satisfactory references by two of their peers and one registered medical referee.

Chiropractic

1. Completion of the four year full-time course at the Anglo-European College of Chiropractic.
2. The DC qualification.
3. In full-time practice for ten years.
4. Acceptance by the Register of the British Chiropractic Association.
5. Two satisfactory references by their peers and one registered medical referee.

Acupuncture

1. Registered medical practitioner practising full-time acupuncture and with ten years experience.
2. Membership of the British Medical Acupuncture Society.
3. Satisfactory references by two of their peers.

Norwich Union

Our main PMI plans do not provide benefits for complementary medicines. However, we will consider payment for osteopathy, chiropractic, acupuncture or homeopathy treatments on specialist recommendation providing the treatment remains under the direct control of that specialist throughout. Each claim is considered on a case by case basis.

In its policy document *Express Care*, no specific mention is made of complementary therapies, and they are not listed under the benefits and cover available.

Under the exclusions from cover are listed:

treatment received in health hydros, nature cure clinics or similar establishments, or private beds registered as a nursing home attached to such establishments.

BUPA

Whilst complementary medicine is gaining acceptance within the wider medical professions and BUPA is keen to support changes in medical practice which improve the treatments available to our members, we do need to ensure that such treatments are appropriate and improve the health of our members.

The qualifications and therefore eligibility of the person providing the complementary medical treatment is a key factor in determining whether a claim for complementary medicine is eligible. At present, in some areas of complementary medicine there is only limited control over the training of practitioners and therefore our policy is designed to ensure that our members are treated by appropriately qualified practitioners. On the whole we are not questioning the validity of the treatment, our main concern is that the person providing the treatment is appropriately qualified.[4]

Practitioners of complementary therapy who do not have a medical qualification are not eligible to be defined as 'Consultant' for the purpose of BUPA regulations.

If they are medically qualified then they may apply to be a 'Special Eligible' provider on the following basis:

- Registered medical practitioner with post graduate qualification in their field of complementary medicine;
- Practised solely in their field of complementary medicine for a minimum of four years;
- References from two medically qualified consultants;
- Must only treat patients referred by a GP or medical 'Specialist'.

Other factors to support application would include the practitioner having published scientific papers in their field of complementary medicine, holding an NHS post which entails the use of and/or the holding of a teaching post in an area of complementary medicine.

BUPA's definition of a therapist is:

A chartered or state registered physiotherapist, an occupational therapist or orthoptist with state registration or a member of the College of Speech Therapists;
Any other practitioner who holds written confirmation from BUPA specifically notifying its acceptance that the practitioner is of recognised status for the purpose of BUPA's schemes.
Services of 'Other Practitioners' (i.e. health care professionals who do not fall within our definitions of Specialist or Therapist) are provided for within a member's out-patient benefit.

Any claims for payment in respect of the services of any medical or health practitioners who are not 'Specialists' or 'Therapists' will be considered for payment on a purely discretionary basis by BUPA if the following conditions are both fulfilled:

- a specialist had specifically referred the patient to that practitioner before any of the services were provided; and
- all the services were provided as an essential part of an overall course of treatment given personally by that Specialist.

The claim must be eligible in all other areas:

- The condition requiring treatment would normally require treatment by a Specialist, and could not be provided by the patient's General Practitioner.
- The claim is otherwise eligible for benefit and in particular the claim fulfils BUPA's definition of eligible treatment, i.e. an acute illness or injury or an acute episode of illness or injury.
- The particular area of complementary medicine has gained acceptance within the UK as an appropriate treatment.

Legal and General health care

In its *Guide to the Health care Maze*, Legal and General point out that some insurers may offer a cash reserve which you can use during the year to cover expenses such as dental and eye treatment or complementary medicine (such as acupuncture or osteopathy). If you do not use the reserve during the year, then its value may be increased for the next year when you renew your policy. In its own health care plan it includes an added benefit of up to £500 cash per year, depending upon the nature of the membership. From this fund you can claim cash payments towards optical, dental and other medical expenses, including complementary treatments such as homeopathy and acupuncture.

Conclusions

It can be seen from the brief review of some of the main providers of private health care that there is a lack of uniformity in relation to the cover for complementary therapies. However there is evidence of a growing acceptance that such cover will be provided, if only on an individual discretionary basis. The inclusion by BUPA in its criteria that 'the particular area of complementary medicine has gained acceptance within the UK as an appropriate treatment' is an interesting point in view of the difficulties of determining 'acceptance' other than through state recognition.

Interesting too is the fact that often the gateway to complementary therapies is through registered practitioners of orthodox medicine. If complementary therapies can obtain support by the registered medical practitioners (often secured by establishing clear research findings of effectiveness) then referrals may take place to complementary therapists.

THE DEPARTMENT OF SOCIAL SECURITY

To what extent does the DSS recognise complementary therapists as being able to provide evidence as the basis for a claimant's right to benefits. A letter to the DSS elicited the following information:

If a customer makes a claim for benefit and furnishes medical evidence from a source other than a registered general practitioner the case is passed to an adjudication officer to determine whether the medical evidence can be accepted. Adjudication officers act independently from the Department and the Secretary of State. Central Adjudication Services provide guidance for adjudication through their publication *The Adjudication Officer's Guide*. Volume 2 part 18 of the guide states:

'**18170** Evidence other than from a registered medical practitioner can be accepted if
  1. it is unreasonable to require a doctor's statement AND
  2. the evidence shows that the person is unfit for work because of a disease or disablement.
18171 The adjudication officer decides what is reasonable in each case. For example, evidence from alternative therapists such as chiropractic, osteopaths, etc. can be accepted if the person is usually treated by them as well as, or instead of a GP.
18172 Depending on the circumstances, a declaration that a person is incapable of following a particular occupation and is receiving non-medical treatment such as Christian Science treatment may be sufficient proof.'

This guidance only alludes to a couple of examples of the types of other evidence that our officers receive. Other examples would equally be covered by this guidance and would be considered on the individual merits of each case.

The Social Security Medical Evidence Regulations 1976 (SI 1976/No 615) makes provision for evidence from alternative sources. Regulation 2 (1) (d) sets out that

'where it would be unreasonable to require a person to provide a (medical) statement (from a doctor) such other evidence as may be sufficient to show that he should refrain (or should have refrained) from work by reason of some specific disease or bodily or mental disablement'.

CONCLUSIONS

Looking at the overall picture of the NHS, local authorities and the private sector there is evidence that complementary therapies are gradually growing in acceptance. However any further development of this through state funding or private health insurance is dependent upon orthodox medical practitioners supporting the benefits which they can give to their patients. On the other hand many if not most therapists are paid privately by clients on a personal basis and there is no reason why this should not continue to flourish. White papers on the NHS for England, Scotland and Wales were published between November 1997 and January 1998. Resulting legislation may see the abolition of the internal market and the emphasis on primary health consortia or local health groups. These developments may support the increased availability of complementary therapies within the NHS.

Questions and Exercises

1. What considerations should a complementary therapist take into account before agreeing a contract with a General Practice?
2. In what way, if any, is there a difference between a complementary therapist providing services for a GP non-fundholding practice compared with a GP fundholding practice.
3. Are there any disadvantages in your therapy becoming automatically available to those who are covered by private medical insurance?

REFERENCES

1. Report of complementary therapies. Which? November 1992
2. Dimond BC 1997 The legal aspects of care in the community. Macmillan, Basingstoke
3. R v. Newcastle upon Tyne City Council, ex parte Dixon The Times Law Report 26 October 1993
4. Personal correspondence from BUPA to the author 21 May 1997

9

Consent to treatment and giving information

Many practitioners of complementary therapies pride themselves on the fact that their therapies do no harm and they would not treat a person unless that person came willingly for a consultation. However it is important for all such therapists to have a good understanding of the law relating to consent and the giving of information so that they can ensure that their procedures comply with that law. In addition, as more patients are referred to complementary therapists within the NHS, an increasing number of patients/clients may be receiving complementary therapies without having themselves initiated the contact as has been the rule in the past.

This chapter covers the legal issues relating to consent to treatment. It will deal first with those issues which arise in relation to the mentally competent adult. The laws relating to consent in the case of children, mentally ill, elderly and those with learning disabilities will also be covered. The topic of disclosure and access to records is considered in the next chapter.

BASIC PRINCIPLES

There are two distinct aspects of the law relating to consent to treatment. One is the actual giving of consent and the possibility that a trespass to the person has occurred because the patient did not give consent to the treatment. The other is the duty to give information to the patient prior to the giving of consent. The absence of consent could result in the patient suing for trespass to the person. The failure to provide sufficient relevant information could result in an action for negligence. These two different legal actions will be considered separately. The difference between them is significant because in an action for trespass to the person harm does not have to be established and even if the therapist has conferred a benefit on the patient civil action could still be possible; whereas in the case of negligence harm must be shown.

TRESPASS TO THE PERSON

A trespass to the person occurs when an individual either apprehends a touching of her person, (this is known as an assault) or the individual is actually touched, (this is known as a battery) and has not given consent.

The person who has suffered the trespass can sue for compensation in the civil courts (and in criminal cases a prosecution could also be brought).

In the civil cases, the victim has to prove:

- the touching or the apprehension of the touching and
- that it was a (potentially) direct interference with her person.

The victim does not have to show that harm has occurred. This is in contrast with an action for negligence in which the victim must show that harm has resulted from the breach of duty of care (see Chapter 3).

Care should be taken if it is necessary to examine patients or have physical contact with them to ensure that the patient is consenting to this contact, since otherwise the mere touching could constitute a trespass.

Defences

The main defence to an action for trespass to the person is that consent was given by a mentally competent person. In addition there are two other defences in law which are:

1. Statutory authorisation, e.g. Mental Health Act 1983, Children Act 1989
2. The common law power to act out of necessity.

These are both considered below.

NATURE OF CONSENT

Consent can be given by word of mouth, in writing or it can be implied i.e. the non-verbal conduct of the person indicates that she is giving consent. All these forms of giving consent are valid, but where procedures entail risk and/or where there are likely to be disputes over whether consent was given, it is advisable to obtain consent in writing, since it is then easier to establish the facts in a court of law. The writing is not the consent: it is evidence that the consent was given. (There are a few situations where consent must be recorded in writing by law.)

Consent forms

The Department of Health has given guidance on consent to examination and treatment.[1] This guidance gives examples of consent forms and includes a form which is specifically for non-doctors and non-dentists and could be used by a complementary therapist for treatments, whether inside or outside the NHS. In addition some of the associations for complementary therapies have devised their own consent forms and these are referred to in Section 2 of this book covering specialist areas. There are clear advantages in obtaining evidence of the patient's consent on such a form if there are any risks inherent in the treatment or if there is likely to be a dispute later as to whether or not consent was actually given.

Consent by a mentally competent adult

For consent to treatment to be valid, the person giving it must be mentally competent. In addition the consent must be given without any duress or force or deceit. Individuals must know to what they are consenting, but do not have to have the same amount of information which they need to be given under the duty to inform (see below).

What if someone wishes to stop a course of therapy?

It is a principle of consent that a person who has given consent can withdraw it at any time, unless there is a contractual reason why this is not so. This means that, if people wish to cease undertaking any therapy, they are free to do so even contrary to their best interests, unless the person concerned lacks the capacity to make a valid decision.

Clearly in such circumstances there are advantages in asking the patient to sign a note that the self-discharge or refusal to accept treatment was contrary to clinical advice. Many of the complementary therapies would not result in harm if the client were to cease to undertake them but the ending of care may well not be in the individual client's best interests. For example, a course of psychotherapy may have reached a critical point and it would be unwise for the treatment to cease at that time. However, if mentally competent adults consider that they wish to cease treatment, that is their legal right. The therapist must ensure that adequate information is given of any harmful effects caused by ending the therapy in the middle of the treatment plan.

Refusal to consent

The Court of Appeal set out the basic principles of self-determination of the mentally competent adult in the case of *Re T*[2] but also emphasised the importance of the health professional ensuring that any refusal to give consent to life saving treatment and care was valid. The facts are shown overleaf.

The Court of Appeal dismissed the appeal on the grounds that there was evidence to show that Miss T was not in a physical or mental condition to make a decision, since the influence of her mother was such as to vitiate the decision which she expressed. There was a presumption that an adult mentally competent person had the right to decide on treatment but this presumption could be rebutted. If doctors had doubts about the competence of an adult to refuse life-saving treatment, they should seek a declaration from the court as to whether the proposed treatment would or would not be lawful.

Case 1   Invalid refusal of treatment

Miss T an adult was 34 weeks pregnant and was involved in a road accident. She was admitted to hospital a few days later and was diagnosed as suffering from pleurisy or pneumonia. Her mother was a Jehovah's Witness but she was not herself a member and her paternal family was opposed to that faith. Miss T said that she did not want a blood transfusion. A decision was made that delivery should be by caesarean section. She signed a form of refusal of consent to blood transfusions but it was not explained to her that it might be necessary to give a blood transfusion so as to prevent injury to her health or even to preserve her life, nor was the form read or its contents explained to her. The caesarean was performed but the baby was stillborn. Miss T deteriorated and she was transferred to intensive care. The father of the child and cohabitee obtained a declaration from the High Court that it would not be unlawful for the hospital to administer a blood transfusion to Miss T despite the absence of her consent, because that appeared to be in her best interests.

It would be difficult to envisage circumstances where it would ever be the wish of a complementary therapist to carry out therapies either without the consent of the client or where there had been a change of mind. The recommended practice, therefore, for any therapist is to withdraw treatment whenever clients indicate that that is their wish and not to compel such a client to receive the treatment, even where the therapist is of the view that this would be in the best interests of that client.

Where there is any doubt over the competence of the client to give a valid consent, it is strongly recommended that the practitioner should not give treatment until a third person, unconnected with the therapist or the care of the client, clarifies the competence of the client. If such an expert view on competence is obtained it should be recorded in writing.

The existence of a mental illness will not automatically mean that people are incapable of giving a valid refusal of treatment even if such treatment is in their best interests, (*Re C*[3]).

Case 2   Broadmoor patient can refuse treatment

C, a 68 year old patient suffering from paranoid schizophrenia, developed gangrene in a foot during his confinement in Broadmoor. He was removed to a general hospital where the consultant surgeon diagnosed that he was likely to die immediately if the leg was not amputated below the knee. C refused to consider amputation. The hospital authorities were considering whether amputation could be carried out without his consent.

C applied to the court for an injunction to restrain any doctor from carrying out an amputation without his express written consent.

The High Court held that the evidence failed to establish that he lacked sufficient understanding of the nature, purpose and effects of the proposed treatment, but instead showed that he had understood and retained the relevant treatment information, believed it and had arrived at a clear choice. The declaration was made accordingly and an injunction was ordered against any doctors carrying out an amputation on him without his consent.

In practice many therapies and treatments cannot proceed without the co-operation of the patient and consent to the involvement is often implied from the patient's non-verbal communication. In such cases, therefore, trespass to the person actions are unlikely and the focus is more likely to be on the nature of the information which was given (see below).

Children

Aged 16 and 17 years

A child of 16 or 17 has the right to give consent to treatment under the Family Law Reform Act 1969. This is shown in Box 9.1.

Box 9.1   Family Law Reform Act 1969, section 8

(1) The consent of a minor who has attained the age of 16 years, to any surgical, medical or dental treatment, which in the absence of consent, would constitute a trespass to the person, shall be as effective as it would be if he were of full age; and where a minor has by virtue of this section given an effective consent to any treatment it shall not be necessary to obtain any consent for it from his parent or guardian.

(2) In the section 'surgical, medical or dental treatment' includes any procedure undertaken for the purposes of diagnosis and this section applies to any procedure (including, in particular, the administration of an anaesthetic) which is ancillary to any treatment as it applies to that treatment.

(3) Nothing in this section shall be construed as making ineffective any consent which would have been effective if this section had not been enacted.

The definition of treatment under section 8(2) would probably cover most treatments given by a complementary therapist where these are under the aegis of a doctor. However there is an interesting debate on whether other complementary therapies which are not the result of a referral from a registered practitioner of orthodox medicine would be properly regarded as coming under the scope of section 8(2). Even if a narrow interpretation is taken of section 8(2) it would still be possible for the child to give consent under the ruling laid down by the House of Lords in the *Gillick* case[4] (concerning a girl of under 16 consenting to contraceptive advice and treatment without her parent's knowledge).

Section 8(3) covers two situations: the giving of consent by a parent on behalf of the child of 16 or 17 and the giving of consent by a child below 16 years.

It does not follow that a child of 16 or 17 cannot be compelled to have treatment and the Court of Appeal in the case of *Re W*[5] upheld the decision of the High Court judge to order a child of 16 years who was suffering from anorexia nervosa to undergo medical treatment against her will.

The circumstances in which complementary therapy is given to a child of 16 or 17 against his or her will are probably extremely rare. Usually the philosophy behind a complementary therapy will be one of co-operation and client involvement and any coercion would not only be counterproductive but entirely contrary to the spirit within which complementary therapy is practised.

The child under 16

The parent has a right at common law to give consent on behalf of the child (this includes any child up to 18 years). In addition, as a result of the House of Lords ruling in the *Gillick* case, children under 16 years who have sufficient understanding and intelligence to be capable of making up their own mind can give a valid consent to treatment.

In life saving situations, however, it is unlikely that children under 16 years would be able to make decisions contrary to their best interests (see *Re W* above).

Even where the child and parents both agree that treatment should not be given, as in the case of a Jehovah's Witness family, the court can order treatment to proceed, if it is considered to be in the best interests of the child (the case of *Re E*[6]). The author is not aware of any case where it has been ordered that complementary medicine therapy be given to a child against both the child's and the parents' wishes. As stated above compulsion would seem to be contrary to the philosophy of most complementary therapists.

Parental responsibility and the criminal law

It must be emphasised that the parents have a statutory duty to take reasonable care of the child. Failure therefore on the parents part to seek the advice of an orthodox doctor which led to the death of the child could result in criminal proceedings being brought. Therefore parents who seek assistance only of complementary therapists concerning their children instead of seeking conventional medical help run the risk of criminal prosecution (see Chapter 5).

Disputes between parents

Even when parents are divorced or separated both parents retain parental responsibility for their children under the Children Act 1989, section 2(1). Under section 2(7) where more than one person has parental responsibility for a child each of them may act alone and without the other (or others) in meeting that responsibility. Even where one parent has a residence order in his or her favour, the other still retains parental responsibilities and can exercise these to the full. It also follows that one parent does not have the right of veto over the other's actions. If, however, there has been a specific order by the court relating to a decision affecting the care or treatment of the child, then a single parent cannot change this or take any action which is incompatible with this order unless the approval of the court is obtained.

Prohibited steps order It therefore follows that, if there is a dispute between parents over treatment decisions in respect of the child, either can go to court for a specific issue or prohibited steps order to be made. This can prevent the other parent taking action which the parent seeking the order does not consider is in the interests of the child. The order can be made under section 8 of the Children Act 1989 and means that no step which could normally be taken by a parent in meeting parental responsibility for a child but which is of a kind specified in the order can be taken without the leave of the court. Thus if one parent feared that the other was likely to agree to a mentally impaired daughter receiving acupuncture, then that parent could obtain a prohibited steps order preventing consent being given without the leave of the court.

Children who are considered to be Gillick competent and who disagree with actions which their parents are intending, can also seek the leave of the court to obtain a prohibited steps order. The child would have to apply to the High Court.[7] The court must be satisfied that the child has sufficient understanding to make the proposed application (section 10(8)).

The mentally incapacitated

Many clients with learning disabilities and mental illness may still have the capacity to make decisions on their own account. Clearly the client's capacity must be related to the nature of the decision to be made. The client may be able to choose what clothes to wear or to buy but may not have the capacity to decide whether or not to receive aromatherapy or hypnotherapy. A decision for a person under 18 years can be made by the parents provided that it is in the best interests of the child. At present, however, for adults of 18 and over who lack the capacity to make their own decisions, there exists a vacuum in law. No person has the legal power to make such decisions in their name.

The Law Commission, following an extended period of consultation on the issue of decision making and mental incapacity, has prepared draft legislation[8] which, if implemented, would set up a statutory framework for decisions to be made in accordance with their seriousness. Court approval would be required for decisions relating to sterilisations, abortions, etc. while at the other end of the scale simple decisions, e.g. to go on a coach trip, could be made by a carer with specific statutory power to make them.

The Lord Chancellor has published a consultation document (Who decides, 1997) in response to the Law Commission's recommendations. In the meantime, carers and health professionals giving treatment and care to those who do not have the capacity to give a valid consent are protected by the common law powers to act out of necessity (the case of *Re F*[9]), provided that they act in the best interests of the client and follow a reasonable standard of care (see below).

There would appear to be no reason why complementary therapy could not be provided in the best interests of an adult mentally incapacitated person who is incapable of giving consent under this common law power. Adults with learning disabilities, elderly mentally infirm persons, unconscious persons in intensive care may benefit from such therapies as aromatherapy, reflexology and others. Complementary therapists could therefore give treatment to such patients in their best interests. Where the patients are being cared for in the NHS this would be with the agreement of the responsible medical officer for that patient. In the private sector therapists themselves would have to decide if treatment was in the best interests of a mentally incapacitated client. No person in law has the right to give or withhold consent for a mentally incapacitated adult.

Where, however, the mentally incompetent person is physically resisting such treatment, it is doubtful if any therapist would consider that it could be in the best interests of that client to force the treatment upon him or her.

EXCEPTIONS TO THE NEED FOR CONSENT

The Mental Health Act 1983

Compulsory treatment for mental disorder can be given under the Act to the patient detained under specified sections. Special procedures must be followed in relation to

- medication after the first three months
- electro convulsive therapy
- surgery destroying brain cells and
- hormonal implants to reduce sexual drive.

All other treatments for mental disorder (i.e. those which come under section 63) can be given compulsorily under the direction of the registered medical practitioner in charge of the patient.

Medical treatment is defined in the Act as including 'nursing, and also includes care, habilitation and rehabilitation under medical supervision'. (Section 145(1)).

In a recent decision it was held[10] that initial treatment given to enable the specific treatment for mental disorder to be given was covered by section 63. Thus a detained patient who was anorexic could be given tube-feeding even though that was not the treatment that justified admission under section 3.

This definition would of course cover many of the complementary therapies which in theory could therefore be given compulsorily under section 63 to certain detained patients. However there are very few treatments offered by therapists which in practice can be given compulsorily, against the will of the patient. The patient might be persuaded to accept some of the behavioural conditioning therapies which may be under the supervision of a complementary therapist but, for the most part, the treatments rely for their success upon the active involvement and participation of the patient. There are considerable difficulties in persuading acutely ill or chronically sick patients to accept attendance at therapy sessions.

In addition it must be noted that all treatments must be given under the direction of the responsible medical officer for the patient. Therefore only if the patient's doctor refers the detained patient to a complementary therapist or practitioner would complementary therapy be available to be given without the consent of the patient under the provisions of the Mental Health Act 1983.

Complementary therapies could of course be given to any detained patient with the consent of the patient. However they would still have to be given on the direction or with the agreement of the doctor in charge of the patient's treatment.

Necessity

The other exception to the requirement that consent must be given otherwise an action for trespass to the person could be brought is a situation of necessity.

Case 3   Sterilisation

In one case there was concern amongst the professionals over who could give consent to an operation to sterilise a woman with learning disabilities. (As we have noted above, there is at present a vacuum in law in relation to the situation where a mentally incapacitated adult is incapable of giving consent: no one has the power in law to give consent on that person's behalf.) The issue was therefore brought to court.

The House of Lords[11] recognised the vacuum in law but stated that a professional had the duty to act in the best interests of the adult person who lacked the necessary mental capacity and follow the Bolam test in providing the reasonable standard of care. The House of Lords recommended that a decision relating to an operation for sterilisation or similar treatment should be brought to the court and a practice direction[12] has been issued to that effect.

The House of Lords therefore gave approval to the right at common law (i.e. judge made law) to act out of necessity in the best interests of the mentally incompetent person. Where the patient lacks the capacity to give consent to treatment, treatment can proceed on the basis that it is in the best interests of that individual and is given according to the reasonable standards of the profession. In such circumstances, the health professional would not be committing a trespass to the person.

There is no reason why a complementary therapist could not act out of necessity in caring for a mentally incapacitated adult. In such situations therapists must ensure that they are acting in the best interests of the client, and are following the standard of care which would be recognised and approved by other competent practitioners of that therapy. The therapist should not rely upon the carer to give consent, but of course would wish the carer to be involved in any discussion about that person's care and treatment. There are forms in the Department of Health guidelines referred to above which cover the situation where treatment and care is given to an adult who is mentally incapacitated but who is not detained under the Mental Health Act 1983, and these could be used in respect of complementary therapies.

Can a carer give consent?

Situation   Therapy on the unconscious patient

A registered nurse who was also qualified in aromatherapy wished to provide aromatherapy to patients in ITU (Intensive Therapy Unit). The Trust protocol permitted the use of such complementary therapies provided that the nurse was qualified and that the patient consented. The nurse claimed that patients in ITU are usually admitted in an unconscious state and wanted to ignore the trust stipulation about consent or else obtain the consent of a relative.

The nurse, in this situation, should accept the Trust's protocol. The trust is entitled to require the patient's consent before complementary therapy is given to the patient.

The nurse cannot rely on the consent from the relative, except in the case of consent by a parent for a child. No other relatives have a right in law to give consent on behalf of another person. Only if conscious patients are admitted to ITU and give their consent to aromatherapy, would the nurse be able to provide that therapy. The situation may change in the future if aromatherapy and other complementary therapies are considered to be part of basic nursing skills and therefore can be given to a patient in the patient's best interests as part of the usual duty of care owed to the patient.

INFORMATION GIVING AND WARNINGS

The duty to inform

It was mentioned at the beginning of this chapter that there are two aspects to consent: an action for trespass to the person if there is a touching or apprehension of a touching without consent or other lawful justification; and an action for negligence if there is a breach of the duty to inform the client/patient of any significant risks of substantial harm and specific harm arises.

As part of the duty of care owed in the law of negligence the therapist has to inform the patient about the significant risks of substantial harm which could occur if treatment were to proceed.

If the harm has not been explained to the patient, and the harm then occurs, the patient can claim that had she known of this possibility she would not have agreed to undergo the treatment. She could then bring an action in negligence. To succeed the patient would have to show:

- that there was a duty of care to give specific information;
- the defendant failed to give this information and in so doing was in breach of the reasonable standard of care which should have been provided;
- as a result of this failure to inform the patient agreed to the treatment; and
- the patient subsequently suffered the harm.

Case 4   Paralysis from alleviating surgery

Mrs Sidaway who suffered from intractable pain in her right arm and shoulder sought the advice of a neuro-surgeon who operated to relieve the pain. This was initially successful, but the pain returned and the neuro-surgeon diagnosed pressure on the nerve root. He decided to operate to relieve the pressure and Mrs Sidaway agreed to the surgery. As a result of that operation she became severely disabled by partial paralysis. She sued the neuro-surgeon and the hospital alleging that she had not been told of the risk of injury to the spinal cord (1% risk). She had been told of the risk of damage to the nerve root (2% risk). There was no allegation that the operation was not properly performed. Whilst the case was proceeding the neuro-surgeon died.

The High Court judge held that she had consented to the operation and therefore her claim of trespass to the person failed. Her claim for failure to inform her of the risk of paralysis also failed. Mrs Sidaway lost her appeal to the Court of Appeal. The House of Lords applied the Bolam test to the giving of information to the patient and found that, whilst some neuro-surgeons might warn patients of the risk of damage to the spinal cord, many chose not to do so. The normal test of professional negligence was applied i.e. the standard of the reasonable practitioner following the accepted approved standard of care. Her appeal therefore failed.

To ensure that the patient understands the information which is given, there are considerable advantages in a written handout being provided (checking of course that the client is literate). This would also assist if there were any dispute over the information having been given.

What information?

The duty placed upon therapists is that they should ensure that the patient is given information about the significant risks of substantial harm which could arise from treatment. They would be judged by the standard of the reasonable practitioner in that situation with that specific patient (further discussed in Chapter 3 on negligence). This requires therapists to ensure that they maintain their competence and knowledge about current issues and research. This may also include knowledge of alternative therapies and orthodox medicine and readiness to answer any questions raised by the client.

In determining the information which should be given to the client before commencing treatment, therapists must have a clear understanding of any significant risks associated with their specific therapy. Are they able to give a clear explanation of the philosophies and theories within the treatment they provide? Do they understand how their treatments actually work? This is of significance because the information which the therapist gives and the expectations of the patient/client could be the basis of legal action if it is alleged that the therapist was in breach of the duty of care to inform the patient of relevant information affecting the decision to be made by the patient in consenting to treatment.

RECORDING CONSENT

It was noted above that many complementary therapy treatments will be given without any written evidence of consent. Where, however, it is feared that there may be significant risks of substantial harm or there is likely to be any dispute as to whether consent was given, it is advisable for consent to be obtained in writing.

NHSME guidance

The NHS Management Executive has issued guidance which gives sample forms in the appendix.

One can be used to evidence consent for treatments other than by a doctor or dentist. This should ensure that all the requisite information is recorded.

It also recommends a second form that could be completed when an adult who lacks mental capacity to give consent to treatment is provided with care in the absence of consent.

These forms could be adapted for completion by the therapist.

The information required

The following information could be recorded:

- information identifying the client
- the nature of the problems elicited
- the course of action suggested
- the aims of the therapy
- the proposed media
- the date of review.

The client should read through the information recorded and, if satisfied, sign the consent form. Therapists should give their full name, title and signature, together with the date, and this should be on the form before the consumer signs it. It is also suggested that, if necessary, additional time should be given for discussion or consideration before the client signs to give consent.[15]

The use of leaflets

A record should also be kept of information given to the client about the proposed treatments. Where this is set out in leaflet form, a record could be made that the client has been given a copy of the leaflet.

CONCLUSION

The therapist must accept that the law recognises the autonomy of the mentally competent patient to decide whether or not to participate in treatment activities. The onus is on the therapist to inform the patient fully about the benefits and risks of the treatment.

Questions and Exercises

---

1. Analyse your practice in relation to obtaining consent from the patient and decide if it could be improved.
2. Draw up a form for consent to your particular therapy.
3. Prepare a hand out for the client/patient giving information about the nature of any specific treatment which you provide, setting out any inherent risks.

REFERENCES

1. NHS Management Executive 1990 A guide to consent for examination and treatment (HC(90)22) Department of Health
2. Re T (Adult: Refusal of Medical Treatment) [1992] 4 All ER 649
3. Re C (Adult: Refusal of Medical Treatment) [1994] 1 All ER 819
4. Gillick v. West Norfolk and Wisbech Area Health Authority [1986] 1 AC 112
5. Re W (a minor) (Medical Treatment) [1992] 4 All ER 627

6. Re E (a Minor) (Wardship: Medical Treatment) Family Division [1993] 1 FLR 386
7. See further the rights of the child as applicant in: Wyld N 1995 When Parents Separate. Children's Legal Centre, London
8. Law Commission 1995 Report No 231 Mental Incapacity. HMSO, London
9. F. v. West Berkshire Health Authority and another [1989] 2 All ER 545 (also known as Re F)
10. B. v. Croydon Health Authority [1994] The Times Law Report 1 December 1994
11. F. v. West Berkshire Health Authority and another [1989] 2 All ER 545
12. Practice Note October 1989, updated [1993] 3 All ER 222
13. Sidaway v. Bethlem Royal Hospital Governors [1985] 1 All ER 643
14. NHS Management Executive 1990 A guide to consent for examination and treatment (HC(90)22) Department of Health.
15. Suggestions taken from the College of Occupational Therapy 1993 Standards, policies and proceedings Consent for Occupational Therapy (Standard 5). College of Occupational Therapy, London

Client information

This chapter discusses the legal issues which arise from all aspects of personal client information. In particular it considers the law relating to confidentiality and the law relating to access to personal health information. The rules relating to records and record keeping and giving evidence in court are considered in Chapter 14.

CONFIDENTIALITY

All therapists, whether working in the public or private sector have a duty to maintain the confidentiality of information obtained from or about the client. This part of this chapter explores the source of this obligation and the exceptions to the duty recognised in law.[1]

The nature of the duty

The duty to respect confidentiality arises from a variety of sources which are set out in Box 10.1.

Box 10.1   Sources of duty of confidentiality

---

1. Duty set out in the Code of Professional Conduct
2. Duty in the contract of employment/contract with client
3. Duty as part of the duty of care owed to the patient in the law of negligence
4. Duty set out in specific statutes
5. Duty as part of the trust obligation between health professional and patient

---

The Code of Professional Conduct

Many therapists belong to an organisation which requires them to follow a code of ethics and professional practice. Those organisations which come under the umbrella of the British Complementary Medicine Association recognise certain professional obligations which are enforceable through its professional conduct machinery. These obligations include the duty of confidentiality. The specific chapters on individual therapies in Section 2 look at the contents of some of these codes of ethics and practice. Therapists who are also registered with the UKCC or the GMC will in addition have a Code of Professional Conduct to follow issued by their registration body.

Duty in contract

The employed therapist also has an obligation enforceable by the employer which derives from the contract of employment to observe the confidentiality of client information. This will usually be set out expressly in the contract of employment but, even if the contract is silent on the topic, the courts may imply into the contract such a term. Should the therapist be in breach of this expressed or implied term, then the employer can take appropriate action through the disciplinary machinery. This may be simply counselling, or an oral warning or any of the stages in the disciplinary procedure may be invoked, depending on the circumstances. In serious cases, the employer may be considered justified in dismissing the employee. In such a case, if the employee has the necessary continuous service requirement (see Chapter 7) the employee could challenge this action by an application to an industrial tribunal for unfair dismissal.

Those self-employed therapists who employ assistants to work for them should ensure that the duty of confidentiality is understood and respected.

Those who work as self-employed professionals do not have an obligation to an employer but they would have a contract for services with their clients which may impose conditions relating to confidentiality. Should the therapist be in breach of these contractual conditions, then the client could bring an action in the civil courts and obtain the usual remedies for breach of contract.

Duty of care in negligence

Therapists owe a duty to clients to retain information given to them in confidence. Should the therapist be in breach of this duty, then the client could bring an action against the therapist personally or, if the therapist is an employee, against the employer on the basis of vicarious liability for the actions of an employee acting in course of employment (see Chapter 3).

One weakness with the client's right of action in the law of negligence is that the client has to prove harm. There may be potential for harm to arise following unauthorised disclosure, but until it does the client cannot obtain compensation. He could, however, obtain an injunction seeking that the disclosure be prevented. Another difficulty is that if a client is wishing to preserve secrecy of information, then the danger of a court action is that the dispute will be brought into the open and the publicity then will defeat the client's main objectives. This perhaps explains why there are very few decided cases on confidentiality.

Case 1   Injunction and the case of X .v. Y[2]

The court ordered an injunction to be issued to prevent the disclosure by the press of the identity of doctors suffering from AIDS. Two general practitioners were diagnosed as having contracted AIDS. They received counselling in a local hospital, continuing with their medical practice. A journalist heard of the situation from an employee of the health authority and wrote an article for a national newspaper. The health authority sought an injunction to prevent any further disclosure of the information obtained from the clients' records.

The judge granted the injunction on the grounds that the records of hospital patients, particularly those suffering from this appalling condition should be as confidential as the courts can properly make them in order that the plaintiffs may be free from suspicion that they are harbouring disloyal employees. He rejected the defendant's argument that it was in the public interest for the public to know the identity of these doctors.

The judge did not however agree to the health authority's application for the name of the employee who had disclosed the information to the journalist. He held that the exceptions under section 10 of the Contempt of Court Act 1981 to the principle that the court cannot require disclosure from a journalist did not apply to the situation and the journalist was entitled to protect his source.

Duty set out in specific statutes

The following statutes make it an offence to disclose specified information:

- Abortion Regulations 1991 made under the Abortion Act 1967
- NHS (Venereal Disease) Regulations 1974
- Human Fertilisation and Embryology Act 1990 as amended by the Human Fertilisation and Embryology (Disclosure of Information) Act 1992
- Data Protection Act 1984

Where information is disclosed in breach of these statutory provisions, the holder of the records or the patient can initiate the appropriate enforcement machinery. In the case of unauthorised disclosure of information kept in computerised form, the Data Protection Registrar could remove from a data user his right to be registered under the Act and to hold personal information in computerised form (see also below on the Data Protection Act provisions in relation to subject access.)

Duty as part of the trust obligation

This duty was acknowledged by the House of Lords[3] in the case known as the Spycatcher case. It was accepted that as a broad principle a duty of confidence arises:

- if information is confidential; and
- comes to the knowledge of a person where he or she has notice, or is held to have agreed, that the information is confidential,
- with the effect that it would be just that he or she should be precluded from disclosing the information; and
- it is in the public interest that the confidentiality should be protected.

Clearly these principles would apply to information which the therapist was given by or about a client. The principles were applied in the case of *Stephens* v. *Avery*.[4]

Case 2   Unconscionable disclosure

The plaintiff and the first defendant were close friends who freely discussed matters of a personal and private nature on the express basis that what the plaintiff told the first defendant was secret and disclosed in confidence. The first defendant passed on to the second and third defendants, who were the editor and publisher of a newspaper, details of the patient's sexual conduct, including details of the plaintiff's lesbian relationship with a woman who had been killed by her husband. The plaintiff brought an action against the defendants claiming damages on the grounds that the information was confidential and was knowingly published by the newspaper in breach of the duty of confidence owed by the first defendant to the plaintiff. In an action by the defendants to strike out the claim as disclosing no reasonable cause of action, the defendants failed and appealed to the Chancery Division.

They lost on the grounds that although the courts would not enforce a duty of confidence relating to matters which had a grossly immoral tendency, information relating to sexual conduct could be the subject of a legally enforceable duty of confidence if it would be unconscionable for a person who had received information on the express basis that it was confidential subsequently to reveal that information to another.

Exceptions to the duty

All the sources of law which recognise that there is a duty of confidentiality also recognise that there will be exceptions where it is lawful to disclose confidential information. The main exceptions are shown in Box 10.2.

Box 10.2   Exceptions to the duty of confidentiality

- Consent of the client
- Disclosure in the clinical care or in the interests of the client
- Court order (Subpoena and under the Supreme Court Act 1981)
- Statutory duty to disclose
- Disclosure in the public interest.

Consent of the client

The duty of confidentiality is in the interest of the client and the client therefore can give consent to disclosure which without that consent would be unlawful. The client should be competent to give consent. In the case of a mentally incompetent adult, consent to disclosure could be given on the client's behalf in the client's best interests by a representative guardian or carer of the client. Where the client is a child under 16 years, then the principles of the *Gillick* case (see Chapter 9) would apply and a mature competent child under 16 could give consent to disclosure of confidential information.

The consent of the client or her representative would be a defence against any potential proceedings being brought against the therapist. It is essential that evidence is available that consent has been given. There are therefore considerable advantages to obtaining this information in writing.

The client has the right to withdraw consent unless the terms of the disclosure are contrary to this.

Situation 1   Training video
A client agrees that a video could be made about her care and treatment. Considerable expense was incurred for the video to be produced. The client then decided that she does not wish the video to be shown.

Whether or not this can then be prevented will depend upon the terms on which her agreement to the disclosure was obtained.

Where clients specifically refuse to give their consent to the disclosure of their diagnosis to others, such as relatives, this request should as far as possible be respected under the duty of confidentiality and only if a specific exception to the duty applies could the information be passed on.

Clinical care or in the interests of the client

Therapists may work in a multi-disciplinary setting and so need to share information about the client in order to fulfil their duty of care to the client. Indeed it could be said that if relevant information were not passed to professionals caring for the client and harm were to occur to the client as a result of that failure, then the professional and her employer could be answerable to the client in a negligence action.

Where information is disclosed to colleagues as part of the duty of care to the client, care should be taken to ensure that it is relevant to and necessary for their responsibilities.

Situation 2   A closed book
A client requests the assistance of a therapist, but refuses to allow the therapist to contact the general practitioner or give full information about his history.

The client has made it extremely difficult for the therapist to treat him. Many therapists have a Code of Conduct which requires them to work in conjunction with the client's doctor. If, following an explanation from the therapist, the client still refuses to allow the therapist to be in contact with the general practitioner and refuses to give sufficient information about his past health, then the therapist may have to refuse to provide treatment.

It is rarely permissible to breach confidentiality in the client's own interests. However the following situation shows a problem that could arise.

Situation 3 Potential suicide
A therapist learns that a client wishes to commit suicide. What action should be taken?

In these circumstances it is essential for an assessment to be made of the mental competence of the client. If, for example, the client is suffering from mental disorder and the therapist failed to take action to protect the client against his or her suicide wishes, the therapist would be failing in the duty of care to the client. The therapist may wish to refer the client to a health professional. If, on the other hand, the therapist takes the view that the client is mentally competent, and the client refuses to agree to a referral to another practitioner, there is little action that the therapist can take, other than provide as much support as possible. To attempt suicide is not a criminal offence.

Court order

Subpoena The court has the right to ensure that all information relevant to an issue being decided before it is made available in the interests of justice. Both criminal and civil courts therefore have the right to issue a subpoena for the necessary information to be produced before them. Other quasi judicial proceedings such as inquiries may also have a right to subpoena information depending upon the statutory provisions which enable them to be established.

Where a court requires information, a therapist cannot refuse to comply on the grounds that the information was received in professional confidence. The courts do not recognise any privilege from disclosure attaching to the doctor or health professional. The only exceptions recognised by the courts to their right to order disclosure are: legal professional privilege and privilege on grounds of the national security (see below).

Legal professional privilege This covers communications between clients and their legal advisers. The judge cannot order disclosure of such communications. The reason is that it is in the interests of justice for a client to be able to confide fully with legal advisers without fear that such communications would be ordered to be disclosed in court. Reports to legal advisers are also privileged from disclosure if the principal purpose for which they were written is in contemplation of litigation.

Sometimes there may be several purposes behind the preparation of a report, as in a report following a health and safety accident where the report can be used for both management purposes in order to prevent a similar accident arising again and can also be used for legal purposes. This was the situation in the case of *Waugh* v. *British Railway Board.*[5] In this case the House of Lords held that if the predominant purpose behind the report was for advice and use in litigation, then it will be privileged from disclosure.

In *Lask* v. *Gloucester*[6] the court applied the test in *Waugh* in the situation where the health authorities claimed legal professional privilege in respect of confidential reports completed following an accident. The court held that, in spite of declarations by the health authorities and solicitors to this effect, the documents were not actually covered by legal professional privilege, the preparation for litigation not being the predominant purpose.

Public interest immunity The other exception to the right of the judge to order disclosure of any document relevant to an issue before the court is that of public interest immunity. This covers such interests as national security. The privilege from disclosure is given under the sworn affidavit of a Minister and can be overruled by the judge. Public interest immunity is currently under review following the report of the Scott inquiry on the excessive use of this privilege by Ministers in the 'arms for Iraq' case and it is likely that changes will be recommended on this constraint on disclosure in future, especially in relation to its use in criminal proceedings.

Disclosure ordered under the Supreme Court Act 1981   This Act enables disclosure to be made in two distinct circumstances:

- where disclosure can be ordered against a prospective party to a case involving a claim in respect of personal injury or death prior to the writ being issued (details in Box 10.3) and
- where disclosure is ordered against a third party (i.e. not directly involved in the case) where the writ has been issued in a case involving a claim in respect of personal injury or death (details in Box 10.4).

Box 10.3   Supreme Court Act 1981, section 33

Under section 33 of the Supreme Court Act 1981, disclosure can be ordered against a person likely to be a party in a personal injury case before the writ is issued. Disclosure can be ordered to be made to the applicant's legal advisers and any medical or other professional advisers of the applicants or, if the applicant has no legal advisers, to any medical or other professional adviser of the applicant.

From Box 10.4 it is clear that if a client is suing in relation to an incident during the care by a complementary therapist it can be ordered that the therapist's records be disclosed to the legal advisers or professional advisers of the client.

Box 10.4   Supreme Court Act 1981, section 34

After litigation has commenced, i.e. after the writ has been issued, under section 34 of the Supreme Court Act 1981 disclosure can be ordered against a person who is not likely to be a party to a case, if that person has information likely to be relevant.

Section 34 could cover a situation where the client was being cared for by a therapist. The client is involved in a road traffic accident and sues the driver of the vehicle which caused the accident. This driver wished to have access to information about the client held by the therapist relating to her care in order to determine the likely prognosis of the client. If for example there was concern that the client was unlikely to make a full recovery as a result of the road accident, but that he suffered from severe disabilities anyway, these existing disabilities could affect both liability and quantum.

Statutory duty to disclose

Several statutes require disclosure to be made, whether or not the patient gives consent. These are as follows:

Notifications of Communicable Diseases

- Public Health Act 1936
- Public Health (Infectious Diseases) Regulations 1988 (SI 1988/1546)
- Public Health (Control of Disease) Act 1984
- Public Health (Aircraft) Regulations 1979 (SI 1979/1434)
- Public Health (Ships) Regulations 1979 (SI 1979/1435)

Notifications of Abortions

- Abortion Act 1967, Section 2
- Abortion Regulations 1991 (SI 1991/499)

Notifications of Drug Addicts

- Misuse of Drugs Act 1971, Section 10
- Misuse of Drugs (Notification of and Supply of Addicts) Regulations 1973 (SI 1973/799)

Notification of Births and Deaths

- National Health Service Act 1977, Section 124
- National Health Service (Notification of Births and Deaths) Regulations 1982 (SI 1982/286)

Notification of Poisonings and Health and Safety matters

- Health and Safety at Work Act 1974
- Reporting of Injuries, Diseases and Dangerous Occurrences Regulations 1985 (SI 1983/2023)
- Reporting of Injuries, Diseases and Dangerous Occurrences (Amendment) Regulations 1989 (SI 1989/1457)

Notifiable diseases If therapists are aware that a client they are treating appears to be suffering from a notifiable disease, then they should ensure that the appropriate person is notified. Normally the GP would be the person making the notification which is made to the Community Medical Officer of Health. A client's reluctance to see a doctor should be overruled. Diseases which are notifiable are shown in Box 10.5.

Box 10.5   Notifiable diseases

Category A cholera, plague, relapsing fever, smallpox and typhus

Category B acquired immune deficiency syndrome (AIDS), acute encephalitis, acute poliomyelitis, meningitis, meningococcal septicaemia, anthrax, diphtheria, dysentery, paratyphoid fever, typhoid fever, viral hepatitis, leprosy, leptospirosis, measles, mumps, rubella, whooping cough, malaria, tetanus, yellow fever, ophthalmia neonatorum, scarlet fever, tuberculosis, rabies and viral haemorrhagic fever

---

Who notifies?   Under section 11 of the 1984 Act registered medical practitioners have a duty to notify the proper office of the local authority if they become aware, or suspect, that a patient whom they are attending within the district of a local authority is suffering from a notifiable disease or from food poisoning. The duty does not apply if they believe, and have reasonable grounds for believing, that some other registered medical practitioner has complied.

What information must be notified?   Box 10.6 shows the information which must be notified.

Box 10.6   Information which must be given

1. Name, age and sex of the patient and the address of the premises where the patient is
2. The disease or, as the case may be, particulars of the poisoning from which the patient is, or is suspected to be, suffering and the date or approximate date of its onset
3. If the premises are a hospital, the day on which the patient was admitted, the address of the premises from which he came there and whether or not, in the opinion of the person giving the certificate, the disease or poisoning from which the patient is, or is suspected to be, suffering was contracted in hospital.

Powers of a Justice of the Peace   Under Section 37 of the Public Health (Control of Disease) Act 1984, if the Justice of the Peace is satisfied that:

- a person is suffering from a notifiable disease, *and*
- that his circumstances are such that proper precautions to prevent the spread of infection cannot be taken or that such precautions are not being taken, *and*
- the risk of infection is thereby caused to other persons, *and*
- accommodation is available in a suitable hospital

the JP can order the person to be removed to the hospital.

Under section 38 the JP can order the detention of a person suffering from a notifiable disease in a hospital for infectious diseases.

Disclosure in the public interest

This is the most difficult exception to the duty of confidentiality. State registration bodies all recognise that in certain circumstances disclosure without the client's consent and contrary to his wishes may be justified. Organisations for complementary therapists which require a Code of Practice to be followed also recognise that the duty of confidentiality is subject to an exception where disclosure is necessary in the interests of the safety of the client or any other person.

Case 3   Damaging report[7]

A psychiatrist, who had been asked for a report by a patient who was seeking his discharge from detention under the Mental Health Act 1983, considered that the patient, if no longer detained, represented such a risk to the public that he sent his report to the Mental Health Review Tribunal and the hospital without the consent of the patient who then sued him for breach of confidentiality.

In this case on the issue of disclosure in the public interest the Court of Appeal held that the psychiatrist was justified in his action.

Other situations where disclosure in the public interest would be justified would include a situation where harm is occurring or likely to occur to a child or another person.

Certain professional groups including the Council of the Professions Supplementary to Medicine have participated with the British Medical Association and the Royal College of Nursing in drafting legislation to cover the use and disclosure of personal health information. In their report[8] public interest is defined as follows:

It shall be lawful for a qualified health professional to disclose personal health information where:

a. it relates to a patient for whom he [or she] has clinical responsibility, and
b. in the opinion of that professional disclosure is necessary in the public interest.

Disclosure in the public interest is necessary only where:

a. it relates to the prevention, detection or prosecution of a serious offence; or
b. it relates to the protection of public safety; or
c. failure to disclose would expose the patient or some other person to a real risk of death or serious harm.

Most complementary therapists would accept this exception to the duty of confidentiality.

If a therapist decided that confidential information should be disclosed in the public interest, an attempt should be made to obtain the client's consent to the disclosure. If this is not successful, then the therapist should carefully record the reasons and legal justification for the disclosure.

Implications for the therapist

A procedure is necessary for therapists to ensure that they preserve the confidential nature of information about the client. This would also include safe storage of the records which are kept and should also cover any sharing of records on a multi-disciplinary team basis (see Chapter 14 on record keeping). In addition the exceptions to the duty should be clarified, so that therapists can be confident that they are acting within the law and retain the trust of the client. They should have a clear understanding of what is meant by the public interest so that they recognise the situations which give rise to an exception to the duty of confidentiality.

ACCESS TO RECORDS AND INFORMATION

Patients have a statutory right to see their health records, whether they are held in computer or manual form, subject to only a few exceptions. The definition of health records covers records kept by a wide list of health professionals. However the health records kept by a complementary therapist do not appear to come within the definition. Where, however, the complementary therapist is also a health professional, as defined in the Act, then a statutory right of access exists. This would also be the case if the complementary therapist is not a health professional but is working for a health professional. For example, if a GP employed an aromatherapist to work in the practice, the records of the aromatherapist would probably come under the provisions of the Access to Health Records Act.

A distinction therefore has to be made. There are those complementary therapists not coming under the statutory definition of health professionals and who work on their own, whose clients therefore do not have a statutory right of access to records kept in manual form. On the other hand, the records of complementary therapists who work under the aegis of a health professional and whose records can be considered to be made by or on behalf of that health professional, would come under the statutory provisions covering manual records. If the records are on computer, the Data Protection Act applies.

Even if the client does not have a statutory right of access, access could be the subject of agreement between client and therapist. The contractual conditions could not however limit any statutory right which existed. Separate statutory provisions cover the records held by those who work for social services departments. Therapists' records may also become relevant to reports written by the client's doctor for insurance or employment purposes and therefore come under the rules relating to disclosure of such reports.[9]

In addition to the statutory rights of access to health records and personal files kept by social services departments there is also a right at common law for the client to receive, as part of the duty of care owed by the health professional to the client, information which is relevant to decisions which the client may be required to consider in relation to her treatment and care. This is discussed in Chapter 9 on the law on consent. The rights at common law of the client to obtain information are set out in the leading case of *Sidaway*[10] which is considered in that chapter.

The legislation giving the statutory rights is as follows:

- Data Protection Act 1984
- Access to Medical Reports Act 1988
- Access to Health Records Act 1990
- Access to Personal Files Act 1987

The Data Protection Act 1984

The Data Protection Act 1984 gives rights of access to automated processed personal health information subject to the conditions laid down by statutory instrument.[11] Clarification is given of the statutory provisions by the Department of Health.[12]

Principles

The Data Protection Act 1984 regulates the collection, processing and storage of information in automated form from which an individual can be identified. Data users are required to register with the Data Protection Registrar their recording and use of personal data and must comply with the Data Protection principles. These are shown below in Box 10.7.

The Act covers only those records which consist of information relating to a living individual who can be identified from that information (or from other information in the possession of the data user), including any expression of opinion.[13]

Box 10.7   Principles in the Data Protection Act

Personal data shall:
1. be collected and processed fairly and lawfully
2. only be held for specified, lawful registered purposes
3. only be used for registered purposes or disclosed to registered recipients
4. be adequate and relevant to the purpose for which they are held
5. be accurate and, where necessary, kept up to date
6. be held no longer than is necessary for the stated purpose
7. have appropriate security surrounding them
8. be subject to right of access by the data subject to records held about himself.

Provisions on access

The data subject, i.e. the person about whom the information is recorded, has a right of access under the 1984 Act. He has the right to be informed by the data user as to whether any personal identifiable information about him is being held and, if so, he has the right to be supplied with a copy of that information.[14] Children have the right of access if they have the maturity to make a valid application. The concept of being 'Gillick Competent' would apply (see Chapter 9 on children).

The Act provides for regulations to be made to enable those who are responsible for the management of the affairs of an incompetent adult to have access, but no regulations have yet been passed. This may occur if the recommendations of the Law Commission on decision making and the mentally incapacitated adult are implemented.[15]

Exceptions

Under statutory instrument, the access provisions are modified in the case of access to personal health records.[16] This applies to data held by a health professional or data held by a person other than a health professional where the information constituting the data was first recorded by or on behalf of a health professional. Health professional is defined as shown in Box 10.8.

Box 10.8   Definition of health professional[17]

- registered medical practitioner
- registered dental practitioner
- registered chemist
- registered optician
- registered pharmaceutical chemist or druggist
- registered nurse, midwife or health visitor
- registered chiropodist
- dietitian
- occupational therapist
- orthoptist
- physiotherapist
- clinical psychologist, child psychotherapist
- speech therapist
- art or music therapist employed by a health authority
- scientists employed by a health authority as head of department
- osteopath (added by the Osteopaths Act 1993)
- chiropractor (added by the Chiropractors Act 1994)

Access is not permitted where subject access:

- would be likely to cause serious harm to the physical or mental health of the data subject; or
- would be likely to disclose to the data subject the identity of another individual (who has not consented to the disclosure of the information) either as a person to whom the information or part of it relates or as the source of the information, or enable that identity to be deduced by the data subject either from the information itself or from a combination of that information and other information which the data subject has or is likely to have.

This second exception does not apply where the other individual is a health professional who has been involved in the care of the data subject and the information relates to him in that capacity.

A data user, who is not a health professional, is required to consult the appropriate health professional before permitting or refusing access. The appropriate health professional is defined as:

- the medical practitioner or dental practitioner who is currently or was most recently responsible for the clinical care of the data subject in connection with the matters to which the information which is the subject of the request relates; or
- where there is more than one such practitioner, the practitioner who is the most suitable to advise on the matters to which the information which is the subject of the request relates; or
- where there is no practitioner available falling within the definitions above, a health professional who has the necessary experience and qualifications to advise on the matters to which the information which is the subject of the request relates.

If the exclusion provisions apply, the data user does not have to notify the applicant that information is being withheld. It is sufficient for the data user to notify the applicant that there is no information being held which has to be revealed to the data subject.

Procedure for application

The application is made in writing to the data user, i.e. the person who holds the personal data, giving sufficient information for the relevant data and the data subject to be identified, together with the appropriate fee.

Rights of the data subject

- Unless the exclusion provisions discussed above apply, the data subject is entitled to be supplied with a copy of the information requested within 40 days of the date on which the application, giving all the necessary information is received.
- If the information supplied to the data subject is inaccurate the subject can request that the information is rectified or erased and has the right to enforce this in the Court.
- If the inaccuracy causes distress to the data subject, then the data subject has the right to claim compensation for the harm which he has suffered. The data user has a defence if the inaccurate information was received from the patient or a third person or that the data user took such care as was reasonably required in the circumstances to ensure the accuracy of the data at the material time.
- If the data subject is refused the information, he can either make an application to the County or High Court or to the Data Protection Registrar for the enforcement of his statutory rights.

Data protection and European directives

A recent European Directive is aimed at strengthening the protection of individuals with regard to the processing of personal data and on the free movement of such data and in ensuring common standards across the European Community.[1] The Government has, following a consultation exercise, published its proposals on how the Directive should be implemented in this country.[2] At the time of writing legislation is awaited.

The Access to Medical Reports Act 1988

Basic principles

This Act enables a patient to see and if necessary suggest corrections where an insurance company or employer requests a medical report from the patient's own doctor for insurance or employment purposes. The records to which the doctor might refer may include information received from complementary therapists. The right of access can be withheld in similar circumstances to those stated in the Data Protection (Subject Access Modification) (Health) provisions (see above). Therefore if, in the unlikely circumstances that the complementary therapist is concerned that any information is likely to cause serious harm to the physical or mental health of the patient or identify a third person who has requested not to be identified, then she should ensure that the information which she passes to the doctor is suitably annotated.

Access to Health Records Act 1990

Principles

After the implementation of the Data Protection Act an anomaly existed in that there was a statutory right to identifiable personal information, including health records, held on computerised records, but not to health records held in manual form. Since most health records were and still are held in manual form, the statutory right had little impact. Legislation was therefore introduced to enable patients to access their health records even if held in manual form.

The Access to Health Records Act 1990 came into force on 1 November 1991 and only applies to records kept after that date, although earlier records could be shown if they were necessary to make sense of those kept after that date. Guidance was issued by the Department of Health.[20]

The Act gives the applicant the right to seek access from the holder of the records. This phrase is defined as:

- in the case of a record made by the general practitioner, the general practitioner, or, where there is no GP, the Health Authority;
- in the case of the provision of health services by the health service body, on whose behalf the record is held;
- in any other case, the health professional who made the records.

Health professional

This is defined in exactly the same way as under the Data Protection Act (see Box 10.10 above). This does not, therefore, include most complementary therapists unless they also have a qualification in orthodox medicine.

Health record

A record is defined as a health record if:

- it consists of information relating to the physical or mental health of an individual who can be identified from that information, or from that and other information in the possession of the holder of the record; and
- it has been made by or on behalf of a health professional in connection with the care of that individual.

Who can apply

The following have the right of access:

- The patient.
- A person authorised in writing to make the application on the patient's behalf.
- Where the patient is a child (a person under 16 years), a person having parental responsibility for the child. The patient must either consent to the application or the patient must be incapable of understanding and the giving of access would be in his best interests. (Refer to Chapter 9 for the law relating to children.)
- Where the patient is incapable of managing his own affairs, a person appointed by the court to manage his affairs.
- Where the patient has died, the personal representatives of the patient (i.e. the people appointed as executors by the will or, where there is no will, the relatives authorised to deal with the estate) or any person who may have a claim arising out of the patient's death. Access under this subsection can be prevented if the record includes a note, made at the patient's request, that he did not wish access to be given on such an application. Information need not be disclosed if the patient's death is not subject to a claim.

If the applicant is a child (i.e. a person under 16 years), then the holder must be satisfied that the child is 'Gillick competent', i.e. is capable of understanding the nature of the application. (See chapter 9 on children)

Procedure

The patient has the right to make an application for access to a health record or any part of a health record. The application is made to the holder of the record and, if not the same person, the observations of the health professional by or on behalf of whom the record was made must be sought. No fee can be charged unless access is required to records which were made more than 40 days before the application. A charge could be made for postage and copying. The 40 days is calculated from an acceptable application. If the applicant has provided insufficient information, then the holder has 14 days within which to write to the applicant asking for any necessary information.

Nature of access

Where an application is made the holder of the record must (unless the exceptions exist) allow the applicant to inspect the record or a part of the record and if requested supply a copy of the record or extract.

Exclusions

The holder of the records can refuse access on similar grounds as exist in relation to computerised records:

- If any part of the health record would disclose information likely to cause serious harm to the physical or mental health of the patient or of any other individual.

- If the health record would disclose information relating to or provided by any other individual, other than the patient, who could be identified from that information (unless that individual has consented). This does not apply where the individual is a health professional who has been involved in the care of the patient.
- If the health records were made before 1 November 1991 (unless access is necessary in order to make intelligible any part of a later record to which access is required to be given).

Right to request the correction of inaccurate records

Section 6 of the 1990 Act enables a person who considers that any information contained in a health record or part of a health record is inaccurate, to apply to the holder of the record for the necessary correction to be made. If the holder is satisfied that the information is inaccurate, he must make the necessary correction. If he is not so satisfied, he must make a note in the part of the record containing the disputed information of the matters in respect of which the information is considered to be inaccurate. In both cases, he must supply the applicant with either a copy of the correction or the note. A fee cannot be charged. The Act defines 'inaccurate' as meaning 'incorrect, misleading or incomplete' (section 6(3)).

Request to clarify and explain

Where the information contained in a record or extract which is inspected or copied for the applicant is expressed in terms which are not intelligible without an explanation, an explanation of those terms shall be provided with the record of extract, or supplied with the copy (section 3(3)). This provision prevents health professionals hiding behind professional jargon to keep information secret from the patient.

Means of enforcement

A person with a statutory right of access under the 1990 Act can apply to the County Court or the High Court if the holder has failed to comply with any requirement under the Act. The court must be satisfied that the applicant has fulfilled any requirements laid down by the Secretary of State.

Protection of those with rights of access

Section 9 of the 1990 Act makes any contractual term which compels an individual to supply to another person a copy of a health record to which he has been given access under this Act void. Thus no-one can be compelled to show to another person the record. (This does not of course prevent the court requiring the holder of the record to disclose health information under a subpoena).

Access to Personal Files Act 1987

Provisions comparable to those under the Access to Health Records Act 1990 have been enacted in respect of housing and social services records to enable the person in respect of whom the records are held to obtain access. However access can be withheld if serious harm would be caused to the physical or mental health of the applicant. The fact that the right of access is subject to different statutory procedures can cause difficulties where there is a unified record system in existence with social services records and health records being held on the same file, since the holders of the records are defined differently according to whether they are health records or social services records.

NON-STATUTORY ACCESS

The existence of statutory rights of access for the patient does not mean that the patient necessarily has to apply formally for access. There may be many reasons why the health professional agrees to informal access of the patient to his records and this could then be arranged. The same principle applies to the sharing of information between a complementary therapist and the client.

A decision by the Court of Appeal has established that, if the statutory provisions do not apply, the patient does not have an absolute right of access at common law.

Case 4   Access to health records refused[21]

A former mental patient brought an action against a Family Health Services Authority and Health Authority for their failure to allow him access to his records. He wished to discover the reason why a psychotherapist, who was treating him and with whom he had fallen in love, was taken off his case. He had been haunted by the desire to know why and also to discover the reasons for his detention in 1969 under the Mental Health Act 1959. The Health Authority had said three years before that it would consider disclosure of records but only if it was given an assurance that neither it nor its staff faced legal action. The plaintiff refused to give this assurance.

The High Court Judge Mr Justice Popplewell refused to allow access. He ruled that the Access to Health Records Act 1990 was not relevant since it applied only to records after 1 November 1991. He held that a patient did not have an unconditional right of access at common law to medical records which existed before the commencement of the Access to Health Records Act 1990. On the issue of access as a common law right, the applicant argued that the refusal of access involved a denial of the right of the respect for a person's private life and that a patient of sound mind had a right to receive on request all relevant information which he sought. If he was entitled, quite irrationally, to refuse treatment which would protect his life he was equally entitled, rationally or not, to require information whatever damage it might do to his health. The common law rule was and had been that the confidential relationship between doctor and patient required, subject only to the exception of protecting informants, access as of right to ensure respect for private and family life.

This was not accepted by the High Court Judge who held that there was no right at common law to access any records which pre-existed the 1990 Act.

The Court of Appeal upheld this decision on the grounds that a doctor or health authority was entitled to deny access to the records by the patient on the ground that their disclosure would be detrimental to him. Lord Justice Nourse stated that the doctor's duty and the health authority's duty was to act at all times in the best interests of the patient.

Those interests would usually require that a patient's medical records should not be disclosed to third parties; conversely that they should be usually handed on from one doctor to the next or should be made available to the patient's legal advisers if they were reasonably required for the purposes of legal proceedings in which he was involved.

This principle would not necessarily apply to the situation between a client and complementary therapist in private practice, since the agreement made between them at the time the treatment commenced may have made specific provision for access to the records.

ACCESS AND THE THERAPIST

It is seldom that secrecy of information from the patient can be justified in the case of the treatment provided by the therapist. There are very few situations where the therapist would feel that serious harm could arise to the physical or mental health of the patient if access were to be permitted.

Problem situations

Sometimes, however, the problems which can arise are not of the therapist's making as the following situation illustrates.

Situation 4   Orders to withhold

A consultant physician treating a patient has diagnosed multiple sclerosis. It is his view that the patient could not yet cope with this diagnosis and he therefore instructs the multi-disciplinary team caring for the patient that she should not be told. The doctor refers the patient to an aromatherapist. During the session the patient raises with the aromatherapist her concerns about her illness and asks the therapist directly if she has multiple sclerosis. What is the legal situation?

Although the aromatherapist is a personally accountable professional who should use her own discretion in making health decisions, she may also be part of the multi-disciplinary team usually headed by the consultant responsible for the care and treatment of the patient. Her concerns about openness and disclosure to the patient should have been raised as soon as she was aware of the restrictions ordered by the consultant and she should have taken this up with him.

In the situation which occurs she has the following options:

- refuse to say and suggest that the patient should have an appointment to discuss with the consultant her diagnosis and treatment;
- answer the patient honestly and ignore the consultant's orders; or
- lie to the patient.

It would be hoped that the last option would be unacceptable to all therapists. The first may be appropriate in most cases. Ignoring the consultant's instructions may in exceptional circumstances be justified. However, if the therapist follows this line, then she must be prepared to justify her actions in one or more of the following ways:

- If she is an employee, before disciplinary proceedings should the consultant report her to her managers.
- In civil litigation, for example if the patient reacts to this information by attempting to take (or succeeding in taking) her own life and the employers of the therapist are sued for their vicarious liability for the harm caused by the therapist, or, not being an employee, she is sued personally.
- In professional conduct proceedings if it is decided that she is guilty of misconduct as a qualified aromatherapist.

It may be that before all three forms of hearings, she is able to justify her actions as being in the best interests of the patient. She should ensure that her records are comprehensive and explain clearly why she took the decisions which she did. In deciding whether the option to tell is appropriate she should be mindful of the fact that there is no absolute duty to disclose everything to the patient: under the statutory provisions there is a right to deny access, which the holder of the records can exercise on the basis of the advice of the health professional concerned; at common law, the House of Lords in the *Sidaway* case[10] recognised the concept of therapeutic privilege, the right to withhold information from the patient in exceptional circumstances when it is justified in the best interests of the patient.

There has been no decided case where such a dispute has arisen, so it is not possible to be categorical as to what decision the court would make in such circumstances.

A distinction may also have to be made between those therapists who work in private practice, where the patient may not be directly under any consultant, and the therapist liaises with the GP as the lead medical practitioner responsible for the clinical care of the patient, and therapists who are employees supplying services to an NHS or private health care organisation.

Situation 5   Information denied to the therapist

A variant of the situation discussed above, is where the therapist is not herself told the diagnosis of the patient, either by the patient or by the patient's doctor. Problems can arise for the therapist when she does not know the medical condition of a referral. How, for example, can she decide on priorities? Can the doctor be forced to disclose? What happens if the client does not want the therapist to get in touch with the doctor?

In such a situation each case would have to be treated on its merits and many different legal principles apply. The duty in relation to confidentiality is discussed above where it is noted that the client has the right to refuse to permit the therapist to contact the general practitioner, and this may lead to the therapist declining to treat the client.

Another issue which arises in the situation where the doctor is refusing to give the therapist information about the client, is that of the standard of care to be provided by the therapist. If she is kept in ignorance of certain information about the client's condition, she may make some grave errors of judgment which could cause harm to the patient. The therapist's right to have the relevant information to care appropriately for the patient would be clear, and she should bring up such an issue with the client.

Questions and Exercises

1. Examine your practice in relation to passing on confidential information. What faults would you see in it?
2. A client asks for sight of the clinical records you are keeping on her. What action do you take and what considerations do you take into account?
3. In what circumstances, if any, do you consider that it would cause serious harm to the physical or mental health of a client to see his or her records?

REFERENCES

1. Further information can be obtained from: Darley B, Griew A, McLoughlin K, Williams J 1994 How to Keep a Clinical Confidence. HMSO, London
2. X *v.* Y [1988] 2 All ER 648
3. Attorney General *v.* Guardian Newspaper Ltd (No 2) [1988] 3 All ER 545
4. Stephens *v.* Avery and others [1988] 2 All ER 477
5. Waugh *v.* British Railway Board [1980] AC 521
6. Lask *v.* Gloucester The Times Law Report 13 December 1985
7. W *v.* Edgell [1989] 1 All ER 1089; The Times Law Report 20 November 1989 Court of Appeal
8. Multi-disciplinary Professional Working Group 1994 An explanatory handbook of guidance governing use and disclosure of personal health information. British Medical Association, London
9. For more detailed information see: Cowley R 1994 Access to Medical Records and Reports, a Practical Guide NAHAT Radcliffe Medical Press, Oxford
10. Sidaway *v.* Bethlem Royal Hospital Governors [1985] 2 WLR 480
11. Data Protection (Subject Access Modification) (Health) Order 1987 SI 1987/1903
12. HC(87)14 and HC(89)29
13. Data Protection Act 1984 section 1(3)
14. Data Protection Act 1984 section 21
15. Law Commission 1995 Report No 231 Mental Incapacity. HMSO, London
16. Data Protection (Subject Access Modification) (Health) Order 1987 SI 1987/1903
17. Schedule 1 of Data Protection (Subject Access Modification) (Health) Order 1987 SI 1987/1903
18. 94/46/EC Directive of the European Parliament and the Council of Europe.
19. Data Protection The Government's Proposals July 1997 Command Paper 3725 Home Office
20. HSG(91)6 Access to Health Records Act
21. R *v.* Mid Glamorgan Family Health Services Authority ex parte Martin [1993] Queens Bench Division 137 SJ 153; Times Law Report 2 June 1993, upheld Court of Appeal Times Law Report 16 August 1994; [1994] 5 Med LR 383

Education, research and teaching

In comparison with health professional education within orthodox health care, the education for complementary therapies is funded from private as opposed to public sources. Many organisations which provide complementary therapies either provide their own training in the specific therapy or provide an accreditation system for colleges and other organisations supplying the training. In some cases however the training has had state support. Thus the homeopathic hospitals have had both state recognition and funding for their work. For the most part however the training in complementary therapies has to be provided privately and can vary from a university course to a few days part time training which leads to a certificate of competence or membership of an association which recognises competence to practise. Each specialist chapter covers the particular training and accreditation available to individual therapies. This chapter provides an overview of education, research and the legal aspects which arise from teaching.

EDUCATION

To what extent is state support necessary for training, educational accreditation and the provision of colleges in the field of complementary therapy?

The answer must be 'it depends'. It depends firstly on the extent to which training is relevant to the particular therapy. Some therapies are dependent on natural ability. For example, in the technique of dowsing as a diagnostic aid it appears that the ability is innate and cannot necessarily be developed through training programmes. Some may argue that the skill of healing is also inborn.

It also depends on the extent to which it is seen that the purchase of complementary therapies is considered to be a responsibility of society and therefore be provided within the NHS. In Chapter 1 it was noted from the NAHAT survey that there has been considerable uptake in the purchasing of complementary therapies. Even so, complementary therapy is a minor part of the NHS. If this were to change and more GP fundholders and more health authorities were prepared to purchase complementary therapies for their patients, then there would be a need for the state to subsidise training programmes as there would be a clear shortage of therapists to meet the increased demand.

Does the receipt of state recognition through registration automatically mean that state funding would be available for those who seek to pursue a course in that field?

Certainly in the field of medicine (registration through the GMC), dentistry (registration through the GDC), nursing, midwifery and health visiting (registration through the UKCC), and professions supplementary to medicine – dietitians, occupational therapists, physiotherapists, medical laboratory scientific officers, radiographers, orthoptists and chiropodists – (registration through the CPSM) the training programmes are funded either through local government support to students, or through government grants to purchasers of health care education. This is also true, however, of professions which are recognised as part of orthodox health care but are not at present state registered e.g. clinical psychologists, clinical scientists, physicists, speech therapists and social workers.

At present there appears to be no automatic right of students for state registered professions to have access to funding for training. The current review of higher education chaired by Sir Ronald Dearing, which recommends a contribution to fees by students, does not draw a distinction between fees for courses which lead to state registration and those which do not. It does recognise, however, that students from low income families may be exempt from payment of tuition fees.

Does the accreditation of courses give rise to potential legal liabilities?

Situation 1   Negligent accreditation

An organisation which as part of its activities assessed courses for accreditation which enabled successful students to secure membership as complementary therapists was under pressure because of lack of resources. A student who obtained membership of the association has now been informed that the course she undertook was defective since it provided inadequate supervision during clinical practice and the lecturers were not of the appropriate standard. What remedies does the student have and could any one harmed by the student claim against the organisation which gave accreditation to the course?

The student may have a case against the training institution both in contract and in negligence. The student would have paid fees to the college. It could be assumed that there was an express or implied term that the course would be properly accredited. Failure by the training organisation in this respect could make it liable to the student for breach of contract or misrepresentation.

There is no contract between the accrediting body and the student but, if it is the case that the student obtained a list of allegedly accredited courses from that body and in reliance on that list entered into the contract with the training organisation, it is arguable at least that there was a duty care, breach of that duty and harm or loss arising from it, hence liability in negligence.[1]

Any causal connection between the accrediting body and a client harmed by the student may be too remote with too many other factors intervening (see Chapter 3 on the difficulties in proving causation).

How can a potential NHS employer or a client determine if a therapist is properly qualified?

The chapters on individual therapies in Section 2 give an outline of some of the main accreditation bodies and organisations giving approval to a variety of courses. In the absence of a National Complementary Therapy Board with the function of giving state recognition to training and courses each individual claim to qualification by a therapist has to be looked at individually. West Yorkshire Health Authority has issued guidelines to its trusts on the employment of complementary therapists within the NHS covering professional status, insurance and qualifications.[2] It suggests that an employer should check the evidence shown in Box 11.1 and obtain the information shown in Box 11.2 before employing a complementary therapist.

Box 11.1   Evidence to be seen by employer

Therapist's certificates; copy of the syllabus studied; details of school/college providing training; copies of written assignments; examination results; evidence of continuing professional development; references from patients, doctors etc.

Box 11.2   Information to be obtained by employer

The length of training; proportion of theory and practice in training; why a particular therapy was chosen; what treatment involves; number of treatments generally required; contraindications for the therapy; how the therapy works; details of training in first aid, interviewing and counselling; number of years in practice; keeping clinical records; disclosing content to GP with patient's consent; how overall results are monitored; details of research carried out in the therapy; the communication strategy between therapist and referring health care professional.

RESEARCH

How is research into complementary therapies funded? Does the Research Council for Complementary Therapies (RCCM) have government backing?

The RCCM is a charity founded in 1983 which relies on individual and corporate benefactors. It provides the research services shown in Box 11.3.

Box 11.3 Functions of RCCM

1. To encourage practitioners of complementary medicine to undertake vigorous research
2. To teach skills in research to complementary medicine practitioners
3. To guide and assist in research projects
4. To develop a data base on research published on complementary medicine – Centralised Information Service for Complementary Medicine (CISCOM)
5. To assist in the evaluation and synthesising of research results
6. To encourage the implementation of research findings
7. To work closely with conventional practitioners in increasing their knowledge of complementary medicine
8. To advise practitioners on the audit and evaluation of their services
9. To provide an information service.

In addition to the services shown in Box 11.3 the RCCM also holds conferences and colloquia for researchers and practitioners, sponsors first time researchers and encourages government funding of research into complementary medicine. The CISCOM currently has access to over 40 000 references and is able to provide assistance in literature searches.

What other bodies contribute to funding of research into complementary therapies?

Individual charitable trusts or education foundations have made available research grants to complementary therapies. Thus the Wellcome Foundation has just made available a grant for research in healing to take place at Exeter University. Government funding for research through the Medical Research Council and other research bodies and specific projects is also available for research into complementary therapies.

Post-graduate medical education is organised through several regional centres which provide both financial support and approval of courses as meeting the criteria for post-graduate medical education. Support can be given to participants on courses in complementary therapies. For example the Dean of Post-Graduate General Practice Education South Thames Region (West) at the University of London replied to the author's query about the recognition of complementary therapies as part of post-graduate training as follows:

Each application for support to educational fees for doctor's involvement in higher professional development is considered on its own merits and the degree of support will vary according to funding available.

Complementary therapies are not excluded and there are no special conditions attached to any recognition for funding purposes. At the present time I am supporting one such initiative.

Another opportunity which is available for GPs in relation to higher professional development is Prolonged Study Leave whereby a GP may apply to the NHSE for locum support for up to 12 months' leave of absence from his or her practice, or on a pro rata basis. In these circumstances I am merely asked to make a recommendation and not a decision. Complementary therapy training would be eligible for consideration and again there are no special circumstances which apply for recognition. One such application has recently received my support and is being considered by the NHSE.

Are all complementary therapies susceptible to modern scientific techniques?

One of the dilemmas for many complementary therapies is that, since they are holistic (see Chapter 39) and therefore closer to a philosophy of life or religion, their claims for their work in developing a person's full potential and well being are not susceptible to the usual research methods applied to science.

The placebo effect may weaken the claims made for some orthodox medicines, yet some therapists may actually rely upon the placebo effect for their value. Thus those who believe in the power of 'the mind over matter' use this power explicitly in healing techniques.

In an article in the *Sunday Times* Margaret Driscoll[3] reviews the work of Andrew Weil a Harvard trained doctor who sees the future of medicine in combining western science and alternative remedies. Margaret Driscoll writes

Arguments still abound over the standards of evidence required for the weird and wacky remedies to become acceptable to the medical establishment.

She quotes Andrew Vickers of the Research Council for Complementary Medicine:

I need more evidence that there's a unicorn in my garden than I do for a sheep.

Ultimately it will have to be accepted that there are some complementary therapies which can never be validated in the way in which orthodox medicine requires. This does not necessarily render them valueless, but it does mean that different criteria will have to be applied if they are to be purchased within the NHS.

TEACHING

In what circumstances could a teacher be liable in law?

In Chapter 3 the principles relating to negligence are considered and it is noted that liability can arise for negligent advice. This could therefore apply to the instruction given by a tutor, teacher, trainer, instructor or any other person giving advice to another.

The following elements would have to be proved to establish a claim:

- A duty of care was owed by the giver of the information to the other to ensure that care was taken in the advice offered.
- It could be expected that there would be reliance upon this advice so that a special relationship was created between the parties.
- The giver of information failed to take reasonable care in ensuring that the information was correct.

● In reliance upon this information, reasonably foreseeable harm was caused to the recipient of the information.

Situation 2 Incompetent teaching

Mavis, a student of herbal medicine, was given instructions about certain plants used in Chinese medicine. On completing the course, she set up in practice and implemented some of the lessons which she had learnt in her classes.

Unfortunately one of the herbs she recommended caused kidney failure in one of her patients, who is threatening to bring legal action against her. Mavis is now wondering whether she has any right of action against her instructor and whether the patient could sue the teacher directly.

To succeed against the instructor, Mavis would have to show that the instructor was in breach of the duty of care owed to Mavis by giving negligent advice and that in reliance on the advice Mavis caused harm to the patient. Her loss would therefore be any compensation which she has to pay the patient.

Her main difficulty will be in establishing the causal link, because it could be argued that there are other sources of advice that a student should use, not simply one teacher. If, therefore, she could have obtained the correct information by referring to recommended text books, then there should not have been sole reliance upon the instructor. Had she referred to these other sources and realised that there was a conflict, then maybe she would not have given that particular herb to the patient. There is considerable uncertainty therefore over the likelihood of a successful outcome to her claim against the teacher.

In contrast the patient would have a much stronger case against Mavis if it can be established that no reasonable herbalist would have prescribed that particular herb.

What of a direct action by the patient against the instructor? This would hinge not only on causation, i.e. whether the harm which resulted to the patient was a direct and reasonably foreseeable result of the negligence of the instructor, but also upon whether an instructor owes a duty of care to those persons who could be harmed as a result of his giving negligent instructions to a student. There has been no decision by the courts on the exact issue, but from recent cases where the courts have had to decide whether a duty of care exists, it is unlikely that a duty would be owed by the teacher to a client injured by the student.[4]

To what extent does a teacher have a duty outside his main responsibilities of teaching?

Situation 3 A wider responsibility

A student tells a teacher on a complementary therapy course that he is concerned about a therapist he has met on his work placement who does not appear to be following ethical guidelines in the care he is providing for patients. Does the teacher have any legal responsibility to take action?

In the civil law of negligence, the courts do not recognise the duty of any person to volunteer their services. Unless there is a pre-existing duty, an individual does not have to be a Samaritan and offer assistance, even when he or she has the relevant skills. There would therefore be no duty upon the teacher to take action in this case, unless such action has already been defined as included within the scope of the duty of care owed to the student or as part of the duties which he is paid to perform. He may however give advice to the student on what action he should take as part of his work within that clinical placement.

Whilst there may be no legal duty on the teacher, there may be an ethical duty as a practitioner within a specific therapy if he learns of information relevant to the organisation of which he is a member. This duty may be included within the Code of Ethics and may require any member to bring to the attention of the Association concerns relating to another practitioner or member of that organisation.

Questions and Exercises

---

1. You are aware of many students who would wish to attend, on a full time basis, a course on complementary therapy which your organisation is running. In what circumstances would those students have the fees paid by local education authorities?
2. What criteria would you use to identify a complementary therapy which should not be subjected to research in accordance with modern scientific methods into clinical effectiveness?
3. Draw up a Code of Practice for teachers in any chosen area of complementary therapy.

REFERENCES

1. Hedley Byrne & Co Ltd v. Heller [1964] AC 465
2. News Item 1996 Medical Law Monitor Jan/Feb: 8–10
3. Driscoll M Trust me I'm a guru. The Sunday Times 18 May 1997, p 15
4. OLL Ltd v. Secretary of State for the Home Department The Times Law Report 22 July 1997

Handling complaints

INTRODUCTION

Any well organised business or service should have a clear system for handling complaints and the provision of complementary therapies is no exception to this principle. Where complementary therapies are practised within the NHS or as part of local authority services (e.g. in nursing homes or residential care homes), then they will automatically be subject to the complaints procedures required by statute within those organisations. In addition, membership by the practitioner of a recognised association will usually entail complying with a code of practice which will require a complaints system to be in existence with appropriate guidance being given by the association. Where complementary therapy is offered as a private business service and the practitioner is not subject to the regulatory mechanism of an association or other professional organisation, it will be up to such practitioners to establish their own complaints procedure. This chapter covers the principles which should apply in any complaints procedure and the specific systems which exist in the NHS and Local Authority. It also looks at how therapists working on their own could operate a complaints system.

Why do people complain?

It can take courage to make a complaint. Many people may not bother, preferring not to use that service again and thus not giving that organisation or therapist the opportunity to improve the service or make amends. Complaints should therefore be viewed positively by an organisation or therapist since they create an opportunity for improvement and retention of that client. Nor should it be assumed that the number of complaints is in itself an indicator that one organisation or therapist is worse than another. An organisation or therapist may by its attitude encourage feedback, both negative and positive, from clients and thus have more complaints than a comparable organisation or therapist which inhibits such feedback. The existence of complaints is not therefore necessarily a sign that an organisation or therapist is failing its clients.

The motives of the complainant can determine the speed of resolution. Thus a person who is simply seeking an explanation of what has gone wrong may be satisfied more quickly than a person who is looking for financial compensation where the therapist believes that such a claim is unjustifiable. Some of the motives for complaining are shown in Box 12.1.

Box 12.1   Why people complain

1. To obtain an explanation of what went wrong
2. To obtain an apology
3. To obtain financial recompense
4. To ensure that such events do not occur to another person
5. To ensure disciplinary action or professional conduct proceedings are taken against a therapist
6. Emotional motives such as guilt, revenge, bitterness etc.

Why do people not complain?

What is perhaps of greater interest is knowing why people do not complain. Possible reasons are shown in Box 12.2.

Box 12.2   Why people do not complain

1. There is no reason to complain
2. There is reason to complain but a speedy apology, response or other form of satisfaction resolves the situation
3. There is reason to complain, but
    - the individual does not know of the reason for possible complaint, or
    - it is felt that complaining would be a waste of time, or
    - the individual is too lazy, indifferent, apathetic to complain.

Where therapists are self-employed they may not be aware of the existence of a complaint until the client has failed to return for an appointment. Thus the opportunity to resolve a problem is denied.

Principles to apply for a complaints system

Although legislation was passed in 1985 for each hospital to set up a complaints system, it was clear that complaints in the NHS were not being handled speedily or effectively and therefore an expert committee was set up by the Government under the Chairmanship of Professor Alan Wilson to review NHS complaints procedures.[1] The report reviewed the current situation and set objectives for any effective complaints system. These principles are set out in Box 12.3.

Box 12.3   Principles of an effective complaints system

1. Responsiveness
2. Quality enhancement
3. Cost effectiveness
4. Accessibility
5. Impartiality
6. Simplicity
7. Speed
8. Confidentiality
9. Accountability

All the principles set out in Box 12.3 should be easily implemented, except possibly for impartiality. Single handed therapists who handle their own complaints may not be able to bring the required detachment to investigate a complaint thoroughly. It may be possible for a therapist to arrange with the relevant association for complaints to be channelled through that organisation or for a colleague to be prepared to act as an independent investigator or intermediary.

NHS COMPLAINTS

The Wilson report recommended that the principles shown in Box 12.3 should be incorporated into an NHS complaints system. The areas covered by its recommendations are shown below. The new procedures came into operation on 1 April 1996.

Recommendations of the Wilson report

1. There should be a common system for all NHS complaints.
2. The complaints procedure should not be concerned with disciplining staff.
3. Staff should be empowered to deal with complaints informally.
4. There should be training of staff.
5. Support should be provided for complainants and respondents.
6. The degree of investigation should relate to the complainant's required degree of response.
7. Conciliation should be made more widely available.
8. Time limits should be set.
9. Deadlines should be set for:

   - acknowledging complaints (2 working days)
   - the response to the complaint (three weeks)
   - further action and response (two weeks).

10. Confidentiality should be preserved and complaints filed separately.
11. There should be a system for recording and monitoring.
12. Impartial lay people should take part in the system.
13. Key aspects of the system should be set by the Department of Health but detailed implementation and operation should be left to individual organisations.
14. Three fold procedures:

   - stage 1 immediate first line response
   - stage 2 investigation/ conciliation
   - stage 3 action by chief executive officer.

A panel should be set up to consider those complaints which cannot be resolved in the earlier stages.

15. There should be training in communication skills.
16. Oral and written complaints should receive the same sensitive treatment.
17. Community service staff should have particular training in responding to complaints.
18. Purchasers should specify complaints requirements in their contracts with non-NHS providers.
19. Complaints about policy decisions should be referred to the Health Service Commissioner (HSC) if they cannot be resolved locally by the purchasers.
20. Where more than one organisation is involved it should be the organisation which receives the complaint which makes sure that a full response is sent.
21. Community care: there should be close liaison with local authorities and the government should consider further integration of NHS and local authority complaints procedures.
22. Stage 2 procedures: there should be a screening officer.
23. The jurisdiction of the HSC should be extended to GPs and the operation of the service committees.
24. Recommendations on implementation.

The new complaints procedure emphasises the importance of resolving the complaint at local level. If this fails, the complainant has the right to apply to the non-executive director of the trust or board who acts as the complaints convenor. The director determines whether there are grounds for the complaint to proceed to the independent panel. This is made up of lay persons, with medical assessors if appropriate, who can examine the complaint further. Should the complainant still be dissatisfied, the complainant can apply to the Health Service Commissioner.

The Health Service Commissioner is the final stage in the NHS Complaints system and the jurisdiction has been extended following the Wilson Report recommendations and now includes the right to consider complaints relating to clinical judgment, formerly excluded from the range, and also the right to investigate complaints against family practitioners as well as the health authority administering those services.

Whilst the Health Service Commissioner is the final stage in the complaints procedure for the NHS, it would be possible to seek a judicial review of the decision or investigation of this office if it were felt that the principles of natural justice were not followed. Judicial review would also be available to a complainant who considered that other stages of the complaints system had been operated without following the principles of natural justice.

LOCAL AUTHORITY SOCIAL SERVICES COMPLAINTS

Complementary therapy services may be provided as part of social service provision. In this case, clients, if they are not satisfied with the services provided, would have the right to utilise the statutory complaints procedure which must be established by each local social services authority.

The first stage in requiring action or remedial action to be taken is a representation and/or complaint to the relevant authorities; the National Health Service and Community Care Act 1990 makes an important feature of the right to make representations about social service provision.

Under the 1990 Act section 50 added section 7B to the Local Authority Social Services Act 1970, which enables the Secretary of State to require the local authority to set up a procedure to hear representations and complaints. As a result of directions issued under this section, each local authority is now required to establish a procedure to hear representations and complaints from persons entitled to receive services. The operation of the procedures must also be monitored. Policy guidance has been issued in *Caring for People: Community Care in the next decade and beyond*, pages 59–72.[2]

The guidance defines the essential requirements of a complaints procedure and these are shown in Box 12.5.

Box 12.5   Requirements of a complaints procedure

1. The designation of an officer to co-ordinate the consideration of complaints.
2. The key stages to be identified together with staff responsibilities.
3. Members and staff of the authority to be familiar with the arrangements, responsibilities and key stages.
4. Every registered complaint should be considered and responded to within 28 days of receipt and, if that is not possible an explanation should be given with a full response within 3 months.
5. They respond to the complainant and advise on further options for the complainant.
6. The review panel meets within 28 days of the complainant's request.
7. The review panel's decision to be recorded within 24 hours of the completion of their deliberations and sent formally to the authority, the complainant and anybody acting on his behalf.
8. The authority should decide on its action on the review recommendation within 28 days of the receipt of the recommendation with appropriate notification to specified persons.
9. They should keep a record of all complaints received and the outcome in each case, and identify separately those cases where the time limits imposed by the directions have been breached.

The guidance requires that the final stage in the hearing of complaints and representations should be before an independent person/panel. If the procedure operates effectively it is likely to reduce the extent of litigation before the courts over assessments and the provision of services.

PRIVATE PRACTICE COMPLAINTS PROCEDURES

Many complementary therapists working on their own or in association with other similar professionals in a consortium might find that the guidance for general practitioners provided by the Department of Health[3] could be usefully followed in their own practice. The criteria recommended for practice based complaints are shown in Box 12.6.

Box 12.6   Criteria for practice based complaints

The procedure should be owned by the practice.
One person should be nominated to administer the procedure.
The procedure must be publicised and written information should be made available.
Complaints should be acknowledged in two working days.
An explanation should normally be provided within ten working days.

The procedures should be simple and easy to understand.

First response to a complaint

Many complaints which may be unfounded are dealt with so badly, that the handling of the complaint itself becomes a subject for complaint. It is essential therefore that the therapist is prepared to be as open and receptive as possible in responding to the complaint; prepared to make changes and investigate the client's concerns. It is also essential that, where the complaint is of a clinical nature, action should be taken to ensure that medical or other advice is obtained for the client to prevent any deterioration of the client's condition. Thus any alleged pain, allergy, or other adverse condition following the treatment should be investigated vigorously and an appropriate referral made for the client.

Obtaining the use of an independent person

It is essential that clients should be able to approach an independent intermediary since they may find that it is difficult to discuss matters directly with the person against whom they have a complaint. Therapists could therefore negotiate through their professional association or with colleagues in a similar profession for an independent person to be appointed to discuss the complaint with the complainant and to investigate it. Obviously an independent person could not be brought into the handling of the complaint without the consent of the client, because of any problems about confidentiality.

Complaints on behalf of the client

It may be that a person other than the client makes the complaint on the client's behalf. Thus a parent may complain about how a child has been treated or a daughter may complain about the service provided for her elderly mother.

Where the complainant is complaining on behalf of a person over 16 years it is essential to obtain the written agreement of the client to the complaint being handled by that other person. It could be, for example, that information of a confidential nature becomes relevant during the investigation of the complaint and to disclose that information to a relative without the consent of the client could be a breach of confidentiality.

Time limits

For complaints brought about NHS and LA services there is a six month time limit during which it is expected that they would be raised. However it might be unwise for a private therapist to insist upon such a time limit being applied. It may be that the complaint could be the subject of legal action, where there would be much more generous time limits (e.g. a three year time limit in cases of negligence leading to personal injury or death from the date of knowledge that harm has been caused as a result of a negligent act (see Chapter 3)). It would not be in the interests of therapists to refuse to investigate a complaint about their practice if the outcome was a civil action being brought.

Use of a leaflet

A simple leaflet explaining how any client could complain and the procedure to be followed could be made available in a waiting area. This could include the topics shown in Box 12.7.

Box 12.7   Topics for a therapist's leaflet

- Aim and Philosophy of the therapist
- Practice complaints procedure
- How to make suggestions for improvement
- What action then takes place
- Complaining on behalf of someone else
- What happens if you are dissatisfied
- Useful addresses

Records

It is essential that the therapist keeps very full records of any complaint which is made and how it is handled. Any correspondence with the complainant should also be retained, until such time that it is clear that the complaint has been completely resolved (see Chapter 14 on record keeping).

Handling complaints and preventing litigation

It is essential that a therapist deals comprehensively and effectively with any complaint, since sympathetic handling involving an independent person might result in possible litigation being avoided. In addition the possibility of using alternative dispute resolution mechanisms should be borne in mind.

Mediation

This form of alternative dispute mechanism is growing in importance and is now being introduced as a legal requirement in matrimonial disputes. In appropriate situations, it may resolve a complaint speedily, cheaply and completely. The other advantage of mediation as opposed to other dispute resolution mechanisms is that both parties have to agree to the outcome. No party can be compelled to accept a solution. The result is that both parties are more likely to be satisfied with the outcome. Principles which could apply in a mediation and could be agreed by the parties at the outset are shown in Box 12.8.

Box 12.8   Principles for mediation

The aim of mediation is to secure an agreement between the parties and the following principles will assist in achieving this objective.
   Principles to be accepted:
   1. Both parties will conduct themselves with courtesy and civility to the other.
   2. Submissions will be made briefly and to the point.
   3. Every effort will be geared to resolving the impasse.
   4. The mediator will not 'rule' or make any attempt at arbitration but will attempt to effect a resolution between the parties.
   5. Either party can request an adjournment at any time and this will be granted.
   6. Either party can at any time request to speak to the mediator alone.
   7. Either party can at any time withdraw from the mediation.
   8. Either party can at any time, bring to the attention of the mediator any point which is not acceptable to it or raise any issue with the mediator over the manner in which the mediation is conducted.
   9. Any further rules can be requested by either party and will be considered by the mediator.
   10. Each party will recognise the duty to keep confidential any information disclosed on that basis during the mediation hearing.

SITUATIONS WITH LEGAL SIGNIFICANCE
Disgruntled client

Situation 1   Disgruntled client

A client visits a reflexologist and later complains to a colleague of the reflexologist that she was dissatisfied with the care provided. What action can be taken?

Gossip rumour and disgruntled clients can harm a practice and there would therefore be advantages in the reflexologist attempting to make contact with the client to attempt to resolve this complaint. The complaint may not amount to a legal claim, but it could result in significant harm to the practice if it is not successfully settled.

Complaints on behalf of a relative

Situation 2   Complaints on behalf of a relative
A son complains about the treatment of his elderly father. When the therapist spoke to the father he said that he did not wish to upset any one and showed no interest in pursuing the complaint himself.

It is always essential where complaints are made on behalf of others for therapists to clarify whether the client himself wishes to proceed with the complaint, since there is a danger that confidential information could be disclosed to the relative, without the consent of the client. This consent to proceed should be requested in a sensitive way so that a further complaint does not arise. Even if the complaint does not proceed there would still be value in therapists examining their practice to ensure that any improvements could be made.

Sexual harrassment

Situation 3   Sexual harassment
A client complains to the GP that an aromatherapist employed by the GP was guilty of sexual assault.

Genders issues are a problem for therapists who practise on their own and therefore where a therapist is confronted with caring for the opposite sex then it is essential that the client is informed as to what would be required, e.g. in terms of undressing, so that the client's consent is obtained. Where therapists practise entirely on their own it may not be possible to obtain a chaperone. Any doubts about the situation may be resolved by refusing to accept a client for treatment and recommending a colleague of the same gender to the client (see Chapter 13 on health and safety).

Dispute over fees

Situation 4   Dispute over fees
A client complains about paying the fees after having attended three sessions of hypnotherapy in order to give up smoking. He complained that he had believed that the therapy would have worked far quicker, and at the present time he was still smoking, plus buying patches and also paying for hypnotherapy.

Agreement at the beginning of the client/therapist relationship over the terms of treatment is essential. This is considered in Chapter 4. If a dispute does arise, it is preferable to resolve it through the use of the complaints system making use of an independent person or through mediation. This is likely to be far cheaper and faster than any court action. Sometimes, however, the therapist might consider that the grievance against the client is such that legal action should be taken to recover payment due. It should be remembered that there is little point pursuing a person, which will cost money, if that person would not have the resources to pay what is due.

CONCLUSION

The final stage in any effective complaint procedure is the monitoring and audit of the effectiveness of the procedure and the implementation of any recommendations following the review. Any complainants who remain disgruntled should be advised of any further action which is available to them. This may include the final stage of a statutory procedure, e.g. Health Service Commissioner, or it might be a court action. The possibility of using mediation to resolve outstanding issues should be considered since this could prove a cheaper and more satisfactory means of reaching an agreed outcome. In contrast with arbitration, mediation aims at reaching an actual agreement between the parties. The agreement is not imposed upon the parties by the mediator.

Questions and Exercises

1. Design a simple form to obtain feedback from clients, which gives an opportunity for both positive and negative comments to be made known to the therapist.
2. A complementary therapist who works for an NHS trust has been told that a patient has complained about her care. What procedure can she expect to be followed and what are her rights as a therapist under the procedure?
3. A patient complains to a therapist that she has suffered extreme pain since her last session. What action should the therapist take?

REFERENCES

1. Being Heard. The report of a review committee on NHS Complaints procedures May 1994 Department of Health
2. Policy guidance Caring for People: Community Care in the next decade and beyond p 59–72. HMSO 1990
3. Department of Health practice-based complaints procedures January 1996

13

Health and safety laws

INTRODUCTION

The complementary therapist must ensure that she observes the laws relating to health and safety. If she is an employer, then she will have specific duties as an employer both under the common law (judge made law) and also under statute. As a self-employed practitioner she will also have specific duties under health and safety legislation. If she practises in complementary therapy as an employee then there are both common law and statutory provisions which apply to her in that capacity. This chapter seeks to provide therapists with the legal framework relating to health and safety so that they can understand their responsibilities and duties in whichever context they practise. The topics to be included are shown in the Box above. It is impossible to cover each topic fully in a book like this, so a brief outline has been given of the basic principles and books for further reading are listed in the Bibliography.

STATUTORY PROVISION

Some of the Acts of Parliament which make provision for health and safety in the workplace or which could apply to the therapist working as an independent practitioner are enforced through criminal proceedings (see Chapter 5). Others can be the subject to action in the civil courts for compensation. The basic duties under the Health and Safety at Work etc. Act 1974 do not give rise to civil action for compensation, but breach of the regulations may do so. Thus if a person is injured through manual handling at work as a result of the employer's failure to implement the manual handling regulations, she could bring an action in the civil courts for compensation. The litigant could also rely on an action based on the employer's duty at common law (judge made law) to take reasonable care of the health and safety of employees (see below).

Most of the laws shown in the contents box are implemented through the criminal courts. In contrast the Occupier's Liability Acts 1957 and 1984 are both enforceable through actions being brought in the civil courts where compensation is payable if it can be shown that an occupier has failed to fulfil the duty of care owed to visitors on his premises (the 1957 Act) or to trespassers (the 1984 Act) (see Chapter 15).

HEALTH AND SAFETY AT WORK ETC. ACT 1974

The Health and Safety at Work etc. Act 1974 is enforced through the criminal courts by the health and safety inspectorate who have the power to prosecute for offences under the Act and the regulations and who have also powers of inspection and can issue enforcement or prohibition notices. Since the abolition of the Crown's immunity in relation to the health and safety laws (by the National Health Service Amendment Act 1986), prosecutions and notices can be brought against the health authorities. Trusts do not enjoy any immunity from health and safety legislation, nor do general practitioners. Social services departments can also be prosecuted under health and safety legislation.

Some protection is given to employers who employ only a small number of employees. In addition, where a duty has to be carried out so far as is reasonably practicable, in assessing the reasonableness of the actions of the employer regard would be had to the size and turnover of the organisation: it may be expected that the employer of a large concern should carry out a particular form of protection, but this may be quite unreasonable for the small employer. This difference does not apply when the duty is absolute e.g. the duty to provide a general statement of health and safety policy applies whatever the size of the workforce.

The basic duty on the employer is set out in Box 13.1.

Box 13.1   Duty under the Health and Safety at Work etc. Act 1974

Section 2(1) It shall be the duty of every employer to ensure, so far as is reasonably practicable, the health, safety and welfare at work of all his employees.

Section 2(2) of the 1974 Act gives examples of the various duties which must be carried out but these do not detract from the width and comprehensiveness of the general duty.

The Act also places a specific responsibility upon the employee. This is shown in Box 13.2.

> **Box 13.2** Statutory duty of the employee under section 7 of the Health and Safety at Work etc. Act 1974
>
> (a) to take reasonable care for the health and safety of himself and of other persons who may be affected by his acts or omissions at work; and
> (b) as regards any duty or requirements imposed on his employer or any other person ... to co-operate with him so far as is necessary to enable that duty or requirement to be performed or complied with.

It is also a criminal offence for an employee to interfere with health and safety measures (Box 13.3).

> **Box 13.3** Health and Safety at Work etc. Act 1984, section 8
>
> No person shall intentionally or recklessly interfere with or misuse anything provided in the interest of health, safety or welfare in pursuance of any relevant statutory provisions.

New regulations came into force on 1 January 1993 as a result of European Directives. These are shown in Box 13.4.

> **Box 13.4** Health and Safety Regulations which came into force on 1 January 1993
>
> 1. Management of Health and Safety at Work Regulations 1992 (SI 1992 2051)
> 2. Provision and Use of Work Equipment Regulations 1992 (SI 1992 2932)
> 3. Manual Handling Operations Regulations 1992 (SI 1992 2793)
> 4. Workplace (health, safety and welfare) Regulations 1992 (SI 1992 3004)
> 5. Personal Protective Equipment at Work Regulations 1992 (SI 1992 2966)
> 6. Health and Safety (Display Screen Equipment) Regulations 1992 (SI 1992 2792)

THE MANAGEMENT OF HEALTH AND SAFETY AT WORK REGULATIONS 1992

These make rules relating to the assessment of risk in the work place. The basic principles are valuable across a wide range of activities. A Code of Practice has been approved in conjunction with these regulations.[1] This Code does not have legal force but the preface states:

Although failure to comply with any provision of this Code is not in itself an offence, that failure may be taken by a Court in criminal proceedings as proof that a person has contravened the regulation or sections of the 1974 Act to which the provision relates. In such a case, however, it will be open to that person to satisfy a Court that he or she has complied with the regulation or section in some other way.

Risk assessment

Regulation 3 on risk assessment is set out in Box 13.5.

Box 13.5   Regulation 3

This requires every employer to make a suitable and sufficient assessment of —
(a) the risks to the health and safety of his employees to which they are exposed whilst they are at work; and
(b) the risks to the health and safety of persons not in his employment arising out of or in connection with the conduct by him of his undertaking,
for the purpose of identifying the measures he needs to take to comply with the requirements and prohibitions imposed upon him by or under the relevant statutory provisions.

The duty also applies to those in private practice and is shown in Box 13.6.

Box 13.6   Risk assessment in private practice

Regulation 3 paragraph (2) requires
every self-employed person to make a suitable and sufficient assessment of —
(a) the risks to his own health and safety to which he is exposed whilst he is at work; and
(b) the risks to the health and safety of persons not in his employment arising out of or in connection with the conduct by him of his undertaking,
for the purposes of identifying the measures he needs to take to comply with the requirements and prohibitions imposed upon him by or under the relevant statutory provisions.

There is a duty under regulation 3(3) to review the assessment when there is reason to suspect that it is no longer valid or there has been significant change in the matters to which it relates.

Where more than five people are employed there must be a record of the findings of the assessment; and any group of employees identified as being especially at risk.

The Guidance, which is not the law but of assistance in interpreting the legal duties, emphasises that risk assessment must be a systematic general examination of work activity with a recording of significant findings rather than a de facto activity.

The definition of risk includes both the likelihood that harm will occur and its severity. The aim of risk assessment is to guide the judgment of the employer or self-employed person, as to the measures they ought to take to fulfil their statutory obligations laid down under the Health and Safety at Work etc. Act 1974 and its regulations.

'Suitable and sufficient' is defined in the Guidance as being able to —

• 'identify the significant risks arising out of work.'
• 'enable the employer or the self-employed person to identify and prioritise the measures that need to be taken to comply with the relevant statutory provisions'
• and as being 'appropriate to the nature of the work and such that it remains valid for a reasonable period of time'.

How is the risk assessment to be carried out?

Box 13.7 gives the requirements of a valid risk assessment set out in paragraph 16 of the Guidance.

Box 13.7   Requirements of valid risk assessment

(a) to ensure that all relevant risks or hazards are addressed:
   (i) the aim is to identify the significant risks. Do not obscure those risks with an excess of information or by concentrating on trivial risks;
   (ii) in most cases, first identify the hazards, i.e. those aspects of work (e.g. substances or equipment used, work processes or work organisation) which could cause harm;
   (iii) if there are specific Acts or Regulations to be complied with, these may help to identify the hazards;
   (iv) assess the risks from the identified hazards; if there are no hazards there are no risks;
   (v) be systematic in looking at hazards and risks;
   (vi) ensure all aspects of the work activity are reviewed.
(b) address what actually happens in the workplace or during the work activity;
   (i) actual practice may differ from the works manual;
   (ii) think about the non-routine operations
   (iii) interruptions to the work activity are a frequent cause of accidents.
(c) ensure that all groups of employees and others who might be affected are considered;
(d) identify groups of workers who might be particularly at risk (e.g. young or inexperienced workers, those who work alone, any disabled staff);
(e) take account of existing preventive or precautionary measures.

It may be possible for several employers or independent practitioners engaged in the same activity to share model risk assessments. Thus guidance on the implementation of risk assessment could be provided by the organisations of individual complementary therapies.

Recording

The record should represent an effective statement of hazards and risks which then leads management to take the relevant actions to protect health and safety. It should be in writing unless in computerised form and should be easily retrievable. It should include:

- the significant hazards
- the existing control measures in place
- the persons who may be affected by those risks.

Preventive and protective measures

The basic principles of risk management are set out in Box 13.8.

Box 13.8 Basic principles of risk management

1. Identify the risk
2. If possible avoid the risk altogether
3. Combat risks at source rather than by palliative measures
4. Whenever possible, adapt work to the individual
5. Take advantage of technological and technical progress
6. Risk prevention measures need to form part of a coherent policy and approach having the effect of progressively reducing those risks that cannot be prevented or avoided altogether.
7. Give priority to those measures which protect the whole workplace and all those who work there, and so yield the greatest benefit.
8. Workers, whether employees or self-employed, need to understand what they need to do.
9. The avoidance, prevention and reduction of risk at work needs to be an accepted part of the approach and attitudes at all levels of the organisation and to apply to all its activities, i.e. the existence of an active health and safety culture affecting the organisation as a whole needs to be assured.

Risk management and the complementary therapist

For the most part, the complementary therapist would share common health and safety hazards with other hospital community or social services based employees and thus models of risk assessment and management which applied to other health professionals would also apply to complementary therapy. Thus hazards relating to the safety of equipment, to cross-infection risks, to safe working practices or to violence at work would all apply to complementary therapists who should be involved in the system of the assessment of risk.

Each complementary therapist should therefore be able to carry out a risk assessment of health and safety hazards in relation to both colleagues, clients, carers and the general public.

MANUAL HANDLING REGULATIONS

Back injuries have been recognised as a major reason for sickness and staff retiring early on grounds of ill health. Whilst there are no reported cases of claims brought by complementary therapists, they are vulnerable to the possibility of back injury because of the work which they undertake in the movement of clients and the lifting of equipment. It is essential therefore that they should have a good understanding of the regulations relating to manual handling and the employer's duties and their own. Often manual handling is undertaken as part of therapeutic practice. This is still included within the regulations, since the definition of manual handling includes all movement or supporting of loads including persons.

Guidance

Guidance on the Regulations is provided by the Health and Safety Executive.[2] The guidelines are not themselves the law and the booklet advises that the guidelines set out in Appendix 1 should not be regarded as precise recommendations. They should be applied with caution. Where doubt remains a more detailed assessment should be made.

A working group set up by the Health and Safety Commission has also produced a booklet on *Guidance on Manual Handling of Loads in the Health Services.*[3] This document is described as

an authoritative document which will be used by health and safety inspectors in describing reliable and fully acceptable methods of achieving health and safety in the workplace. Part of this health services specific guidance material relates to staff working in the community.

The two guides are thorough and informative and provide invaluable guidance for any complementary therapist who works with disabled patients or whose work otherwise encompasses manoeuvering heavy loads.

Content of the regulations

The duty under the regulations can be summed up as follows:

1. If possible avoid the hazardous manual handling.
2. Make a suitable and sufficient assessment of any hazardous manual handling which cannot be avoided.
3. Reduce the risk of injury from this handling so far as is reasonably practicable.
4. Give general indications of risk and precise information on the weight of each load; and on the heaviest side of any load, where the centre of gravity is not positioned centrally.
5. Review the assessment.

Avoiding the risk The Guidance asks the question, as an example of this, 'Can a treatment be brought to a patient rather than taking the patient to the treatment?' It may be that in the case of some complementary therapies it would be very difficult to remove the risk of injury entirely without reducing patient choice to unacceptable levels.

Carrying out the assessment Appendix 2 of the Regulations gives an example of an assessment checklist for management use: Section A covering the preliminary stages, Section B the more detailed assessment where necessary and Section C identifying the remedial action which should be taken.

Taking appropriate steps to reduce the risk For example in carrying out the assessment of risk and deciding how to minimise the risk, it might be concluded that it might be preferable to install hoists. This may include the possibility of installing a hoist for a domiciliary confinement, even though temporarily.

Giving general and specific information Where manual handling cannot be avoided appropriate steps have to be taken to provide employees with precise information on:

- the weight of each load
- the heaviest side of any load whose centre of gravity is not positioned centrally.

Review Regulation 4(2) requires the employer to review the assessment as circumstances change and it is in the interests of all complementary therapists who are not self-employed to ensure that their employer is reminded when a review becomes necessary under the above provisions.

Who is covered by the provisions

The duty which is owed by the employer is owed not only to employees but also to temporary or part-time staff such as a complementary therapist called in by GPs to provide a weekly session. All such employees are entitled to be included in the risk assessment process since, as has been seen, the assessment must take into account the individual characteristics of each employee. Complementary therapists who are unusually small in height or not so strong as the average might require special provision in relation to manual handling.

Enforcement

What action can be taken if the employer ignores these regulations? The regulations are part of the health and safety provisions which form part of the criminal law. Infringement of the regulations can lead to prosecution by the health and safety inspectorate. The inspectorate has the power to issue enforcement or prohibition notices against any corporate body or individual. A health authority no longer enjoys the immunity from the criminal sanctions which it once did as a crown authority and therefore these enforcement provisions are available against it. Similarly an NHS trust is subject to the full force of the criminal law.

Protection of employees who report health and safety hazards

Additional protection has been given by Section 100 Employment Rights Act 1996 against dismissal or victimisation in health and safety cases. Employees must follow the correct procedure using safety committees and safety representatives where they exist.

What remedies exist for compensation?

Section 47 of the Health and Safety at Work etc. Act 1974 prevents breach of a duty under sections 2 to 8 of the Act being used as the basis for a claim in the civil courts. Breach of the regulations can however be the basis of a civil claim for compensation unless the regulations provide to the contrary. Even where what is alleged is a breach of the basic duties, a therapist who suffered harm as a result of the failure of the employer to take reasonable steps to safeguard her health and safety could sue in the civil courts on the basis of the employer's duty at common law (see below). The statutory duty to ensure the Act is implemented is paralleled by a common law duty placed upon the employer to take reasonable steps to ensure the employee's health and safety.

Contracts of employment should state clearly the duty upon the employer to take reasonable care of the employee's safety and also the employee's duty to co-operate with the employer in carrying out health and safety duties under the Act and at common law. It is of course in the long term interest of the employer to prevent back injuries thereby avoiding payment of substantial compensation to his injured employees and also reducing the incidence of sickness and absenteeism.

Training

This is essential to ensure that staff have the understanding to carry out the assessments and to advise on lifting and the appropriate equipment. Regular monitoring should take place to ensure that the training is effective and the policies for review are in place. There is also a duty on the employer to ensure that staff who are not expected to be regularly involved in manual handling are aware of the risks of so doing. A therapist working in the NHS should make sure that she gets training of this type.

An example of the need for training is a recent case where a social worker succeeded in her claim[4] against the County Council.

Case 1   Insufficient training

She was employed as a social worker in the elderly care team. Her duties consisted largely of assessing clients for residential placement and other needs. She was called out to an elderly man's home after referral from his GP. When she arrived she gained access with a neighbour, only to find the man halfway out of his bed. He was in a very distressed state and she felt it was important for him to be lifted back into the bed as she was worried about him being injured. The neighbour, who had some nursing experience, told the social worker how to lift the man. As both of them attempted to lift the man, who weighed around 15 stone, the social worker sustained a lumber spine injury.

She sued on the grounds that the employers had failed to provide her with any training and/or instruction in lifting techniques. The employers denied liability on the ground that it was not a normal part of a social worker's duties to undertake any lifting tasks. The employers alleged that she should have summoned some assistance from the emergency services.

The judge held that it was reasonably foreseeable that the plaintiff would be confronted with emergency situations when working as a social worker in the elderly care team. Although the situation which arose was most unusual, the employers were under a duty to warn her that she should not lift in such circumstances. This duty did not go so far as to impose upon the employer in these circumstances a duty to provide a long training course but certainly to bring to the notice of social workers the risks of lifting. Her claim succeeded without a finding of contributory negligence. The issue as to quantum (i.e. how much compensation) was adjourned.

The implication of this decision is that even staff who are not expected to be involved in manual handling as part of their work, must be trained in risk awareness to protect them should they ever be in the situation where they could be endangered through manual handling.

Instructing others

Therapists may be asked to instruct others such as carers, clients or other health or social service employees, in the carrying out of the regulations in manual handling. Before they instruct others they should be sure that they get the necessary additional training to undertake the task of instruction, since failure to instruct competently could in itself give rise to an action in negligence if harm should occur as a result of negligent instructions.

Complementary therapists in private practice

Independent complementary therapists are not employees and, as self-employed persons, would be responsible for carrying out the assessments and taking the necessary precautions for themselves and any staff whom they employ. Where they work alongside employed health professionals they should ensure that the NHS trust takes into account hazards to their health and safety, and that the agreement which they have with the NHS trust reflects this duty. It is advisable that self-employed therapists have personal accident insurance cover, since if they are injured during their work they would not be able to claim compensation from an employer.

Manual handling in therapy

There are no grounds for assuming that the manual handling regulations do not apply if a person is involved in the movement, lifting, supporting, pushing, pulling etc. another person as part of therapeutic care. Thus if a therapist undertaking acupressure assisted the client onto the couch or lifted the body as part of the treatment, that is covered by the definition of manual handling in the regulations. It is therefore essential that the therapist carries out the four stage assessment:

- avoid the manual handling if reasonably practicable;
- carry out a sufficient and suitable assessment of any manual handling which cannot be avoided;
- reduce the risk of harm arising from that manual handling so far as is reasonably practicable; and then
- revise the assessment whenever a significant change of circumstances arises.

RIDDOR 1995

The Reporting of Injuries, Diseases and Dangerous Occurrences Regulations 1995 were introduced in their original form in 1985 governing the reporting of injuries, diseases and dangerous occurrences. The new regulations, which came into force on 1 April 1996, are now one set of regulations in place of the four sets under the 1985 regulations. The list of reportable diseases has been updated as has the list of dangerous occurrences. It is also legally possible for reports to be made by telephone.[5]

The health and safety legislation and the regulations under it are enforced by the health and safety inspectors employed by the Health and Safety Executive which reports to the Health and Safety Commission. Extensive powers are available for the inspectors to investigate any incident and to ensure that reasonable standards of health and safety protection are in place.

CONSUMER PROTECTION ACT 1987

This Act was enacted as a result of the European Community Directive No 85/374/EEC. It enables a claim to be brought where harm has occurred as a result of a defect in a product. It is a form of strict liability in that negligence or fault by the supplier or manufacturer does not have to be established. The plaintiff will however have to show that there was a defect. The existence of the defect would be judged against what was known at the time. The parts of the Act are set out in Box 13.9.

Box 13.9   Consumer Protection Act 1987 – Part headings

  I Product liability
 II Consumer safety
III Misleading price indications
IV Enforcement provisions
 V Miscellaneous and supplementary

Part I on product liability covers the sections shown in Box 13.10.

Box 13.10   Consumer Protection Act 1987 – product liability

1. Purpose and construction of Part I
2. Liability for defective products
3. Meaning of defect
4. Defences
5. Damage giving rise to liability
6. Application of certain enactments
7. Prohibition on exclusions from liability
8. Power to modify Part I
9. Applications of Part I to the Crown

The Consumer Protection Act 1987 enables a claim to be brought where harm has occurred as a result of a defect in a product. It is a form of strict liability in that negligence by the supplier or manufacturer does not have to be established. The plaintiff will however have to show that there was a defect. The supplier can rely upon a defence colloquially known as 'state of the art' i.e. that the state of scientific and technical knowledge at the time the goods were supplied was not such that the producer of products of that kind might be expected to have discovered the defect.

A product is defined as meaning any goods and includes a product which is comprised in another product, whether by virtue of being a component part or raw material or otherwise.

Who is liable?

The producer   Section 2(1) states that

where any damage is caused wholly or partly by a defect in a product, every person to whom section (2) below applies shall be liable for the damage.

Section 2(2) includes the following as being liable:

- The producer of the product
- Any person who by putting his name on the product or using a trade mark or other distinguishing mark, has held himself out to be the producer of the product
- Any person who has imported the product into the EEC in the course of business.

The supplier In addition to the persons set out under section 2(2) section 2(3) provides that the person ('the supplier') who has supplied the product to the person who suffered the damage, can be liable if:

(a) the person who suffered the damage asks the supplier to identify the producer(s) (as set out above);
(b) that request is made within a reasonable period after the damage occurs and at a time when it is not reasonably practicable for the person making the request to identify all those persons; and
(c) the supplier fails, within a reasonable period after receiving the request, either to comply with the request or to identify the person who supplied the product to him.

This provision makes it essential for therapists to keep records of the suppliers of any goods (including both equipment and drugs) which they provide for or use on their clients. In the absence of their being able to cite the name and address of the supplier or producer, they may become the supplier of the goods for the purposes of the Act and therefore have to defend any action alleging that there was a defect in the goods which caused harm. Harm includes personal injury and death and also loss or damage to property.

Where a social services authority or health service body supplies equipment for use in the community then that body can become the supplier for the purposes of the Consumer Protection Act. If harm results from a defect in the equipment the appropriate supplier must provide the client with the name and address of the firm from which the equipment was obtained otherwise it will become itself liable for the defects. Records of the sources of all equipment are therefore essential in order that the client can be given this information.

What is meant by a defect?

Section 3 provides that

There is a defect in a product for the purposes of Part I of the Act, if the safety of the product is not such as persons generally are entitled to expect; and for those purposes, 'safety', in relation to a product, shall include safety with respect to products comprised in that product and safety in the context of risks of damage to property, as well as in the context of risks of death or personal injury.

The phrase 'what persons generally are entitled to expect' is further defined (section 3(2)) as taking into account all the circumstances, including:

(a) the manner in which, and purposes for which, the product has been marketed, its get-up, the use of any mark in relation to the product and any instructions for, or warnings with respect to, doing or refraining from doing anything with or in relation to the product;

(b) what might reasonably be expected to be done with or in relation to the product; and
(c) the time when the product was supplied by its producer to another.

Defences

Certain defences are available under section 4 and are shown in Box 13.11.

Box 13.11   Consumer Protection Act 1987, section 4

(a) that the defect is attributable to compliance with any requirement imposed by or under any enactment or with any Community obligation; or
(b) that the person proceeded against did not at any time supply the product to another; or
(c) that the following conditions are satisfied, i.e.:
    (i)   that the only supply of the product to another by the person proceeded against was otherwise than in the course of a business of that person's; and
    (ii) that section 2(2) above does not apply to that person or applies to him by virtue only of things done otherwise than with a view to profit; or
(d) that the defect did not exist in the product at the relevant time; or
(e) that the state of scientific and technical knowledge at the relevant time was not such that a producer of products of the same description as the product in question might be expected to have discovered the defect if it had existed in his products while they were under his control; or
(f) that the defect
    (i)   constituted a defect in a product (the subsequent product) in which the product in question had been comprised; and
    (ii) was wholly attributable to the design of the subsequent product or to compliance by the producer of the product in question with instructions given by the producer.

What damage must the plaintiff establish?

Compensation is payable for death, personal injury or any loss of or damage to any property (including land) (section 5(1)). The loss or damage shall be regarded as having occurred at the earliest time at which a person with an interest in the property had knowledge of the material facts about the loss or damage (section 5(5)). Knowledge is further defined in section 5(6) and (7).

There have been few examples of actions being brought under the Consumer Protection Act 1987 in health care cases and only a handful of cases brought under it have been reported.

Case 2   Defective scissors[6]

In March 1993 Simon Garratt was awarded £1400 against the manufacturers of a pair of surgical scissors which broke during an operation on his knee, with the blade being left embedded. A second operation was required to remove it.

Had Simon Garratt relied on the law of negligence (see Chapter 3) he would have to show that the manufacturers were at fault in their manufacture of the scissors and were in breach of the duty of care which they owed to him. Under the Consumer Protection Act 1987 all he had to show was the harm, the defect and the fact that it was in something produced by the defendant.

In a report by the National Consumer Council[7] in November 1995 it is recommended that consumers should be assisted in using their rights under this Act. Amongst other recommendations they suggest that the Department of Trade and Industry should review its collection of home accident statistics to alert those responsible to dangerous products on the market; that the Act should be amended so compensation can be claimed for damage costing less than £275 caused by unsafe goods; and that the Act should further be altered to reverse the burden of proof and to amend the development risk defence.

CONTROL OF SUBSTANCES HAZARDOUS TO HEALTH REGULATIONS 1988

Responsibilities are placed upon those who handle substances which are potentially dangerous under these regulations relating to the Control of Substances Hazardous to Health (COSHH). Therapists who use different substances in their work should be specifically alert to the need to ensure that the regulations are implemented. The five stages set out in the guide issued by the Health and Safety Executive[8] are shown in Box 13.12.

Box 13.12   Stages in COSHH assessment

1. Gather information about the substances, the work and the working practices
2. Evaluate the risks to health
3. Decide what needs to be done
4. Record the assessment
5. Review the assessment

Where the therapist works on NHS premises or with others in, for example, a health centre, there must be clarity over who has the responsibility of carrying out the assessment, but the guidance emphasises the importance of involving all employees in the assessment.

All potentially hazardous substances must be identified: these will include domestic materials such as bleach, toilet cleaner, window cleaner and polishes; office materials such as correction fluids as well as the more obvious medicinal products in the treatment room and materials and substances used in therapy.

- An assessment has to be made as to whether each substance could be inhaled, swallowed, absorbed or introduced through the skin, or injected into the body (with needles).
- The effects of each route of entry or contact and the potential harm must then be identified.
- There must then be an identification of the persons who could be exposed and how.

Once this assessment is complete, decisions must be made on the necessary measures to be taken to comply with the regulations and who should undertake the different tasks. In certain cases, health surveillance is required if there is a reasonable likelihood that the disease or ill-effect associated with exposure will occur in the workplace concerned. Therapists should be particularly vigilant about any substances used in their activities such as oils in aromatherapy, paraffin and oils in art therapy and cleaning fluids. They must ensure that a risk assessment is undertaken and its results implemented.

Managers should also ensure that the employees are given information, instruction and training. Records should show what the results are of the assessment, what action has been taken and by whom, and regular monitoring and review of the situation.

DUTY IMPLIED IN EMPLOYMENT CONTRACT

In addition to the statutory enactments, there are decided cases which have set precedents (as described in Chapter 2) which lay down principles which apply in relation to the duties of the employer and employee. These common law duties are for the most part parallel to the duties set down in Act of Parliament but as will be seen they sometimes go far beyond the statutory duties. Some of the duties derive from common law principles relating to the contents of the contract of employment (see Chapters 4 and 7).

Some terms in the contract of employment are implied by common (judge made) law. These include an obligation on the part of the employer to safeguard the health and safety of the employee by:

- employing competent staff
- setting up a safe system of work and
- maintaining safe premises, equipment and plant.

The employee on the other hand must obey the reasonable instructions of the employer and take reasonable care in carrying out the work. Thus as has been seen in the discussion on manual handling above, the employee may have a claim for breach of contract by the employer if her back has been injured as a result of failures by the employer's part in not providing the appropriate training or equipment, but equally she may have her compensation reduced if she contributed to the accident by not taking reasonable care.

Failure by the employer to take reasonable care of the health, safety or welfare of the employee could result in the following actions by the employee:

1. Action for breach of contract of employment.
2. Action for negligence, where the employee has suffered harm. The employee could use as evidence breach of specific health and safety regulations.
3. Application in the industrial tribunal for constructive dismissal, if it can be shown that the situation was so extreme that the employer was in fundamental breach of the contract of employment and the employee was justified in leaving.

Examples of cases brought in relation to the employer's duty of care at common law are the manual handling case above and the stress case below.

SPECIAL AREAS

Violence

Unfortunately there are more and more reports of attacks on health service and other professional employees and practitioners, not just from strangers in the streets but also from carers and even clients. The rules relating to the terms of service of general practitioners have recently been changed to enable them to arrange for the removal from their list of any patient who threatens them with violence. In a case in 1983,[9] a voluntary patient at a mental hospital, was charged with assault occasioning actual bodily harm to an occupational therapist employed at the hospital. An occupational therapist has also been killed by a mentally ill patient in the Edith Morgan Unit at Torbay. An inquiry was set up following this death.[10]

Where the practitioner is an employee working within the NHS or private sector, the employer has a duty to take reasonable care of the employee in relation to reasonably foreseeable violence. A risk assessment (see above) would therefore be required of this possibility and as a result any reasonable means to protect the employee should be adopted. Where practitioners are self-employed, working on their own, special precautions may be necessary to protect health and safety. Many complementary therapists work on their own, often from a consulting room in their own home. They should take special precautions before inviting strangers for treatment to their home. The following questions should be answered:

Is it possible to remove the risk altogether? If the answer to this is 'yes, but …', for example, 'only by stopping all visits to the practitioner's home', this may not be reasonably practicable. However if the situation is serious the practitioner may have to consider ceasing to work from home, and work instead in a centre with other practitioners and some minimum security.

What preventive action or protective measures can be taken? The answer to this might include the provision of two-way radios, personal alarms or, in very dangerous areas, ensuring that there is help immediately available. An important point in receiving a new client is to obtain as much information as possible from any referral agency.

Is the situation changing – for better or worse? Review the situation to ascertain if the nature of the risk has changed (e.g. is the district more violent than it was formerly assessed to be? Has the nature and condition of clients deteriorated?) and the extent of the success of the measures taken to prevent harm in the past. Are any further measures necessary?

This type of risk analysis can relate not only to the violence but could be part of a wider assessment of all risks which are reasonably foreseeable.

Where practitioners work as employees or employ persons themselves then they should ensure regular monitoring of potentially violent situations. The Health and Safety Commission published in 1997 guidance on assessment and management of violence and aggression to staff in the health services. This provides practical and constructive advice.

Stress

Concern with stress at work is now recognised as part of the employer's duty in taking reasonable care of the health and safety of the employee.

Case 3   Stress at work[11]

A social worker in charge of a team dealing with child abuse obtained compensation when his employers failed to provide the necessary support in a stressful work situation when he returned to work following an earlier absence due to stress.

The employers were not liable for the initial absence, but that put the employers on notice that the employee was vulnerable and their failure thereafter to provide the assistance he needed was a breach of their duty to provide reasonable care for his health and safety as required under the contract of employment.

Many therapists will be involved in providing care for their clients because the latter are suffering from stress related illnesses. The therapists should not ignore the fact that they, and also any employees they may have, are also vulnerable to stress, and they should take appropriate action to identify this as part of a wider risk assessment.

Sexual harassment

It is essential that complementary therapists are sensitive to the dangers of sexual harassment and make every effort to avoid potentially difficult situations. On the one hand they must be aware of the Sex Discrimination laws (see Chapter 7) and must ensure that they do not discriminate either directly or indirectly. On the other hand they must ensure that they are chaperoned in any situation which could lead to accusations of harassment by the client or by the therapist against the client. Planning in advance for potentially hazardous situations is essential. For example does the treatment session involve the removal of clothes? If so, written information could be given in advance to potential clients, advising them of this fact, and suggesting that, if they wish to, they could bring a friend or colleague with them.

CONCLUSIONS

A risk management strategy is at the heart of any policy relating to health and safety, not just for employees but also for the clients and general public. Regular monitoring of the implementation of a risk management policy should ensure that harm is avoided and that a quality service is maintained for the public. This should be accompanied by clear, comprehensive documentation.

Questions and Exercises

1. Undertake a health and safety risk assessment of your premises. To what extent are there any hazards and how could they be reduced?
2. To what extent are you or your staff or colleagues involved in manual handling in relation to the care of the client? Are there any other areas of your working life, where the manual handling regulations are relevant?
3. What system do you have for recording untoward incidents. How are these monitored and remedied?

REFERENCES

1. Health and Safety Commission 1993 Management of health and safety at work approved code of practice. HMSO, London
2. Health and Safety Executive 1992 Manual handling guidance on regulations. HMSO, London
3. Health and Safety Commission 1992 Guidance on manual handling of loads in the Health Services. HMSO, London
4. Colclough v. Staffordshire Country Council Current Law No 208 October 1994
5. Enquiries can be made to Health and Safety Executive Information Centre, Sheffield. Tel 0114 2892345; Fax 0114 2892333
6. Dimond BC 1993 Protecting the consumer. Nursing Standard 7 No (24): 18–19
7. National Consumer Council 1995 Unsafe products: how the Consumer Protection Act works for consumers. London National Consumer Council
8. Health and Safety Executive 1993 A step by step guide to COSHH assessment. HMSO, London
9. R v. Lincolnshire (Kesteven) Justices, ex parte Connor [1983] 1 All ER 901 QBD
10. Blom-Cooper L, Hally H, Murphy E 1995 The falling shadow – One patient's mental health care 1978–1993. London (Report of an Inquiry into the death of an Occupational therapist at Edith Morgan Unit, Torbay 1995) Duckworth
11. Walker v. Northumberland County Council QBD Times Law Report 24 November 1994

Records, reports and evidence

Complementary therapists, particularly those in private practice, will find they have to keep a multitude of records. Some of the more obvious ones are shown in Box 14.1. This chapter will however concentrate upon the principles to be followed in client record keeping and the use to which these records may be put. The chapter will also cover issues which arise in relation to record keeping within a multi-disciplinary team setting, since some therapists work as employees within general practice or in secondary care.

Box 14.1   Records kept by complementary therapists

1. Client treatment: notes, correspondence, referrals, outcomes.
2. Income tax and therefore
    - income: invoices, fees received, unearned income.
    - expenditure: rent, electricity, gas, rates, postage, equipment, car expenses (petrol, service charges, road tax).
3. VAT (if appropriate): details as above.
4. Property: correspondence, deeds, lease, mortgage, rent etc.
5. Insurance: professional indemnity insurance, buildings and contents, car, personal accident.
6. Professional association: papers, supervision records, links with other professionals.
7. Car documents: insurance, MOT, road tax etc.
8. Financial documents: mortgage, life insurance, loans, savings etc.

CLIENT RECORDS

The principle purposes of record keeping in respect of client treatment are to ensure the quality of care provided for the client, to facilitate communication between professionals and to maintain a record of the diagnosis, treatment and future plans for the client. A good standard for documentation would be that if any therapist were to be called away in an emergency, her colleagues would be able to provide continuity of care on the basis of full comprehensive clear records.

If high standards of record keeping are maintained, then, should a report be required, should litigation commence, a prosecution be initiated or a complaint be made, therapists would be able to protect themselves on the basis of the comprehensive clear records which have been kept.

STANDARDS TO BE FOLLOWED

Professional duty to the client, includes the responsibility of keeping records of the care and treatment provided. If this duty is properly fulfilled then therapists will be better able to defend their practice should any litigation or other court proceedings arise.

What information should be recorded?

This is a most difficult question for therapists and there may be a reluctance by some therapists to record any confidential client information. (The special problems for psychotherapists are considered in Chapter 35 which covers the specific legal issues which arise in that area.) Some therapists may find it possible to have only basic client information: name, address and date of attendance, but most therapists would wish to have a record of the information listed in Box 14.2.

Box 14.2   Client information to be recorded

1. Name
2. Address
3. Date of birth
4. Marital status and children
5. General practitioner name and address
6. Source and date of referral
7. Personal health history including known allergies and contraindications
8. Reason for consultation
9. Treatment plan (see Box 14.4)
10. Records of each consultation: date, treatment and outcome
11. Client agreement to the contract

Some of the basic principles relating to recording client treatment are shown in Box 14.3. These are taken from the NHS Training Directorate booklet *Just for the Record*.[1]

Box 14.3 Principles of clinical record keeping
Documents related to the central care plan should: 1. Assess and identify a patient's or client's problems/needs 2. Plan the expected outcome and the treatment/interventions/care required to achieve it 3. Put the planned treatment/interventions/care into practice 4. Evaluate the actual outcome with the expected outcomes, changing care or treatment where required

Guidelines for recording

Box 14.4 sets out some of the basic points to follow in writing the actual records.

Box 14.4 Principles to follow in record keeping
1. Records should be made as soon as possible after the events which are recorded 2. They should be accurate, comprehensive and clear 3. They should be written legibly and be jargon-free 4. They should avoid opinion and record simply the facts of what is observed 5. They should be signed by the maker 6. They should not include abbreviations 7. They should not be altered, unless the changes are made so that the original entry is clearly crossed out, but still readable 8. Any alterations should be signed and dated

Reference should be made to the publications of the NHS Training Authority on standards for record keeping.[2] The UKCC guidelines *Standards for Records and Record Keeping*[3] is also of value to all health professionals, including complementary therapists.

Changing records

Records should not be altered. If the writer discovers that the wrong information was recorded, a line should be put through that information, it should be initialled and then the correct information written down. Any attempt to cover what was previously written by tippex or heavy blocking out will arouse suspicion. What was erroneously recorded should still be legible.

Case 1 Changing the notes of a sick baby
It was reported in the *Times* in 1995[4] that a casualty nurse who told the parents of a sick baby that he probably had a sniffle and that they should take him to the family doctor, altered the notes when the baby died one hour later. She changed the words 'extremely pale' to 'quite pale', and added a pulse reading, although she had not taken his pulse.

Even though an independent inquiry found that her actions probably had no bearing on the child's outcome, she faced internal disciplinary proceedings and was dismissed.

Computerised record keeping

Many therapists may have personal computers and put their client information and records straight onto their computer. The points shown in Box 14.5 should be noted.

Box 14.5   Computerised records

1. Exactly the same principles in terms of content apply as to manually held records
2. Information should always be backed up on floppy discs
3. Floppy discs should be kept in secure conditions separately from the main system
4. Data Protection Act Provisions of registration, and use of the information should be followed (see Chapter 10)

THE OWNERSHIP AND SECURITY OF RECORDS

NHS records are owned by the Secretary of State and responsibility is delegated to the statutory health authorities. This also applies to the NHS records kept by general practitioners as part of their terms of service. Under the arrangements since April 1996 the health authorities are responsible for arranging the transfer of the records to a new general practitioner where patients have indicated their wish to transfer and for collecting the records from a general practitioner when a patient has died. General practitioners have a duty under their terms of service to keep appropriate records of patients and to return these to the health authority when the patient dies or is transferred to another GP.

For NHS trusts and health authorities the ultimate decision on disclosure to others rests with the chief executive officer of the health authority or NHS trust. Thus statutes such as the Data Protection Act 1984 and Access to Health Records Act 1990 give to the holder of the records the ultimate decision making on whether access should be permitted. The holder should, however, consult the health professional who cared for the patient (see Chapter 10). Where the therapist works for a private hospital then ownership of the records would be subject to agreement between the private hospital and the therapist.

Records relating to private practice are owned by the therapist who made them. It can be agreed between the therapist and the client before assessment and treatment commences as to what access is to be arranged and whether there should be client-held records. The agreement could also transfer ownership to the client. Since complementary therapists do not come under the definition of health professional for the purposes of the Access to Health Records Act and Data Protection Act (apart from osteopaths and chiropractors following the relevant legislation (see Chapters 22 and 33)), the client does not have a statutory right of access. However it would be seen as good professional practice for therapists to be as open as possible with clients and enable them to access any records on an informal basis. The therapist should bear in mind that if records are to be seen by the client then any jargon or illegible script would have to be deciphered (see Chapter 10).

All records whether kept in manual or computerised form should be kept securely. A therapist could be sued if a breach of confidentiality arose as a result of failure in ensuring that client records were kept secure (see Chapter 10). The Audit Commission in its report on hospital records[5] considered that patients were being put at risk because their medical records are kept in a mess and sometimes lost. Failure to find records led to consultations being cancelled and to operations being postponed. It recommended that hospitals set up one main records library with good security. Hopefully standards of record keeping are higher in the private practice of individual therapists.

Where records are in computerised form failure to ensure that personal information is kept secure could lead to prosecution under the Data Protection Act. Unauthorised access to the computer should be prevented. Dangers of keeping records in the car or at home are obvious; not so obvious, however, is negligent practice in having records around a consulting room where they could be seen by others. Any persons employed by the therapist must also recognise the duty of confidentiality and the importance of keeping records secure.

TIMES FOR STORAGE

Where litigation is a possibility, it would be extremely unwise ever to destroy records until the case is finally disposed of or the time passed when it could be begun. From Chapter 3 it can be seen that cases can be brought many years after the incident which is the subject of the dispute took place. In the case of those under a mental disability no time limit on bringing an action for negligence exists and records should be kept until the person dies. Where a child has suffered harm, the time limit of three years does not commence until the child becomes an adult at 18 years.

In addition the judge has a discretion to extend the statutory time limits in actions for personal injury, taking into account the extent to which one party would be prejudiced by the extension.

In potential actions for breach of contract records need to be kept for at least six years as that is the time limit within which an action for breach of contract can be brought.

Therapists in private practice have to make their own decision on the extent to which records should be kept. There are the considerations relating to likely litigation, and other factors such as space, cost and workload will also influence the decision. Where the therapist is working within the NHS then their records will be covered by the policy of that hospital; where the therapist is working in a private hospital or nursing home then keeping the records will be subject to the agreement between the hospital or home and the therapist.

Where the records are so old as to amount to historical documents then the Public Records Act 1958 comes into play and legal advice should be taken on circumstances in which these must be held.

DESTRUCTION OF RECORDS

Even though any critical time limits have been passed, most therapists would prefer to transpose records onto microfilm rather than destroy them completely. However this is expensive and time consuming and might not always be justifiable. Whatever the individual therapist's policy, it is essential to ensure that the storage is secure so that there is no unauthorised access to the records. When destruction is undertaken this should be done with confidentiality in mind, any documents being burned or shredded or disposed of through a specialist contractor.

LEGAL STATUS AND EVIDENTIAL VALUE

It will be apparent from Chapter 3 on negligence and the discussion on the times within which an action can be brought that, since cases can take many years before a hearing takes place, it is inevitable that there must be considerable reliance upon documentation rather than on memory. Therapists can be compelled to disclose their records even though they are not personally involved in the litigation (see Chapter 10 on confidentiality). It must be emphasised, however, that records are essentially hearsay evidence. It does not follow that what is contained in any record is necessarily accurate or true. It is possible for a completely fictitious account to be recorded. In determining the weight to be attached to the records and to determine their evidential value, the judge would listen to the makers of the record being cross-examined and, in the light of those answers, determine how much value can be placed upon what the records say.

It may sometimes be asked, when does a document become a legal record? The answer is that any evidence which is relevant to an issue arising before the court can be subpoenaed. (The only exception is information protected by legal professional privilege and by the public interest, such as national security – see Chapter 10.) Thus not only client records but correspondence, bus tickets, odd jottings on scrap paper may all be relevant depending on the issues arising in a case.

CLIENT HELD RECORDS AND CLIENT FRIENDLY RECORDS

Many different professionals are increasingly allowing clients to hold their own records. There are considerable advantages in complementary therapy practice if clients are encouraged to keep their own records and become responsible and involved in their progress.

There are some fears associated with the client acting as custodian of the records. However the fears that records could be lost if the therapist ceases to be in control of their care could lead to the setting up of a second system of record keeping at a central point. The dangers of this dual system are that neither might be complete and there might not be consistency in what is recorded in each place.

There is also a fear that if records in the custody of the client go missing and litigation is commenced, then professionals will be at a disadvantage in defending themselves. The burden is, however, on the person bringing the case (i.e. the patient as plaintiff) to establish negligence, and this may be difficult to do if the documentation is missing and it is the plaintiff who is responsible for that loss.

The NHS training authority has given guidance on 'patient friendly' records.[6]

Audit of record keeping

Since high standards of record keeping are so important both to client care and also to the protection of the therapist against any complaint, litigation or professional conduct hearing, good practice should ensure that at regular intervals the therapist carries out a simple audit on the record keeping to ensure that high standards are maintained.

The audit should cover the areas shown in Box 14.6.

Box 14.6   Audit of record keeping

1. Content of records
2. Clarity of records: legibility and also meaning
3. Security and controlled access
4. Robustness in covering all aspects of client care and providing good protection in the event of legal action
5. Has follow up action been clearly set out?

REPORTS AND STATEMENTS

Complementary therapists may be asked to appear as expert witnesses in litigation or prepare a report for litigation or other purposes. Expert witnesses will normally be asked to prepare a report by a solicitor representing one of the parties to the case. This report is vital since, if it is unfavourable to the party seeking it, the outcome may be that the case is settled or even withdrawn.

Principles of report writing

Box 14.7 illustrates some of the principles to be followed in report writing.

Box 14.7   Principles to be followed in report writing

1. Identify the purpose of the report, likely readership and the kind of language which can be used; and therefore the appropriate style to be used.
2. Identify the main areas to be included.
3. Decide the order to be followed: sometimes chronological order is appropriate, at other times subject order may be preferable.
4. Sign and date it but only after reading it through and being 100% satisfied with it.
5. Identify the different kinds of information used in the report and state the source of the material e.g.
   • hearsay evidence
   • factual evidence observed or heard by the author of the report
   • evidence of opinion of another person
   • statements by others
   • similar fact evidence.

Common errors

Typical mistakes in report writing are:

Lack of clarity
Failure to follow a logical order
Inconsistency
Ambiguities
Lack of signature and/or date
Lack of dates within the report
Wrong names included
Confusing account
Mix of evidence and sources
Inaccuracies
Opinion without facts
Failure to cite facts to support statements
Too complex a style for reader
Use of inappropriate jargon
Use of misleading abbreviations
Failure to give conclusions
Failure to base conclusions on the evidence
Failure to have it checked through by someone else

Style

For most purposes the style likely to be of greatest use is one of simplicity, with short sentences, clear paragraphing and sub-paragraphing, and avoiding jargon and meaningless clichés. The report should begin with the statement as to its purpose, the person(s) to whom it is addressed, and the name and status of the writer. Other documents which are relevant should be carefully referenced.

Statement writing

Witnesses can refer to any contemporaneous records and statements in giving evidence and therefore since it takes many years for some court hearings to take place, it is vital that comprehensive clear records have been kept and statements made. If therapists are asked to prepare a statement they should ensure that they obtain advice from a senior colleague and, if possible, a lawyer. Many NHS trusts now have solicitors who would provide assistance in the making of any statement. The statement should be made with reference to the records which they have kept.

GIVING EVIDENCE IN COURT

At present there are very few reported cases involving complementary therapists. However there is considerable increase in the number of NHS cases in which patients are seeking compensation for harm and this trend may spread as the practice of complementary therapy becomes more popular. In addition many therapists are developing their role in giving expert evidence in court. This section covers both aspects and also looks at some of the rules of evidence and the terminology which is likely to be encountered. The following topics will be covered:

- Witness of fact
- Expert witness
- Procedure
- Rules of evidence

Witness of fact

Any one who can give evidence on a matter relevant to an issue before the court can be summoned to appear. The only grounds for refusing to attend and give evidence is if the evidence is protected by legal professional privilege against disclosure in court or if, on grounds of national security or other public interest, a minister of state has signed a public interest immunity certificate that the information should not be disclosed. (Legal professional privilege is considered in Chapter 10 on confidentiality.)

As witnesses of fact therapists may be required to give direct evidence over matters with which they have been involved. They should ensure that they keep to the facts and do not offer any opinion. In some cases they may be asked to pronounce upon the prognosis of the client: they should not magnify the extent of any disability and a poor prognosis in order to obtain more compensation for the client. Therapists have to ensure that their professional standards are maintained and they tell the client and if necessary the court honestly the nature of the prognosis as they see it. They may need guidance and training in how to withstand cross-examination. It is vital that they do not express views outside their competence. Thus whichever party calls them as witness, they should not alter the facts or emphasis to support that party but should give their evidence according to professional standards of integrity.

Key points for witness of fact

Preparation

1. Ensure that the records are available, identify with stickers significant entries, but do not mark or staple or pin anything to the records. Read them through so that you are familiar with them.

2. Try to obtain assistance from a lawyer or senior manager in preparation for the court hearing, so that you are prepared for giving evidence in chief and answering questions under cross-examination.

3. Try to visit the court in advance to familiarise yourself with its location, car-parking, toilet facilities etc.

At the court before the hearing

1. Be prepared for a long wait and take work to do or something to occupy yourself with.

2. Dress appropriately and comfortably but not too casually.
3. Try to relax.

Giving evidence

1. Keep calm.
2. Give answers clearly and without exaggeration.
3. Tell the truth.
4. Do not feel that you are there to represent only one side; you must answer the questions honestly even though it might put the side cross-examining you in a good light.
5. Take time over your answers and do not make up replies if you are unable to answer the question raised.
6. Do not answer back or allow yourself to be flustered during the cross-examination.
7. If you do not understand any legal jargon which is used, ask for an explanation.
8. Keep to the facts and do not express an opinion.
9. Ask for time to refer to the records if this is necessary.

Expert witness

An expert witness can be invited to give evidence of opinion on any issue which is subject to dispute. It might be on what would be the appropriate standards of care which would have been expected according to the Bolam test (see Chapter 3); it may be an opinion on the prognosis of the patient where the amount of compensation is disputed.

Expert witnesses should not change their views according to the side which calls them. They may be asked to edit their report to make it more favourable to the side asking for their opinion. They should only agree to any amendments if they are satisfied that the changed report accurately represents their opinion and they are able to support it by oral evidence in court.

One essential rule for therapists to follow is to give an honest reasoned opinion whichever side call them. They must not be partisan, nor should they exaggerate or belittle the amount of compensation due. If they always give an honest and professional view, they will be respected by the solicitors who will know that they will be able to trust them to withstand cross-examination as an expert witness and will know them to be reliable. They personally will not see the court battle as involving them and thus, whichever side wins, they will be able to feel that they have given an honest opinion. A carefully prepared report, well substantiated, can reduce the length of a court hearing and enable many matters to be agreed by the parties, thus avoiding court time.

Duty of expert witness to the court

In the case shown below (Ignorant expert) the court held that the expert witness had a responsibility to approach the task of giving evidence seriously and an expert should not be surprised if the court expressed strong disapproval if that was not done.

Case 2 Ignorant expert[7]

An expert in his report had stated that 'as far as I am aware no other previous seal manufacturer had used such a system'. In fact it became apparent not only that that system was used by others in the trade but that the witness neither knew what coding systems were used by such others nor had made any effort to find out.

The lesson from this is that an expert must not express an opinion unless it is clearly based on fact and where possible on established authorities or research. A further lesson is that the experts should know and keep within their field of competence.

Points which as an expert witness you should remember are:

1. Do not take sides.
2. Outline your professional credentials (status, experience, appointments and academic qualifications).
3. Give a professional, not personal opinion.
4. Understand on what issues and topics you have expertise.
5. Provide a logical report (see above).
6. Always support opinion with fact.
7. Avoid confusing, technical language and jargon.
8. Avoid being verbose.
9. Give concrete understandable examples and use everyday analogies.
10. Keep facts and opinions relevant to the issues before the court.
11. Ensure that you understand the purpose of the proceedings.
12. Date and sign the report.

Dos and Don'ts of the expert witness

As expert witness you should follow these guidelines:

1. Find out where the court is and turn up.
2. Make sure that the case has not been adjourned before travelling.
3. Do not stand on your dignity.
4. Be acquainted with court procedure and the role of the judge, jury and counsel.
5. Know how to address the judge and others.
6. Dress appropriately.
7. Do not get emotional and forget what to say.
8. Know your report and the facts contained in it.
9. Do not deviate from the report or introduce new material.
10. Believe what you have written and what you are saying.
11. Be dispassionate about the outcome.
12. Do not take an adversarial stance.
13. Prepare for cross-examination.
14. Remain calm under cross-examination.
15. Do not exaggerate.

16. Keep to the facts.
17. Do not try to be humorous.
18. Do not try to hasten the case along.

Conflicting evidence

What is the situation if there is a clash between evidence given by expert witnesses, who both purport to speak on behalf of a body of competent professional opinion? This was the situation which arose in the *Maynard* case[8] which is mentioned in Chapter 3. The House of Lords held that where the sides were supported by equally competent professional opinion, then the plaintiff had not established its case.

Cross-examination

This is the term applied to the opportunity of the one side (A) to question the witnesses called by the other side (B) (and *vice versa*). There are two distinct objectives in cross-examination. The one is to discredit the witness or show that their evidence is irrelevant to the point being established. The other is to use this witness to strengthen the case of one's own party.

Discrediting the witness In pursuing the first aim, the barrister or solicitor conducting the cross-examination will attempt to:

- undermine the confidence of the witness
- show up inconsistencies, ambiguities and anomalies in their evidence
- show how the evidence being given is contradicted by other witnesses
- show how the witness is unreliable and unintelligent.

Strengthening one's own case In pursuing the second aim, the cross-examiner will attempt to ensure that the witness (for side A) gives evidence helpful to side (B), praises side (B), corroborates evidence being given by side (B). The witness may also be used to testify on professional/expert matters and may be brought to express opinions useful to the other side.

Preparation and a genuine belief in the opinions expressed in your report are essential for cross-examination.

Rules of evidence

This is a complex area and the rules depend upon the nature of the court hearing.
    Some of the issues which are covered by the rules include:

- rules on relevance and admissibility and hearsay
- weight of evidence
- burden of proof
- degrees (standard) of proof
- presumptions
- judicial notice

- competence of witness
- compellability of witness
- corroboration
- doctrine of privilege (see Chapter 10).

It is not possible in a work of this kind to give full details of the significance of the rules of evidence on the above topics and reference must be made to one of the specialist books listed in the appendix on further reading.

The future

Lord Woolf has published a report on access to civil justice.[9] This is discussed in Chapter 10. One of the consultation papers relates to the use of expert evidence. Lord Woolf considered that the uncontrolled adversarial nature of the present system of civil litigation was the main cause of excessive cost, delay and complexity. He therefore recommended a new system in which the courts would have an active role in case management, including control over the use of expert evidence. He recommended a 'fast track' for cases below £10 000 where experts would normally be jointly appointed by the parties and would not be required to give oral evidence in court. Cases above £10 000 would be allocated to a multi-track, in which the court would have wide powers to define the scope of expert evidence and prescribe the way in which experts should be used in particular cases. His proposals include the following:

- Appointment of court experts and expert assessors
- A clearer role for experts and guidance which emphasises their independence and their duty to the courts
- Appropriate choice and use of experts
- Better arrangements for expert evidence at trial.

At the time of writing the present government's intention on the implementation of the Woolf proposals are still awaited.

CONCLUSIONS

Some therapists may consider that with a single handed practice there is no necessity to keep either clinical records of clients or any correspondence relating to the client. However it must be accepted that as complementary therapy becomes more popular and more this inevitably leads to more complaints and litigation; therapists who fail to keep any records could find themselves in a vulnerable situation. The importance of maintaining high standards of record keeping may become more and more evident.

There are considerable fears about giving evidence in court and it is vital that any witness, whether expert or witness of fact, should be properly prepared for the occasion. Even though they are not on trial themselves, their professional standing and integrity is being put to the test and it is therefore essential, that they follow the highest standard of professional practice.

Questions and Exercises

1. With some colleagues carry out an audit of the standards of record keeping amongst yourselves. Imagine that you were having to answer questions on the records in ten years time.
2. What abbreviations do you consider could be usefully used in record keeping within your own particular sphere of complementary therapy? What steps would you take to ensure that there was no confusion arising from their use?
3. If you keep records on a personal computer, what particular legal requirements must you implement?
4. You have been asked to appear as a witness in a case. Draw up a list of your fears and try to work out ways in which these fears could be resolved.
5. Try to attend a court hearing and analyse the way in which it operates, the procedure followed and the actions of judge, jury (if present), barristers, solicitors, court clerk, court usher, witness, and any other person taking part in the court proceedings.
6. Prepare a protocol for the preparation of a report as an expert witness.

REFERENCES

1. NHS Training Directorate 1994 Just for the record: A guide to record keeping for health care professionals. Bristol NHS Training Directorate
2. NHS Training Directorate 1992 Keeping the record straight. Bristol NHS Training Directorate
3. United Kingdom Central Council 1993 Standards for Records and Record Keeping. UKCC, London
4. Wilkinson P Notes on dead baby altered by nurse. Times 7 November 1995
5. Audit Commission 1995 Setting the records straight: A Study of Hospital Medical Records. HMSO, London
6. NHS Training Directorate 1994 Just for the record: A guide to record keeping for health care professionals. Bristol NHS Training Directorate
7. Autospin (Oil Seals) Ltd v. Beehive spinning (A firm) Times Law Report 9 August 1995
8. Maynard v. West Midlands Regional Health Authority [1985] 1 All ER 635
9. Woolf Access to Civil Justice Inquiry Interim Report June 1995 and Consultation paper January 1996. Lord Chancellor's Office, London

Premises and the law

Many complementary therapists may use their own homes, whether they own or rent it, as their business premises, possibly in conjunction with the use of a room in a health centre or similar property. Others may rent premises for business use to conduct their practice. This chapter sets out the basic laws which apply to the use and occupation of premises and indicates further sources of information. The chapter will cover briefly the topics in the box above.

Box 15.1 shows the different forms of landholding.

Box 15.1   Different forms of landholding
Owner occupier: leasehold or freehold Tenant: domestic or business Licensee: with no security

USING DOMESTIC PREMISES

Restrictive covenants

Many therapists, particularly those who do not need to have substantial equipment or space, may choose to use their own homes for the purpose of their practice. Before they do so, they should ensure, if they are the freeholder, that there is no restrictive covenant which would prevent their property being used for business purposes. If so, it may be that their particular business would not be caught by the restrictive covenant. If the property is registered with the land registry (as most property now is) any restrictive covenant will be recorded as part of the registration. In unregistered property, the title deeds should indicate any covenants limiting the use of the property. Even when the property is described as being for residential purposes, there may be an exclusion for a doctor's surgery and this may be interpreted as including the use of premises for complementary therapy practice.

Should a restrictive covenant be in existence which restricts the use of the property to residential purposes, and the complementary therapist, regardless of this restriction uses the property for his or her professional practice, in theory those neighbours or other persons who are entitled to the benefit of this restrictive covenant could enforce this through the courts. However this is likely to be a costly and slow procedure and any disgruntled neighbour is more likely to apply to the local authority alleging breach of planning laws, claiming that there has been an unauthorised variation in the use of the land (see below).

Where the premises are a flat or maisonette, and therefore almost certainly owned under the terms of a long lease, it is very likely that there will be some covenants restricting the use that can be made of the premises. Details of these will be in the lease itself, a copy of which can be obtained from the Land Registry (if the property is registered) and which will also be with the title deeds. Neighbours will know of these covenants as they probably hold their property under leases which are almost identical and there may be provision for application to be made to the managing agents (who collect the rent and deal with the service charge) to deal initially with any dispute as to enforcement.

Where the therapist is not the owner of the property, but a tenant, then the landlord should be informed of the intended use of the property for business purposes, since the landlord may be aware of some reason preventing this use (see below).

Planning laws

The complementary therapist intending to use his or her own home for their practice should also make a check with the local authority to ensure that there are no planning permissions necessary to conduct a business in that particular area and also to check that there are no local by-laws which restrict the current use or the proposed use of the property. For some therapies it is necessary to obtain a licence from the local authority.

If planning permission for change of use is required an application for this can be made to the local authority. Notices will be posted up outside the premises and delivered to the occupiers of adjoining property to give such interested parties a chance to object. The local planning officer or a solicitor can advise on the procedures and the fees required.

LANDLORD AND TENANT

The law of landlord and tenant is complex and any therapist should obtain expert advice before entering into any agreement to rent property. The following discussion is simply a brief outline of the various arrangements which may be in place and an analysis of the different statutory provisions which apply.

Domestic premises

There may be an express restriction in the lease preventing the property being used for other than residential purposes. Where there is a restriction on the premises being used for residential purposes and the tenant decides to use the premises for the practice of complementary therapy, the landlord could claim that there is a breach of the terms of the agreement. In the absence of an express term in the agreement, and subject to planning requirements and similar restrictions, the tenant may use the premises for any purpose provided it is not illegal or immoral. However there is a danger that any statutory protection which the tenant enjoys through renting premises as a dwelling (particularly if the arrangement began before the late 1980s) could be lost because of the different use of the premises. Advice should therefore be obtained before the tenant risks security of tenure or breach of the tenancy agreement for using the premises for other than residential purposes.

Where premises are leased for business purposes

The main statutory provision covering the lease of premises for business purposes is the Landlord and Tenant Act 1954. This act gives the following protection to business tenants:

- It limits the ways in which a tenancy can come to an end
- It gives security of tenure to the tenant, unless the occupation ends in one of the ways specified in the Act
- It enables the business tenant to apply for a new tenancy at the end of his current tenancy
- The landlord can only oppose the granting of the new tenancy on one or more of the grounds specified in the Act
- Compensation may be payable to a tenant who has to leave.

This Act covers tenants occupying the property for business, professional or certain other purposes. The practice of complementary therapy would come within this definition, unless it was considered to be an interest or leisure activity, rather than a business or profession. The Act does not apply where premises are occupied by virtue of a licence (see below). It will apply however where there are two purposes for which the tenant is leasing the property, e.g. for a residential flat as well as a business, provided the business use is a significant purpose of the tenant's occupation of the premises. Thus where a doctor took a tenancy of a maisonette near his consulting rooms and very occasionally saw a patient there in emergencies, it was held that the 1954 Act did not apply to the tenancy.[1]

Mixed use of premises

Where the premises are used for business as well as residential purposes they come under the 1954 Act rather than the Rent Act 1977 or the Housing Act 1988.

Licence

The distinction between a lease of property and a licence to occupy property is significant in law, since many statutory provisions which protect tenants of residential property or tenants of premises used for business purposes do not apply to persons who only have a licence to use the property. The distinction between a lease and a licence was considered by the House of Lords in the case of *Street* v. *Mountford*,[2] where the existence of exclusive possession was seen as a major factor. If exclusive possession has not been granted then the occupier is not a tenant but a licensee.

However even where exclusive possession has been granted other factors may be evidence of an intention not to grant a tenancy but to grant a licence. For example, there may be simply a family arrangement, with no intention of creating legal relations. An example of a situation which the court held to be only a licence was that where a house was bought by a woman who allowed her brother to occupy it free of charge. She paid the rates. The brother lived there for more than 13 years but the Court of Appeal held that this was a family arrangement which negated any intention to create a lease and the brother was only a licensee.[3]

The implications for the complementary therapist are clear. If as a result of a family or social arrangement which is not intended to create any legal relationship the complementary therapist uses a room, perhaps incurs expense in decorating and other building work and establishes a substantial professional practice, the owner of the property may at any time end the licence, refusing to accept that the therapist has a lease. Thus the therapist has little statutory protection for his continued use of the premises.

It is therefore essential that, where he has no security of tenure the therapist established clearly the basis on which he is to occupy any premises before he commits himself to any significant expenditure.

Situation   No security of tenure

Rachel, a reflexologist approached a hotel and asked if she could have a room to undertake reflexology for hotel clients. This was agreed and she paid a weekly sum of £100 rent for the use of the room. Her business prospered and after three years she had established an excellent practice both amongst the hotel guests and also amongst persons living in the neighbourhood of the hotel. Totally unexpectedly, the hotel manager gave her two weeks notice to leave the hotel. (She subsequently heard that the niece of the hotel manager intended to commence a business as a reflexologist in the hotel.) Rachel is claiming compensation from the hotel, but has been told that she only had a licence which could be ended at any time.

In this situation it is essential that Rachel takes legal advice to ascertain whether her occupancy of the hotel room could be seen as coming within the Landlord and Tenant Act 1954 rather than as being simply a licence. Factors such as who cleaned the room and whether it was used outside the session times are relevant. The situation shows the importance of legal advice being obtained before premises are used, since much work in building up a practice could be lost if a licence to occupy was withdrawn without any compensation.

COMMUNITY CHARGE

Clearly the use of premises for business purposes will affect the rateable value used in the calculation of the community charge payments. Thus in a case before the land tribunal reported in 1996,[4] the judge noted that the premises were let during the season and one of two rooms on the top floor were used by the Colwyn Music Centre. The rate payer stated that he taught music there if requested to do so and also practised alternative medicine and sometimes saw patients at home, using either the dining room or the study for this purpose. The lands tribunal upheld the decision of the valuation officer that for specified periods the property should be classified on the non-domestic rating list.

LIABILITY FOR HARM ON PREMISES

A complementary therapist may be held liable for harm arising to persons who come onto premises in the occupation or ownership of the therapist. Alternatively the therapist may be injured whilst a visitor on premises in another person's occupation, e.g. if she visits a health centre or provides services to clients in their own homes. Both these situations are covered by the Occupiers' Liability Act 1957. Where injury is caused to a trespasser, then liability if governed by the Occupiers' Liability Act 1984.

The 1957 Act establishes the occupier's liability for harm caused to visitors who enter onto his property. The occupier is anyone who has control over the land and premises. It could therefore be an owner of the property, a tenant, a manager or any other person who could be deemed to have some responsibility for the property so that they could be classified as an occupier. There might in fact be several different occupiers who would be held accountable for different aspects of the safety of the premises.

For example a therapist might use a room in a centre run by different practitioners in complementary medicine. Each tenant may have responsibilities under the lease for internal decoration but the landlord and owner may have duties in relation to the structural repairs. In addition there might be contractors on site who are undertaking the internal decoration. They also could be regarded as occupiers for the purposes of the Occupiers' Liability Act 1957. If a client is injured on the premises she might have a claim against any of these depending upon the cause of her injuries. If she were injured by tripping on a threadbare carpet this would be the responsibility of the tenant, who rented and furnished that particular part of the premises; if the client were injured because of the carelessness of the painters in leaving an unsafe ladder in the hallway the contractors would be liable; if she were injured because the stone steps leading to the house were dangerous then it would probably be the responsibility of the landlord. In situations of multi-occupancy of premises it is essential for the responsibility for harm arising to visitors to be defined, and for the necessary insurance cover to be taken out.

In contrast where the therapist is owner occupier of the premises used for the professional practice, he or she will have full responsibility for ensuring that the premises are reasonably safe (see below).

Where the therapist visits a client in the client's home and is injured on the premises there may be difficulties in obtaining compensation for the injuries. The potential defendants (tenant, landlord, independent contractor) may not be able to pay any compensation which was due. Unless they had taken out insurance cover for such an eventuality the therapist might have an excellent case yet little chance of recovering compensation. There are considerable advantages in ensuring that she has her own personal insurance cover for such a risk, since in the absence of this she is unlikely to obtain compensation.

What has to be established under the Occupiers' Liability Act?

The visitor has to show that the person alleged to be the occupier is in breach of the common duty of care which is owed to all visitors. The definition of this is shown in Box 15.2.

Box 15.2   Occupiers' Liability Act 1957, section 2(2)

A duty to take such care as in all the circumstances of the case is reasonable to see that the visitor will be reasonably safe in using the premises for the purpose for which he is invited or permitted by the occupier to be there.

Who is a visitor?

The visitor is any one who is invited by the occupier to be on the premises or would be regarded as a licensee at common law. The latter will include those to whom the occupier has given express permission and also those to whom the occupier has given implied consent. Thus persons such as the milkman and paper boy would be regarded as visitors, but the occupier can of course bar such visitors by an express prohibition. Whether one is a visitor or not is important since the 1957 Act places a duty on the occupier only to the visitor. If a person does not come in this category then the person would be defined as a trespasser and a different duty applies, set out under the Occupiers' Liability Act 1984 which is discussed below. If a visitor refuses to leave, he may become a trespasser and again the different duty applies.

It is only if the visitor stays within the purposes for which he had been permitted to enter the premises that he receives the protection of the 1957 Act. If a client visiting a therapist in the consulting room of the downstairs of the house decided to have a look around the rest of the house and was injured she would probably not be protected by the Act unless she had a genuine reason such as needing to have access to a wash hand basin or toilet.

Notice of dangers

The occupier can obtain some protection from liability by giving notice of any dangers to the visitor. 'Careful when you go upstairs because the carpet on the third stair is frayed.' If this is sufficient for the visitor to be safe, yet in spite of the warning the visitor is injured because she takes inadequate care then the occupier would probably not be liable.

The exact wording of the section is shown in Box 15.3.

Box 15.3 Occupiers' Liability Act 1957, section 2
2(4) (a) In determining whether the occupier of premises has discharged the common duty of care to a visitor, regard is to be had to all the circumstances, so that (for example) where damage is caused to a visitor by a danger of which he had been warned by the occupier, the warning is not to be treated without more as absolving the occupier from liability, unless in all the circumstances it was enough to enable the visitor to be reasonably safe.

In addition an occupier cannot discharge himself of liability for his negligence by putting up a disclaimer notice of the type shown in Box 15.4.

Box 15.4 Typical exemption notice (This is invalid)
The owner accepts no responsibility for any liability for injury or loss or damage to property whilst using these premises.

The notice shown in Box 15.4 is invalid because the Unfair Contracts Terms Act 1977 prevents a person excluding or restricting his liability for negligence where death or personal injury occurs as a result of the negligence.

If the harm which occurs is loss or damage to property liability can be excluded provided it is reasonable so to do. The burden is upon the person seeking to rely upon the contract or notice to show this. Thus in the disclaimer notice shown in Box 15.4 the occupier could not exempt himself from liability for injuries caused by his negligence but the exemption from liability for property loss or damage might succeed (see Chapters 3 and 4).

Different categories of visitors

The occupier's duty varies according to the nature of the visitor: greater care would have to be taken for the safety of children and those who cannot take good care of themselves (e.g. those with learning disabilities). In addition an occupier can expect that any person who enters the premises because of his particular expertise (e.g. an electrician, plumber, sweep etc.) will appreciate and guard against any special risks which are ordinarily incident to it, so far as the occupier leaves him free to do so (section 2(3) (b)).

In the case below (An ambulanceman tripping) the Court of Appeal dismissed the appeal and held that though the lighting was dismal, the judge had found that the ambulancemen were able to see where they were going; they had shortly before the accident ascended the staircase and crossed the landing; they were trained to look for apparent hazards and the plaintiff's colleague had the ability to give a warning if he perceived a potential hazard. In the circumstances, therefore, it was impossible to say that the pile of books gave rise to a reasonably foreseeable risk of personal injury to the plaintiff. Consequently it was unnecessary to consider the application to the facts of section 2(3) (b) of the Occupiers' Liability Act 1957.

Case   An ambulanceman tripping[5]

The plaintiff, an ambulanceman, was in the defendant's house, in dismal lighting conditions, carrying a chair containing the first defendant, who was unconscious. The plaintiff's colleague, who was also carrying the chair, was walking forwards and the plaintiff was walking backwards. The plaintiff knocked over a pile of books onto a landing alongside a wall, trod and slipped on a book and sustained personal injuries. His claim for damages was dismissed by the judge and he appealed to the Court of Appeal, contending amongst other things that the judge had erroneously construed section 2(3) (b) of the Occupiers' Liability Act 1957 in concluding that the pile of books composed a special risk that the plaintiff in the exercise of his calling would appreciate and guard against.

Independent contractors

If the harm that arises has been caused by the negligence of contractors who have been brought onto the site, this will normally relieve the occupier of any liability. He must, however, have taken care in selecting them. (If he knows that they are dangerous and slipshod in their methods and as a result harm occurs, the occupier might still be liable.) In addition the occupier must have taken all steps, if any, that he reasonably should in order to satisfy himself that the contractor was competent and that the work had been properly done (section 2(4) (b)).

If painters leave out a ladder in a dangerous way which falls and injures a visitor then they may well be liable for that harm unless it could be established that the occupier is also at fault.

Shared premises

It is increasingly common for premises to be shared by different occupiers working in the field of health and social services and voluntary agencies. Thus health professionals employed by an NHS community trust might work from premises owned by a fundholding GP practice, which employs a complementary therapist; the community mental health team might work with social worker colleagues in premises owned by the social services and complementary therapists may provide services on the premises, either as an employee of one or other agency or as self-employed practitioners; the NHS trust might share its premises for community services provision with a variety of associated professionals, some employed by voluntary organisations others by GPs or by social services. Alternatively the complementary therapist may share premises with several other therapists as part of a complementary therapy practice.

If harm should occur in this multi-occupation who would be liable?

If there is an agreement between the parties over the sharing of premises this may clarify responsibility over liability for maintenance, structural repairs and furnishings and equipment. If personal injury occurs as a result of failure to fulfil these responsibilities, then that person/organisation would be liable. Unfortunately such responsibilities are not always defined and in this case it would be a question of determining liability on the basis of the person/organisation in control or whose fault caused the harm.

Liability for trespassers

As we have seen the Occupiers' Liability Act of 1957 is only concerned with the duty towards visitors. The Occupiers' Liability Act 1984 was passed to cover the position in relation to trespassers. The Act sets out the rules which determine whether a duty is owed to non-visitors in respect of any risk of their suffering injury on the premises by reason of any danger due to the state of the premises or to things done or omitted to be done on them. It also sets out the nature of the duty.

A duty only arises upon the occupier to those who would not be classified as visitors under the 1957 Act in the circumstances set out in Box 15.5.

Box 15.5   Occupiers' Liability Act 1984

A duty arises on the occupier of premises in respect of a danger on the premises if the occupier is —
(a) aware of the danger or has reasonable grounds to believe that it exists;
(b) he knows or has reasonable grounds to believe that the other is in the vicinity of the danger concerned or that he may come into the vicinity of the danger (in either case, whether the other has lawful authority for being in that vicinity or not); and
(c) the risk is one against which, in all the circumstances of the case, he may reasonably be expected to offer the other some protection.

The Act's primary purpose was to deal with those tragic circumstances where children had been attracted on to premises by dangerous equipment or activities and as a result were harmed. The issue was to determine what was reasonable in terms of the duty of occupiers in relation to such trespassing and also to provide some protection for such trespassers.

Once it has been determined that a duty arises the nature of the duty upon the occupier is set out in Box 15.6.

Box 15.6   Duty of occupier to trespasser, section 2(4)

S.2(4) The duty is to take such care as is reasonable in all the circumstances of the case to see that he does not suffer injury on the premises by reason of the danger concerned.

The occupier can discharge this duty by

taking such steps as are reasonable in all the circumstances of the case to give warning of the danger concerned or to discourage persons from incurring the risk. (section 2(5))

In addition no duty is owed to any person in respect of risks willingly accepted as his by that person (section 2(6)). No liability arises from this Act for loss or damage caused to property.

Application of the Occupier's Liability Act 1984

As managers of premises, the property of complementary therapists may afford certain attractions to trespassers. They may for example have certain equipment which would attract children and which is inherently dangerous. In such circumstances they would have a duty to take such care as is reasonable in all the circumstances of the case to see that the trespasser does not suffer injury on the premises by reason of the danger concerned. If there are fears of burglary, the use of glass on the top of walls or any man traps for the burglar would be unlawful under the Act.

Where the therapist is visiting a client in the client's own home, and is asked to leave, failure to leave when requested would mean that the therapist then becomes a trespasser. The occupier has the right at common law to use reasonable force to evict a trespasser.

The Defective Premises Act 1972

If harm is caused by defects in the structure of the premises and other matters for which the landlord is liable then the person who has been harmed could have a claim under the Defective Premises Act 1972. The Act is summarised in Box 15.7.

Box 15.7 The Defective Premises Act 1972

Section 1 sets a duty of care to any one who takes on the work of providing a dwelling: 'to see that the work which he takes on is done in a workmanlike, or, as the case may be, professional manner, with proper materials and so that as regards that work the dwelling will be fit for habitation when completed'.
Section 2 provides certain exemptions from section 1.
Section 3 states that the duty of care does not end when the premises are disposed of.
Section 4 defines the landlord's duty of care to premises rented out.
Section 5 applies the Act to the Crown
Section 6 gives definitions

INSURANCE COVER

To protect themselves against possible claims in respect of injuries on their premises it is essential that therapists who use their home for consulting purposes check with the insurance company providing cover for their home that the use of the home for therapy purposes does not invalidate the cover provided. In addition they should ensure that they are covered either by their home insurance policy or their professional indemnity insurance cover for injuries sustained by clients and other visitors on their home premises (see also Chapters 4 and 6.)

Questions and Exercises

1. You intend to use a spare room on the ground floor of your house for a treatment room for aromatherapy. You own the house. Do you have to obtain any permission to do this?
2. Since the landlord has discovered that you are using an annexe in your rented bungalow as a consulting room for hypnotherapy he has stated his intention to charge you more rent. How could you check on the validity of his claim?
3. A client slips on the path as she is leaving your house. The path is safe, but autumnal leaves were scattered over it. To what extent do you consider that you are liable for the injury your client has suffered?

REFERENCES

1. Royal Life Saving Society *v.* Page [1979] 1 WLR 1329
2. Street *v.* Mountford [1985] AC 809
3. Cobb *v.* Lane [1952] 1 All ER 1199
4. Hodkinson *v.* Humphreys-Jones (Valuation Officer) Lands Tribunal [1996] RA 69
5. Neame *v.* Johnson and another (1993) Personal Injuries Quarterly Review March p 100

Specific therapies and the law

SECTION CONTENTS

16

Acupuncture

DEFINITION

Acupuncture simply means needle insertion or piercing but it is based on a philosophy of health and healing.[1]

BACKGROUND

Brief history

It is at least 3000 years old and was practised in China. The philosophy which underpins its use is that the body, mind and spirit are seen as a dynamic self-healing whole, fuelled by energy, which flows through a network of invisible channels called meridians. There are 12 main meridians which correspond to the vital organs of the body, together with Governing and Conception Vessels. The meridians have been mapped and measured by modern technology and are the basis for treatment known as touch for health (applied kinesiology) and acupressure (shiatsu). Some practitioners of reflexology believe that the pressure points used in their therapy are the same as the acupuncture points.

The theory is that if these channels are blocked or weakened in any way, then illness can result. When the natural energies are in balance flowing through the body, then health results. The basic energies have been called the Yin and Yang. Yin is associated with qualities such as cold, rest, responsiveness, passivity, darkness, inferiority, downwardness, inwardness and nourishment. Yang is associated with heat, stimulation, movement, excitement, light, upwardness, outwardness and increase.[2] Five elements are also recognised: fire, earth, metal, water and wood. Each of the five elements governs a pair of meridians, one Yin and one Yang (except for Fire which has two pairs).

Acupuncture aims at placing fine needles into the skin to stimulate specific points to restore and maintain good health. The points are located along the meridians and 365 principal acupuncture points are recognised. Because it aims at restoring the self-healing properties of the body the initial discussion and diagnosis by the acupuncturist are an essential part of the therapy. Acupuncture should not, therefore, be seen simply as the relief of symptoms but rather the treatment of the whole person. Some practitioners in acupuncture may also use herbs and acupressure.

In 1979 the World Health Organisation recognised that acupuncture can be effective in treating over 40 diseases.[3]

Acupuncture has been used for the treatment of pain relief, chronic respiratory problems, neurological and musculoskeletal disorders, digestive disorder and chronic menstrual problems. It is also used in the treatment of mental and emotional disturbances and behavioural problems. In February 1996 the National Asthma Council reported research that acupuncture helps in the treatment of asthma. Thirteen of 16 studies into the value of acupuncture showed it to be effective by easing breathlessness and reducing the medication sufferers need. Kim Jobst, a trained acupuncturist who conducted the research stated that drugs and acupuncture combined were more effective than acupuncture alone.[4]

An example of the work of acupuncture and hypnosis to relieve pain in pregnancy is shown by Graham Arthurs[5] who describes past research where acupuncture has been used with effect in a variety of situations in pregnancy and its use for repositioning the fetus in breech position, stimulation of contractions and pain relief in labour, citing Beal (1992).[6] Arthurs concludes:

There is need for more research to be conducted in a controlled way to determine the effectiveness for acupuncture in society, stripped of any mystic and cultural effects.

Links with orthodox medicine

Like other complementary therapies, acupuncture is increasingly being practised by those who are already registered practitioners in other areas of health care. Thus in midwifery the advantages of using acupuncture alongside traditional professional practices of the midwife are shown by Sharon Yelland.[7] For the past six years, she and a colleague have offered acupuncture to over 2000 women at all stages of pregnancy at the Derriford Hospital in Plymouth. She describes the conditions during antenatal, labour and postnatal care and neo-natal care which can be treated by acupuncture (NB Similar conditions to those listed for treatment by homeopathy). She recounts several case studies where acupuncture was effective. Her conclusion is

Acupuncture is safe, cheap, and has no known teratogenic effects. Furthermore it gives greater autonomy to the midwife practitioner, as a midwife able to offer a complementary treatment can enhance her reputation and improve her holistic approach to care.

It was reported[8] that a project was set up in 1993 in a GP practice in Cirencester with funds from the local health authority. The initiative arose from the long waiting list for orthopaedic services in the district. Patients with specific problems – head, neck, and back pain were entered into the programme. If after the initial consultation with a GP (who offered advice, exercises and simple pain relief) the problem or pain persisted, these patients were clinically matched by their symptoms to receive either acupuncture, osteopathy or homeopathy from therapists working in the same surgery. Over 9 months, almost 1000 patients passed through the programme, with about 300 being referred for complementary therapists. More than 60% of those referred for acupuncture for head, neck or upper back pain reported a major improvement. Lumbar or chronic lower back problems were more difficult to treat with acupuncture because they are often caused by poor posture which is difficult to alter in the long term. One of the values of the project was in the cooperation and communication between the doctors and the complementary therapists. The effect of the project was not only the increased knowledge by the GPs of complementary therapy but a change in referral patterns. Early referral to acupuncture for recurrent migraine was one of the effects.

The British Medical Acupuncture Society has been established for doctors qualifying in acupuncture. Membership is restricted to doctors and its aim is to promote a holistic approach within orthodox medicine. In 1993 it had approximately 300 members.[9]

Controlling body

In October 1995 the British Acupuncture Council was officially launched as a single body to govern and regulate the acupuncture profession after the unification of the country's five major acupuncture professional associations. The new body is responsible for every aspect of governing the profession. It maintains and publishes a register of qualified practitioners and works with the British Acupuncture Accreditation Board, an independent body, to monitor educational standards and structures. It can provide advice and guidance to the public and practitioners on matters of professional conduct and ethical standards and will use its Code of Ethics and Practice to take action against those unfit to practise. Registered practitioners bound by this Code can now be identified by the initials MBAcC after their name.

REGISTRATION AND TRAINING

There are five internationally recognised registers representing acupuncture which are shown in Box 16.1.

Box 16.1 Registers for acupuncture specialists

1. British Acupuncture Association and Register (BAAR)
2. Chung San Acupuncture Society (CSAcS)
3. International Register of Oriental Medicine (IROM)
4. Register of Traditional Chinese Medicine (RTCM)
5. Traditional Acupuncture Society (TAS)

Training of acupuncturists in the UK is monitored by the British Acupuncture Accreditation Board (BAAB). This is an independent body which is closely allied to the British Acupuncture Council. The BAAB's procedures involve a rigorous three year process of Accreditation. Colleges apply for candidacy status. If this is granted they then carry out a self-evaluation of their educational methods and standards according to criteria set by BAAB. Graduates of accredited or candidate colleges have automatic right of membership of the Council either as full or associate members, provided that they apply within two years of qualifying. Other applicants are only accepted after thorough evaluation of their training and skills. The list of accredited and candidate colleges is updated every three months.

This system of accreditation does not prevent unaccredited courses taking place, or marketing of videos and other forms of teaching acupuncture. If such claims are fraudulent, then they could be prosecuted for fraud or obtaining a pecuniary advantage by deception. However until there is a system of state registration such unaccredited courses cannot be prevented. It is essential that those bodies who support the British Acupuncture Council educate the general public in how to distinguish the properly qualified acupuncturist from those who have had an inadequate and unaccredited training.

RULES ON PROFESSIONAL MISCONDUCT AND INSURANCE

A Code of Ethics[10] and a Code of Practice[11] have been published by the British Acupuncture Council.

The Code of Ethics covers the topics shown in Box 16.2. The Code of Practice relates primarily to the standards of hygiene, prevention of cross-infection in the management of premises and equipment.

Box 16.2   Code of Ethics of the British Acupuncture Council

1. Conduct in an honourable manner
2. Promotion only in accordance with the guidance of the BAC
3. Compliance with the law and Code of Practice
4. No formal teaching by members unless in accordance with the guidance of the BAC
5. The Code applies to all their professional activities, including those in other therapies
6. Breaking the rules can result in disciplinary action

Members of recognised organisations are required to obtain professional indemnity insurance cover.

LAWS WHICH APPLY

Local authority bye-laws

In 1997 an outbreak of hepatitis traced to an acupuncturist using dirty needles gave rise to questions being asked in the House of Commons about registering and controlling the practices of acupuncture.[12] The Under-Secretary of State for Health answered that registration would not necessarily prevent dirty needles, and anyway might have the side-effect of giving statutory support to the acupuncture profession before it has established itself. He put forward the Health and Safety at Work etc. Act 1974 as existing legislation which could prevent acupuncturists endangering the public, but it was realised that the overworked and small health and safety inspectorate would be unable to enforce the Act by inspecting all the acupuncturists' premises.[13] West Midlands had previously put a Bill before Parliament requesting powers to control standards of hygiene by licensing acupuncturists, tattooists, massage parlours and similar activities. Despite the opposition of acupuncturists who pointed out the lack of evidence that the premises of acupuncturists were unhygienic the Bill was passed.[14]

Under Section 14(7) of the Local Government (Miscellaneous Provisions) Act 1982 local authorities can enact bye-laws which can cover acupuncture. As an example, the bye-laws passed in Cardiff are summarised in Box 16.3.

Box 16.3   Bye-laws in relation to businesses of acupuncture

- Interpretation
- Duties in relation to securing the cleanliness of the premises and fittings
- Duties in relation to securing the cleansing and sterilisation of the instruments, materials and equipment used in connection with the treatment
- Duties in relation to securing the cleanliness of the operators

(Cardiff – made on 28 September 1983)

These regulations are enforced through the environmental health department (see Chapter 6). Similar bye-laws exist in relation to ear piercing, electrolysis and tattooing.

General

In addition of course, like any other complementary therapy, practitioners of acupuncture are subject to the general laws relating to health and safety (see Chapter 13), contract (Chapter 4) and negligence (Chapter 3).

Purchasing contracts

The *Which?* survey on complementary medicine in 1995 found that acupuncture was the fourth most popular therapy.[15] As seen above acupuncture is now being purchased by GPs within the NHS.

The terms of any agreement to purchase acupuncture services are likely to be on a purely sessional basis, so that the therapist will contract to provide so many sessions at a specific cost to the referred patient. There is no further attempt to identify how the practitioner should work in that session.

MATTERS OF CONCERN

Concern about patients being able to refer themselves to an acupuncturist who has no medical training was expressed in a letter to the BMJ.[16]

I believe that the present law, which permits patients to refer themselves to acupuncturists who are not medically qualified, should be reviewed. To safeguard the public, might the BMA consider entering into discussions with the government about this?

Research in Norway has shown that pneumothorax, fainting and increased pain after treatment may be more common than had previously been thought.[17] In the research where 1135 doctors trained in acupuncture and 197 acupuncturists were surveyed, 12% of doctors and one third of acupuncturists reported adverse effects. As the popularity of acupuncture increases with referrals taking place within the NHS, so more complaints and litigation are likely to arise.

SITUATIONS WITH LEGAL SIGNIFICANCE
Referral to registered medical practitioner

Case 1 Referral to registered medical practitioner

Mark Seem in a case study[18] describing the use of acupuncture describes an encounter with a person, reluctant to seek advice from orthodox medicine, who complains of a crushing pain in the chest with discomfort and strange sensations down the inner aspect of his left arm. He was interested in having acupuncture. What would be the situation if the patient was given acupuncture without referral to a doctor?

Mark Seem stated that

I explained that symptoms such as his had to be checked out by an internist or cardiologist to rule out a possible heart condition, and assured him that if, as I suspected, his medical examination proved negative for such a condition, acupuncture probably could help a great deal. I always send a patient with such symptoms to a physician to rule out serious pathology.

What, however, if the confidence of the acupuncturist is such that they are so convinced that the symptoms do not suggest a condition which must be dealt with by practitioners of orthodox medicine but can be treated with assurance by a practitioner in acupuncture and the patient then has a heart attack? Relatives may then bring an action for failure by the acupuncturist to ensure that the patient was treated by a registered medical practitioner. The relatives' success would be in proving on a balance of probabilities that any reasonable practitioner of acupuncture would have referred the patient to a cardiologist or other specialist before carrying out acupuncture.

The difficulty about applying this test to a complementary therapist is that, in many cases, the practitioner of complementary therapy would consider that their art or science is as able if not better adapted to heal the patient than orthodox medicine. If complementary therapists can only undertake care where orthodox medicine has failed, it may reduce the scope of their practice unjustifiably.

One possibility is for the acupuncturist to say to the client, 'I have defined your symptoms as *xyz*. However there is a remote chance that I am wrong in which case you are advised to seek the assistance of a registered medical practitioner'. Such a statement would place the responsibility upon the patient in relying upon the skills of the acupuncturist. This would be in keeping with the philosophy of self-help and personal responsibility of the client, which is central to many complementary therapies. However if there has been negligence by the acupuncturist, such a statement would not necessarily relieve the acupuncturist of responsibility because of the effect of the Unfair Contract Terms Act 1977 (see Chapter 3).

A letter to the editor of the BMJ cited earlier (Peter Baldry) quotes the claims made by acupuncturists to provide assistance in infertility, insomnia, emotional problems, hypertension, and circulatory, respiratory, menopausal, menstrual problems and skin disorders. He says

It must be wrong that people other than doctors are allowed by law to treat conditions that require skilful and systematic investigation before any decisions concerning their correct management can be made. The exclusion of renal disease in patients with hypertension and of uterine carcinoma in women with menorrhagia are two obvious examples.

It should be noted, however, in relation to referral to general practitioners that the Code of Ethics of the BAC[19] considers it good practice to refer patients to general practitioners when appropriate and states that 'cooperation will be improved if the member takes the opportunity to communicate with a patient's doctor whenever necessary'. Failure, therefore, of a practitioner registered with the BAC to refer a patient to that patient's doctor could result in that practitioner facing disciplinary proceedings of his profession. The Code emphasises, of course, the importance of obtaining the patient's consent before the patient's doctor is contacted.

Undiagnosed pregnancy

Situation 1   Undiagnosed pregnancy

A woman sought the advice of an acupuncturist to prevent painful and irregular menstrual bleeding. He agreed to give her standard treatment. Subsequently she complained to him that she had miscarried a very much wanted child, and blamed him. He investigated and discovered that there had been no clear diagnosis. He had not asked her about the possibility of pregnancy, but had asked her about her general health and she had not mentioned to him that she might have been pregnant. She is now intending to sue him for compensation. What are her chances of success?

The chances of the woman obtaining any compensation for the loss of the baby will depend upon the evidence in two areas:

1. Was the acupuncturist following a reasonable standard of care in carrying out the treatment which he did on a woman who may have been pregnant, and should he have checked out this possibility first?

2. Was the actual treatment used by the acupuncturist the cause of the miscarriage? It may be for example that he used moxibustion for certain points and this is known to be contraindicated in pregnancy. (Moxibustion is the use of heat from burning mugwort at the acupuncture points.)

There might also be evidence of contributory negligence of the client in failing to give all the necessary information to the acupuncturist. This might reduce the amount of compensation payable if the patient succeeds in her civil court action (see Chapter 3).

Evidence of the records which were kept will be important in supporting the acupuncturist's defence. There are considerable advantages in using a form to take down the patient's history prior to commencing treatment and to use a comprehensive check list to ensure that a full account is taken of the patient's past and present state of health.

Dirty needles

Case 2   Dirty needles

In 1977 an outbreak of hepatitis was traced to a lay acupuncturist who had previously been denied entry to acupuncture associations. He had been using dirty needles. If similar circumstances arose again what remedies would the affected clients have?

The situation in case 2 gave rise to the legislation authorising a degree of control by local authorities referred to on page 235.

The Code of Practice of the British Acupuncture Council[20] emphasises the importance of sterilising equipment and appendix B gives advice on acute viral infective hepatitis. It emphasises that the absence of a history of the disease when taking account of the patient's health record does not mean that the patient could not be a carrier. The acupuncturist has to work on the assumption that any patient could be a carrier and that the highest standards of care must be employed at all times to prevent cross-infection. Advice is given in the Code of Practice on hygiene in respect of:

- the premises
- the equipment
- preparation of acupuncture equipment
- disposal of equipment
- disinfectants
- clean hygienic procedures
- keeping a register of patients
- health and safety at work legislation

and appendices also give information about sterilisation and home visits by mobile acupuncturists.

Any acupuncturist registered with the BAC would, of course, face disciplinary proceedings if it were established that he had failed to follow the Code of Practice thereby endangering his patients.

However in case 2 the acupuncturist was not a member of a recognised association, therefore he would not have been subject to professional disciplinary proceedings.

He could of course face criminal action under the Health and Safety at Work etc. Act in failing to take reasonable care for the safety of the general public. He could also face civil proceedings in negligence for failing to fulfil his duty of care to his patients and other persons who may be infected by them as a foreseeable result of his negligence. However the value of bringing civil action will depend to a considerable extent on whether he has the funds to meet any compensation award or if he has the necessary insurance cover to pay out the compensation.

Punctured lung

> **Situation 2**   Punctured lung
>
> An acupuncturist was carrying out acupuncture on a child. By mistake he punctured the lung of the child, who then had to be taken by ambulance to hospital. Unfortunately the child died. Can the parents claim compensation?

In situation 2, few would disagree with the view that the acupuncturist was failing to follow a reasonable standard of care in looking after the child. In theory therefore the parents should be able to claim compensation from the acupuncturist. However in the case of the death of the child, where there is no financial dependency, present or future, the amount of compensation is limited by Act of Parliament and is presently fixed at £7500. However, if the parents can prove in addition, that they have themselves suffered post traumatic stress disorder as a result of the loss of the child and the way in which the death occurred they may be able, to claim compensation in their own right. (For example the parents of the children killed or harmed by Beverley Allitt obtained a settlement from the Health Authority for post traumatic stress disorder.)

CONCLUSIONS

Although acupuncture is one of the oldest of the healing arts it is still having to fight for its reputation and status by proving that in comparison with orthodox medicine it can hold its own. Comparative research of acupuncture with orthodox medicine has never been more important.

It was announced in January 1996 that the British Acupuncture Council and the Foundation for Traditional Chinese Medicine which jointly support the Acupuncture Research Resource Centre had published a report on the research carried out recently and its plans for research over the next two years. Its plans include a nationwide audit of acupuncture in the UK. A new Internet World Wide Web service is also described in the report.[21]

A review of acupuncture research was published in the Journal of The Royal Society of Medicine[22] by Andrew Vickers of the Research Council for Complementary Medicine. He reviewed published reports involving just under 2000 patients on the use of acupuncture to prevent and manage postoperative and chemotherapy induced nausea and vomiting and showed that in 11 or 12 conducted trials acupuncture at one single but specific point has a beneficial effect.

Such work is essential to sustain the status of acupuncturists and the contribution which their work can make to health. However as it becomes increasingly popular alongside orthodox medicine, there is greater likelihood of litigation and criminal action following in its wake and further pressure on the professional bodies to regulate conduct and practice.

Questions and Exercises

1. An acupuncturist requests planning permission from the local authority to set up a consulting room, but is refused a license to practice. What are the legal implications and what action can the acupuncturist take?
2. A client complains that following an acupuncture session she suffered considerable pain and is claiming compensation. The acupuncturist believes that this is entirely fictitious and the client is simply trying to obtain money by false pretences. What are the legal implications?
3. What protection does a client have who was not aware that the acupuncturist from whom she was receiving care was not a member of a recognised Association or Society?

REFERENCES

1. Acumedic Ltd London publishes specialist books on acupuncture
2. Stanway A 1987 The Natural Family Doctor. Gaia Publications, Stroud
3. Bannernman RH 1979 Acupuncture the WHO view. World Health December 24–9
4. Laurence J Needles offer asthma relief. The Times 28 February 1996
5. Arthurs G 1994 Hypnosis and acupuncture in pregnancy. British Journal of Midwifery 2(10): 495–8
6. Beal W 1992 Acupuncture and related treatment modalities Part ii, Applications to antepartal and intrapartal care. Nurse-Midwife 37(4): 260–8
7. Yelland S 1995 Using acupuncture in midwifery care. Modern Midwife 5(1): 8–11
8. Dr Abai Berger Needles prove a point. The Times 29 November 1994 p 17
9. BMA Complementary Medicine 1993
10. British Acupuncture Council 1996 Code of Ethics. BAC, London
11. British Acupuncture Council 1995 Code of Practice. BAC, London
12. Hansard 16 December 1977 Column 1174
13. Fulder S 1998 The Handbook of Complementary Medicine. Coronet Books,
14. Hansard 19 February 1980 BD chase up the Act
15. Alternative Medicine Survey Results. Which? November 1995
16. Baldry P 1993 Letter to the editor. British Medical Journal 307: 326
17. Norheim AJ, Fonnebo V 1996 Acupuncture: adverse effects are more than occasional: case reports. Complementary Therapies in Medicine 14: 8–13 Quoted in: Rowlands B 1997 The Which? Guide to Complementary Medicine Consumers, Association, London
18. Seem M 1997 A crushing pain in the chest. In: Acupuncture in Practice Macpherson H, Kaptchuk E (eds). Churchill Livingstone, New York
19. British Acupuncture Council 1996 Code of Ethics BAC, London
20. British Acupuncture Council 1995 Code of Practice. BAC, London
21. Acupuncture Research Centre Research Report Available from Foundation for Traditional Chinese Medicine (FTCM) 122A Acomb Road York, YO2 4EY
22. Vickers A 1996 Report on Acupuncture reports. Journal of Royal Society of Medicine 89(6): 303–311

17

Alexander Technique

DEFINITION

The Alexander Technique is described by the Society of Teachers of the Alexander Technique as

An effective way of addressing the causes underlying the common problems of back pain – the discomfort, the limitations to movement and the effort of keeping the body erect.

By adopting the principles of the Alexander Technique and by learning to prevent interference with these natural mechanisms we can significantly restore their effectiveness and regain poise and vitality, even after injury or surgery. Breathing and speaking become easier, movement becomes freer, lighter and more enjoyable.

BRIEF HISTORY AND CONTROLLING BODY

The Society of Teachers of the Alexander Technique (STAT) was established in 1958 and is the recognised teaching body. The first training course was started in 1931 by F M Alexander in London under the patronage of the Earl of Lytton, Dr Peter Macdonald and Sir Lynden Macassey. Similar courses are run under the auspices of STAT in Holland and by affiliated societies across Europe, Australia, the USA and South America and Africa.

The Constitution of STAT sets out as its first object

To teach expound and propagate the theory and practice of the Alexander Technique of Re-Education (hereinafter called the 'Alexander Technique') as outlined in the four books of F. Matthias Alexander: *Man's Supreme Inheritance, Constructive Conscious Control of the Individual, The Use of Self, The Universal Constant in Living.*

The Society consists of ordinary members, student members, associate members and honorary members. Any person who has attended and completed a teacher's training course in the Alexander Technique approved by the Council of the Society is eligible for certification and to become an Ordinary Member. The Society is able to recognise other organisations for the membership if specific criteria are met. These criteria include the requirement that the organisation embodies similar training standards and rules of conduct and is based and has jurisdiction outside the UK.

The Alexander trust was established in 1990 to advance the education of the public and to promote research and study into all aspects of the Alexander Technique.

REGISTRATION AND TRAINING

STAT requirements in relation to students include that each trainee pupil undertakes, as a condition of acceptance into the relevant training course, to apply to the Society for registration as a Student Member. The student must also complete at least three academic years of three terms each consisting in aggregate of not less than 1600 working hours, each working week should consist of between 12 and 20 hours over four days.

RULES ON PROFESSIONAL MISCONDUCT

The Society of Teachers of the Alexander Technique has issued a Code of Professional Conduct which include regulations last updated in July 1995. These Regulations provide for a disciplinary procedure that is independent of the Council, a tiered system that provides for less serious matters to be dealt with informally; an appeal as an opportunity for the member to clear his or her name or to review a decision made by the Professional Conduct Committee and instructions on how to proceed with an investigation.

The Code of Conduct covers the topics shown in Box 17.1.

Box 17.1   Code of Conduct of STAT

- Introduction
- The teacher–pupil relationship
- The teacher's responsibilities to colleagues
- The teacher's responsibilities to the profession

The introduction emphasises that:

In the absence of a code of professional conduct or ethics, our right to claim to be identified, recognised and treated by the public as a professional association would, to a substantial degree, be forfeited.

PURCHASING CONTRACTS

STAT points out the medical bills insurance from such major providers as BUPA and WPA often covers the cost of lessons when they have been recommended by a consultant as part of a treatment plan. In some cases the NHS is funding lessons (see Chapter 8 on the NHS).

SITUATIONS WITH LEGAL SIGNIFICANCE

In theory the Alexander Technique is not likely to cause harm, because it is essentially a non-invasive, gentle therapy concerned with posture and balance. However it is always possible that a client may fail to seek orthodox treatment of an underlying condition, relying instead on using Alexander Technique and thus reach a stage where the illness or disease is no longer treatable. Teachers of the Alexander Technique should make it clear that they take no responsibility in relation to any illnesses or diseases and that the client should be seeking advice from practitioners of orthodox medicine.

Post surgery

Situation   Post surgery
A student of the Alexander Technique failed to advise the teacher that she had just been discharged from hospital following major surgery. Following the exercises the wound opened. She claims that the teacher should have warned her of the dangers.

In this situation, there would appear to be responsibility on both parties. On the one hand, it could be assumed that the duty of care of the instructor should include ensuring that the students knew when exercises were inadvisable, and such information should be in written form and made available to all students. If it can be established that there were failures by the instructor in this respect, then there may be liability if it can be shown that the wound opened as the result of the exercises which the student should not have been doing. At the same time, there would appear to be some contributory negligence by the student in not appreciating that care should be taken post surgery. (Such information would probably have been given to her by hospital staff. If not there may be some liability there as well.) If there is evidence of a failure by the student, this would be considered to be contributory negligence, the effect of which is to reduce the amount of compensation to which she is entitled in accordance with what would be just and equitable (see Chapter 3).

Questions and Exercises

1. There can be liability for negligent instruction (see Chapter 3). How does the principle apply to the teacher of the Alexander Technique?
2. A teacher of the Alexander Technique uses a hall which is rented to her by the local authority. Whilst she is instructing a class, one of the students slips on a wet surface and breaks her ankle. In what way, if any, is the Alexander Technique teacher liable for the injury? (see Chapter 15 on Occupier's Liability).

18

Aromatherapy

DEFINITION

The Aromatherapy Organisations Council defines aromatherapy as

The systematic use of essential oils in holistic treatments to improve physical and emotional well-being. Essential oils are extracted from plants and possess distinctive therapeutic properties which can be utilised to improve health and prevent disease. Both their physiological and psychological effects combine well to promote positive health.[1]

Essential oils are usually used in conjunction with a carrier oil. For example olive oil, almond oil or grape seed oil are used as carriers and the essential oil applied through that medium.

An aromatherapist is defined as

A person who has been trained to a defined standard in the use of essential oils for therapeutic purposes. An Aromatherapist may also utilise oils for beauty treatment purposes, but a person trained only in their application for beauty purposes is not considered to be an Aromatherapist.

BACKGROUND

History

Aromatherapy is one of the oldest healing arts with evidence that it was used in 4500 BC by ancient Egyptians. The term aromatherapy was first used by Professor

Gattefosse who discovered by chance the healing properties of lavender oil when, after accidentally burning his hand, he plunged it in lavender oil and noticed how the pain ceased and the skin healed without blistering. His work has been developed and extended by Dr Jean Valnet and Marguerite Maury.[2]

Controlling bodies

The Aromatherapy Organisations Council

The AOC was established in 1991, following an initiative from the British Council for Complementary Medicine, as the lead body for the aromatherapy profession in the UK. It is composed of both aromatherapy associations and training schools, but does not have individual membership. It has its own constitution and is governed by a Council which comprises recognised associations and schools. Over 6000 aromatherapist practitioners are indirectly represented on the Council, which covers about 90% of aromatherapists in this country. The aims of the AOC are set out in Box 18.1.

Box 18.1   Aims of the Aromatherapy Organisations Council

1. To unify the profession through bringing together its various organisations.
2. To establish common standards of training, and to ensure that all organisations registered with the Council provide appropriate standards of professional practice and conduct for their members.
3. To act as a public watchdog.
4. To provide for all organisations within aromatherapy a collective voice through which to initiate and sustain political dialogue with government, civil and medical bodies in order to enhance the best interests of professional aromatherapy.
5. To offer a mediation and arbitration service in any disputes involving aromatherapy organisations.
6. To initiate, support or sponsor research into aromatherapy.

In meeting the aims set out in Box 18.1 the AOC sets standards for the training of aromatherapists, holds seminars on topics of general interest, is establishing a research archive and has set up a complaints procedure.

The Aromatherapy Trade Council

The ATC was set up in 1992 by responsible essential oil traders following a seminar organised by the AOC. Its aim was to address common issues of public safety for the sale of essential oils. The ATC is now a separate body from the AOC but is affiliated to the AOC and the chairman of the ATC has a seat on the AOC Executive. The aims and objectives of the ATC are shown in Box 18.2.

The ATC has published a Code of Practice which covers droppers, labelling and responsible marketing.

The ATC is recognised as the regulatory body for the aromatherapy trade. Following a meeting with the Medicines Control Agency (MCA) the ATC was

---

Box 18.2   Aims and Objectives of the Aromatherapy Trade Council

1. To act as a lead body in representing all commercial aspects and interests of manufacturers, suppliers and retailers of essential oils and aromatherapy products.
2. To establish common standards of quality in essential oils and aromatherapy products.
3. To establish guidelines for safety, labelling and packaging for the aromatherapy trade.
4. To promote the responsible use of aromatherapy products.
5. To initiate support or sponsor research into all and any branches of knowledge which are pertinent to the field of aromatherapy products.
6. To publish a register of the names and relevant details of all current membership of the ATC.

---

appointed the Advertising Code Administrators of the aromatherapy essential oil industry. As a result of the discussions between the ATC and the MCA, MAL. 8, a leaflet *Guide to What is a Medicinal Product* was reviewed. The revised MAL. 8 explains the new European legislation which came into force in January 1995.

The ATC controls membership through its membership committee by ensuring that no member is accepted until labels, bottles and literature conform to the ATC's requirements in accordance with the law.

Whilst there are umbrella organisations which have an important part to play in establishing standards and ethical practice for the profession, they do not have the power to prevent any unqualified person setting up as an aromatherapist and selling her services.

EXAMPLES OF USES OF AROMATHERAPY OILS

Pregnancy and childbirth

Sheila Cornwell and Ailsa Dale[3] describe the use of essential oils by midwives at Hinchingbrooke Hospital in their antenatal and postnatal care. Mothers used the oils to relieve perineal trauma, haemorrhoids or lactational problems. The article discusses research designed to answer the question: Do women using lavender oil as a bath additive suffer significantly less perineal discomfort than those not using the preparation? The study showed no statistical evidence to support the practice of adding drops of lavender oil to the bath. However the mothers using the oil find it pleasant to use and there were no unpleasant side effects. They concluded

The pattern of discomfort scores shows no statistical differences between groups. Those using lavender oil showed lower mean discomfort scores, particularly between days 3 and 5. This is a time when the mother finds herself discharged home and permitted discomfort is high. Further studies might explore the effect of varying the amount of oil used or changing the mode of application.

Denise Tiran[4] shows that many of the essential oils which alleviate nausea are contraindicated during the first trimester. Oils which are contraindicated include:

- basil
- cedarwood
- camomile
- clary sage
- fennel
- juniper

- lavender
- marjoram
- peppermint
- nutmeg
- rose
- rosemary.

Oils which could be safely used include:

- ginger
- grapefruit
- lime
- mandarin

- petitgrain
- sweet orange
- tangerine.

She cites a case study where apparently the complementary therapies of acupressure bands, oils, and massage appeared to fail to stop nausea.

There did, however, appear to be psychological factors contributing to the patient's condition. She enjoyed the attention she received from the complementary therapist to such an extent that eventually it was deemed to be detrimental to her recovery. The patient went home after three weeks but, despite several re-admissions, no real resolution of the sickness occurred until delivery.

Maggie Mason[5] states that aromatherapy is a safe effective and enjoyable way of helping women through the pain of childbirth. As a practising midwife and aromatherapist she has been able to help women achieve a drug free labour and drug free babies have been born, a phenomenon which is becoming increasingly rare. She reports on how she set up an alternative preparation for labour service aimed at achieving drug free labour, getting permission from local supervisors of midwives in Southampton, Salisbury, Portsmouth and Winchester.

Jane Harrison[6] discusses the value of aromatherapy for the mother in the postnatal period, of using lavender oil. She lists conditions in new born babies, which can be treated by essential oils:

- nappy rash
- skin troubles
- respiratory ailments
- teething problems
- colic
- sleeping difficulties

Essential oils can be used in the bath, in a massage oil or lotion, or by vaporisation.

She also looks at Bach flower remedies and other complementary therapies such as acupuncture, reflexology, and McTimoney chiropractic. She concludes:

The regular use of essential oils and homeopathy at home can benefit all members of the family and can provide simple-to-use remedies for both parents and children in the postnatal period. Midwives are increasingly seeking alternative ways to support mothers and babies during this time. By adding these therapies to their knowledge, they can often reduce the need for drugs and other more invasive therapies. It would be good to see therapies such as aromatherapy and homeopathy becoming a standard part of midwifery training and an integral part of a midwife's skills.

Stress

Pauline Lim[7] described how essential oils were used in stress relief for health professionals. In a table she lists the oils which appeared to be appropriate to specific conditions such as:

- anxiety
- depression
- emotional fatigue
- headaches/migraine
- poor concentration
- insomnia
- irritability
- reduced immunity
- muscle tension.

Unfortunately like so many articles in this field, there is no accompanying data relating to any controlled trials of the efficacy of the treatment. She does emphasise, however, that qualified advice should be sought to reduce the risks of side effects and to avoid contraindications.

Cramp etc.

Evening primrose oil made from the seeds of *Oenothera biennis* which contain linoleic and gamolenic acid is considered by some to be an extremely useful remedy for treating cramp. When the cramp is accompanied by headaches or nausea it is recommended that the evening primrose oil should be combined with a marine oil supplement.[8] Claims have also been made that evening primrose oil can also be used in the treatment of diabetic neuropathy, eczema, rheumatoid arthritis and the breast pain associated with the pre-menstrual syndrome. Some trials have been carried out which showed that the oil was of benefit when given to patients suffering from rheumatoid arthritis, who were on anti-inflammatory drugs.[9]

Epilepsy

Dr Tim Betts, a consultant neuropsychiatrist at Queen Elizabeth Psychiatric Hospital Birmingham, is reported as using essential oils in the care of patients suffering from epilepsy and is quoted as saying that:

We use them as components to conventional care, rather than as alternatives, but the results are encouraging. Of the first 30 patients, nine became completely seizure free and a further 20 improved significantly.[10]

Research basis for such use

All the above examples point to experienced therapists who have made use of essential oils with evident success. However there is still considerable controversy over the value of essential oils both in general and in particular. Further research is essential to substantiate the claims which are made.

REGISTRATION AND TRAINING

Education standards

The AOC has defined the minimum supervised in-class education and training required to become an AOC recognised Aromatherapist as:

- 40 hours Anatomy and Physiology
- 60 hours Massage (Whole body)
- 80 hours Aromatherapy

The suggested curriculum topics for aromatherapy include: history and development of the use of plants and their essential

- oils (ancient to modern)
- Aromatherapy within the complementary sector and an holistic approach to aromatherapy
- Code of conduct and ethical considerations
- Business organisation and legal considerations
- Basic chemical principles
- Therapeutic properties and safety considerations
- A basic knowledge of common ailments
- consultation procedures
- mixing and blending essential oils
- aromatherapy massage.

These guidelines are not intended to remove from the teaching schools the right to develop their own mode of operation and provide wider studies.

RULES ON PROFESSIONAL MISCONDUCT

The AOC has set out a Code of Ethics and Practice[11] which full members of the Aromatherapy Organisations Council are required to adhere to. Any breach of the Code may render the member organisation liable to disciplinary procedures and clause 9 of the Constitution and appendix 4 of the Rules together lay down the details of the disciplinary procedure.

INSURANCE COVER AND PROFESSIONAL INDEMNITY

The Code of Ethics and Practice of the AOC requires that

Members shall ensure that their Association or School is adequately covered by insurance for both public and professional purposes. Associations shall carry Professional Liability Insurance and make available to their members a group insurance scheme for Professional Malpractice and Public and Products Liability insurance. Schools shall also carry Professional Malpractice and Public and Products Liability insurance.[12]

LAWS RELATING TO THE THERAPY

Medicinal products

If aromatherapy products are advertised as curing or treating ill health they would be defined as Medicinal products and come under the provisions of the Medicines Act 1968. This is discussed in Chapter 5.

Leaflet MAL 8 *Guide to What is a Medicinal Product* produced by the Aromatherapy Organisations Council has recently been revised. The Medicines for Human Use (Marketing Authorisations etc.) Regulations 1994 are considered in Chapter 5 and also in Chapters 26 and 27.

Non-medicinal products

Aromatherapy products which do not come under the definition of medicinal products or herbal remedies may come under cosmetic and other legislation.

Essential oils are not classed as medicines and therefore do not come under the Medicines Control Agency. No instructions are required by statute law on the bottles. However it would be illegal to advertise on the bottles that it can be used to treat a specific disease. If such a claim is made then the product could be defined as a medicinal product because of the claims made about it. Herbal remedies exempt under Section 12(2) of the Medicines Act 1968 and sold without a marketing authorisation may be labelled only by the name of the plant or plants and the process and without any written recommendation as to their use.

The Aromatherapy Organisations Council has published an extremely helpful leaflet setting out the legal issues relating to products used in aromatherapy and gives advice on the wording to be used to prevent products being defined as medicinal products.[13] Thus it suggests that words such as 'balancing', 'cheering', comforting etc. can be used, but not in conjunction with a medical condition such as 'soothes pain'. It advises as follows:

This is a very complicated issue and not one simply of 'this word is okay and this is not'. It depends entirely on how the descriptive word is used. However, if we make a concerted attempt to market aromatherapy products responsibly, we need have no fear regarding government legislation. The ball is very much in our court.

Robert Tisserand states that people should be wary of basil, since there is evidence that basil causes cancer. However there are no restrictions on its sale.[14]

In France there are rules governing the purity of oil.

New Woman in 1994 was pressing for legislation to require aromatherapy bottles to be marked with clear warnings that the contents are not to be used internally, applied undiluted to the skin or left within reach of children. There should be clearly marked instructions and information about what the contents are, where they were grown, how they were extracted and whether or not they have been checked for purity.[15]

LINKS WITH THE NHS

An example is given in a journal for fundholding general practitioners of a West Midlands fundholding practice which is using aromatherapy.[16] In July 1994 the practice of Dr Arun Shah, Dr Prabha Shah and Dr Narider Sahota in Walsall employed an aromatherapist for one session a week especially for patients suffering from osteoarthritis and other chronic pain conditions. The figures for the first six months from August 1994 to January 1995 showed that 104 sessions had been provided at £20 per session. Of the 29 patients attending 15 reported improvements, 9 reported no improvements and 5 were unsure of the effect of the treatments.

The value of aromatherapy in midwifery practice is reported by Lynne Reed and Lynne Norfolk[17] who used it antenatally, intrapartum and postnatally. They concluded from a survey undertaken that there were no risks to the baby in the use of lavender baths and the majority of clients and midwives found the therapy to be of help. They were unable to establish whether or not its use had any effect on the length of labour (see also above).

Fundholding general practitioners are increasingly purchasing aromatherapy treatments for their NHS patients and some are employing full time or part time aromatherapy practitioners. The uncertainty over the rights of the GP fundholders on purchasing non-orthodox forms of treatment gave rise to a question to the editor of the fundholding journal.[18] The question is shown in Box 18.3.

Box 18.3   Can our new Health Authority refuse to pay for aromatherapy?

We have had an aromatherapist on contract for the past six months and we enter the sessions under direct access services 5001 on the fund computer system. A recent boundary change has meant that we come under a new health authority, which refuses to authorise the payments. Can the authority do this and, if not, what should we do?

The answer to the question posed in Box 18.3 is that aromatherapy is a grey area of fundholding. It is not on the approved list of fundholding services but some health authorities (and the old FHSAs) give approval. The reply points out that the fact that the new health authority does not have the moral right to stop a practice agreed with its predecessor for that current year, even though in future years it may not be prepared to fund it.

This issue is of course relevant to many complementary therapists who would like their services to be available to clients through the NHS and is considered further in Chapter 1.

SITUATIONS WITH LEGAL SIGNIFICANCE

It should not be assumed that aromatherapy is a relatively benign complementary therapy. Caroline J Stevensen[19] cites a study which showed that:

Inhalation of various essential oils was found to lead to a change in brain wave activity ... Over stimulation from the oils was found to have a lowering effect on brain waves, which is suggested to be the same effect that oil would have in clinical use. If this is so, then dosage of essential oils may need closer examination through further trials.

Dangers include:

- certain conditions which contraindicate the use of certain specific essential oils such as skin allergies, pregnancy, blood pressure, epilepsy, diabetes
- taking essential oils by mouth or directly onto the skin

Pennyroyal oil

Case 1   Pennyroyal oil

A death occurred in Colorado in 1978[20] when a teenager who wanted to induce a miscarriage drank pennyroyal oil, which is derived from a type of mint.

In case 1 there could be criminal liability on the part of any one who gave that recommendation to the teenager. In this country, failure to obey the provisions of the Abortion Act 1967 (as amended) in ensuring that an abortion only proceeds (except in an emergency) with the signed agreement of two doctors and is carried out under the supervision of a registered medical practitioner could lead to a prosecution under the Offences Against the Person Act 1861 or the Infant Life Preservation Act 1929 (see also situation 2: Abortion wanted in Chapter 37).

Camphor oil

Case 2   Camphor oil

The reporter of the Colorado case described in case 1 above also described a case where camphor oil caused a still birth after a pregnant British woman drank it in a weak solution to fight a fever.

In case 2 if there was no intention or gross recklessness as to whether a miscarriage would result, there is unlikely to be a successful prosecution under the legislation set out in case 1. However there could be liability on any one who recommended that the oil could be successful in treating the fever.

Missing the underlying diagnosis

Situation 1   Missing the underlying diagnosis

An aromatherapist treats a patient with breast pain and fails to diagnose that the patient is suffering from breast cancer. By the time the condition is diagnosed the cancer has spread too far and is inoperable. Can the relatives bring a successful action for the failure to diagnose the cancer?

The success of the relatives suing for the negligence of the aromatherapist in failing to identify the underlying diagnosis and therefore in failing to ensure that action was taken which could have prevented (or at least delayed) the death, will depend upon what evidence is available to show whether the symptoms which the patient told the therapist about were such that any reasonable aromatherapist would have realised that it was necessary for the patient to seek expert medical opinion. It may also be that the aromatherapist was under the mistaken view that the patient was already receiving medical attention although it would have been the aromatherapist's responsibility to clarify this. Expert evidence would be required on what a reasonable aromatherapist would have been expected to do in these circumstances. There may also be an element of contributory negligence – if the patient herself deliberately decided not to seek medical advice on her symptoms.

Patient demands

Situation 2   Patient demands
A patient wishes a certain oil to be used and, against her better judgment, the therapist agrees with the result that harm occurs. Has the patient a possible claim against the therapist?

Whatever the financial advantages no therapist should ever permit practice contrary to professional standards to take place. The aromatherapist in this situation has the choice over which product is safe and appropriate. If she allows her professional judgment to be overruled by the demands of the patient, she must accept the consequences. These could include:

• A successful action in the civil law by the patient – the patient arguing that the therapist had not made clear the dangers of that particular oil
• Professional conduct proceedings held by her professional association because she has brought aromatherapy into disrepute. Even criminal proceedings if the harm she caused was grievous and her actions grossly negligent or reckless.

Consent is not a defence if one person inflicts physical harm upon another.[21]

Silence by the patient

Situation 3   Silence by the patient
The patient fails to inform the therapist of other treatments and medication she is taking and the therapist in ignorance uses oils which are contraindicated by those treatments. As a consequence, harm results to the patient.

Like the situation above concerning patient demands, it is essential that the aromatherapist follows a reasonable standard of care in using her professional skills. The standard of care would include taking a full history of all patients and any past or current medications they have taken. Forms should be available for the therapist to complete during this history taking. It should be pointed out to each patient how important it is for the patient to give a full comprehensive history because of the dangers of the therapist having inadequate information. This may include asking the patient's permission for the therapist to request details from the general practitioner.

If, after such instruction, the patient fails to inform the therapist about specific medication which would contradict some of the oils used by the therapist, and as a result suffers harm, it would not then be the fault of the therapist. Clearly the aromatherapist's records would be extremely important in supporting her defence. The aromatherapist must also take into account the mental capacity of patients to understand the questions and their capability in giving a full medical history. If the patient is mentally incompetent, then information from a carer should be obtained before any possibly harmful treatment is commenced.

Failure to warn

Situation 4   Failure to warn
The therapist fails to warn the patient that after bergamot has been applied the patient should avoid direct sunlight, since bergamot can make the skin photosensitive. As a result the patient suffers from severe skin burn following an aromatherapy session.

In this situation the patient clearly has a very strong case for claiming compensation for negligence:

- the therapist owed a duty of care
- the therapist was in breach of that duty and
- as a consequence of that breach of duty
- the patient has suffered harm.

It may, however, be one person's word against another. What if the aromatherapist did tell the patient to be wary of sunbathing? How can she prove it? If a written leaflet were available giving the appropriate warnings and this had been handed out to the patient, then the therapist would have a better chance of proving a defence. Where it is extremely important that the therapist proves that the necessary information is given, she could ask the patient to sign a tear off sheet on the leaflet acknowledging receipt of the written information and warnings.

Wrong administration

Situation 5   Wrong administration
An oil is drunk rather than massaged into the skin.

Aromatherapists should not assume any knowledge on the part of the patient as to how the oils are administered. It would be unusual for the patient to take oils home but, if this happens, then the therapist must ensure that very precise instructions are given on their use. Warnings about keeping the products out of the reach of children should also be given. If the therapist has failed to give these warnings and harm results there may be some liability on her part although it would have to be shown that the harm was a reasonably foreseeable result of her failures. Again it is useful if the warnings could be given in written form as well as by word of mouth.

Some aromatherapy oils could come under the provisions of the Control of Substances Hazardous to Health. These regulations are discussed in Chapter 13.

Excessive use

Situation 6   Excessive use

A client fails to follow instructions of the aromatherapist when having a bath at home and adds too many drops: an allergic reaction results.

This is similar to situation 5: Wrong administration and the therapist may be liable for the harm which has resulted. It may be however, that it is not the excessive number of drops but the oil itself which has caused the allergy. If the therapist has failed to check for the possibility of an allergic response there could be negligence on her part. It could however be a situation where the allergic response was so unlikely, a chance in a million, that no reasonable therapist could have been expected to take precautions against this possibility. If this can be established, the therapist should not be found at fault.

It should also be noted that the client failed to follow the instructions given. In these circumstances, provided the therapist took all reasonable steps to ensure that the client understood the instructions, any compensation that may be found to be due would be considerably reduced because of this contributory negligence (see Chapter 3).

Patient inhibition

Situation 7   Patient inhibition

A patient fails to tell the therapist that she suffers from asthma, because she is embarrassed about the illness. Had the therapist known this she would have not used certain oils.

Like 'Patient silence' above, the therapist must do all she reasonably can to obtain a full history. If, as a result of the deliberate action of the patient to withhold this information and in circumstances where there is nothing more that the therapist can do, the therapist treats the patient in ignorance of vital information, then the patient must bear the responsibility for the harm which has resulted from the silence. Clearly those therapists who work in GP clinics and have access to patient records, should ensure that their treatment is given in the knowledge of what those records contain.

CONCLUSIONS

Aromatherapy is becoming an increasingly popular therapy and its use within the NHS is expanding. However it is essential that its popularity is paralleled by more research on its clinical effectiveness and that its practitioners do not claim for its potency more success than is justified. Caroline J Stevensen[22] states:

While aromatic substances and oils have been used throughout history, there has been no sound system developed for their use, a fact especially evident while comparing aromatherapy to a system such as Chinese Medicine. Recent research interest in essential oils by both aromatherapists and health care professionals should encourage more research into the science of aromatherapy, so that understanding may be gained as to the importance and worth of this natural therapy. Until a sound scientific base is ascertained, it is believed that aromatherapy will not take a full place beside the more established complementary health care systems.

In addition, as its popularity grows, there is a danger of more complaints and litigation since aromatherapy is by no means a harmless therapy.

Questions and Exercises

1. Following an aromatherapy session, a client decides to buy the essential oils and treat herself at home. Unfortunately she makes a mistake over the oils that the aromatherapist used and causes an allergic skin reaction. Is the therapist in any way liable?
2. A client fails to hear the aromatherapist advising her not to go into the sunlight following treatment. As a result she suffered severe skin burns. Is the aromatherapist liable?
3. A client agrees to pay for 20 sessions of aromatherapy at the suggestion of the therapist who recommended this number for maximum benefit. After three sessions, the client changes her mind. Is she entitled to have her money back? (See also Chapter 4.)

REFERENCES

1. Aromatherapy Organisations Council 1996 Core Curriculum, 4. AOC, Market Harborough
2. Stanway A 1987 The Natural Family Doctor. Gaia Books, London
3. Cornwell S, Dale A 1995 Lavender oil and perineal repair. Modern Midwife 5(3): 31–3
4. Tiran D 1996 Aromatherapy for nausea and vomiting in pregnancy. Modern Midwife 6(3): 19–21 (Extract from her book see Bibliography)
5. Mason M 1996 Aromatherapy in practice. British Journal of Midwifery 4(6): 325–7
6. Harrison J 1995 The use of complementary medicine in postnatal care. British Journal of Midwifery 3(1): 31–4
7. Lim P 1997 Essential stress relief: the use of oils to treat tension. British Journal of Midwifery 5(6): 336–8
8. Stanway A 1987 The Natural Family Doctor, p 171. Gaia Books, London

9. Stuttaford T The primrose path to nowhere? The Times 4 October 1994 p 17 (reviewing an article by Dr Jos Kleijnen in the British Medical Journal October 1994)
10. Lavery S Essential Oils. The Sunday Times 3 March 1996 p 18
11. AOC 1993 Objectives, Constitution and Rules, Appendix 3. AOC, Market Harborough
12. AOC 1993 Objectives, Constitution and Rules, Appendix 3. AOC, Market Harborough
13. Aromatherapy Trade Council 1995 Responsible Marketing and the Medicines Control Agency. AOC, Market Harborough
14. Tisserand R 1994 Essential Oil Safety. Tisserand
15. Nelson F Magic or Poison? The truth about aromatherapy oils. New Woman June 1994, p 141
16. Cresswell J 1995 Sweet Smell of Success. Fundholding 1 November 1995, p 21–3
17. Reed L and Norfolk L 1993 Aromatherapy in Midwifery. International Journal of Alternative and Complementary Medicine 11(12): 15–17
18. Question. Fundholding 15 November 1995, p 11
19. Stevensen CJ 1996 Aromatherapy, Chapter 10 In: Marc M (ed) Fundamentals of complementary and alternative medicine. Churchill Livingstone, New York, also refers to Torri S, Fukuda H, Kanemoto H *et al* 1988 Contingent negative variation (CNV) and the psychological effects of odour In: Van Toller S, Dodd GH (eds) Perfumery: The Psychology and Biology of Fragrance, p 107–121. Chapman Hall, London
20. Nelson F Magic or Poison? The truth about aromatherapy oils. New Woman June 1994, p 141
21. R *v.* Brown and others HL The Times Law Report 12 March 1993
22. Stevensen CJ 1996 Aromatherapy, Chapter 10 In: Marc M (ed) Fundamentals of complementary and alternative medicine. Churchill Livingstone, New York

19

Art, creative and movement therapies

DEFINITION

Art therapists help and encourage clients of all ages to express difficult emotions, promoting physical, mental, social and emotional well-being through the creative use of art materials, music, role play or story telling.[1]

BACKGROUND

History

The scope for the benefits of art in health care has been increasingly recognised over recent years and such therapists have been employed in the NHS since the 1940s. Many trusts, especially those providing services for psychiatric patients and those with learning disabilities, are now employing therapists from the different creative arts to provide services for their patients. The Department of Health has provided career information on art, drama and music therapy for potential applicants. (Psychodrama is considered in Chapter 35, Yoga in Chapter 38 and the Alexander Technique in Chapter 17.)

Art, music, and drama therapies have now been granted state registration and come under the Council for Professions Supplementary to Medicine. The rules relating to this regulatory body are discussed in Chapter 6. The various associations which provide approved training and keep registers of those qualified have come under one umbrella known as Art Therapists for the purpose of state registration (see below). The art therapies are a good example of organisations meeting the criteria for state registration set out by Lord Benson and shown in Box 6.7, Chapter 6. Of great importance was the agreement between the various associations that they would work together to secure state registration.

In a fascinating chapter[2] Ray Rowden describes the many creative arts which can play an important part in the progress of patients, illustrating his account with case studies of patients. He shows how a

creative regime that uses the arts can restore to a person a sense of individuality and reality. In the drab and lonely world of the person in institutional care art can speak of beauty, or emotion, of feeling, of human richness, for the way in which each of us responds to creative stimuli is totally unique.

He looks at the use made of canned music, music systems, walkmans, videos, guest speakers, crafts, sports, gardening, music rooms, live performance and ward based activity.

Art therapy

Shaun McNief[3] begins his book, *Art as Medicine*, by saying that

Whenever illness is associated with loss of soul, the arts emerge spontaneously as remedies, soul medicine. Pairing art and medicine stimulates the creation of a discipline through which imagination treats itself and recycles its vitality back to daily living.

He later states that

Art therapy, like surrealism, focuses on using the creative process to treat and attend to the other, thriving on collaborations with other disciplines.

Art in the NHS

An article in the Times[4] has described the work of the Chelsea and Westminster Hospital as the flagship of the NHS's Art for Health movement in encouraging the creation of attractive surroundings. James Scott, an orthopaedic surgeon is convinced that an art-rich environment is conducive to patient well-being.

So far it hasn't been proved possible to hold controlled clinical trials about the effect of art on ill people. There are too many variables to make scientifically based statistics reliable, although the Americans are trying. But medical staff here and elsewhere share my conviction that the arts in the hospital have transformed the atmosphere.

Uses of art

Rita Page Barton was a leading practitioner of art therapy in Britain. She was a psychoanalyst who trained under Jung in Zurich. She believed that art could be used both diagnostically and therapeutically.

The therapeutic value of the arts in eliciting the patients' own healing powers is constantly shown and never fails to be awe inspiring.

She found that art therapy often works through enabling a patient to take the first steps towards detachment, when more rational methods fail, by 'exteriorization of the unconscious contents of the mind'.[5]

Umbrella organisation

The British Association of Art Therapists was founded in 1964 to develop the recognition of art therapy within health care. Members are required to have a degree in art and design or comply with the core requirements set by the Association. The Department of Health lists the organisations which provide post-graduate training accredited by the British Association of Art Therapists. There are about 600 art therapists in the UK.

Music

Persons who could benefit from music therapy include:

- People with learning, physical and sensory disabilities, including multiple disabilities and neurological conditions.
- People with learning illness or emotional disturbances.
- People with speech and language impairment.
- People with disabilities within the continuum of autism.
- Elderly people.

Music therapy is also increasingly being sought by people who may not have specific difficulties but who would like to gain insight into themselves and their ways of relating to others.[6]

Uses of music

Frances Biley in her article on the use of music in therapeutic care[7] considers the use of background music rather than the use of music therapeutically in controlled situations e.g. for those with learning disabilities. In the background the music may not be able to change a patient's psychological state but it may act as a distracter.

Three things need to be considered. First anybody who is considering playing music outside a strictly family or domestic circle needs to be aware of legislation controlling copyright. The Copyright, Design and Patents Act 1988 protects the interests of composers and artists and two licences are required by anybody wanting to publicly broadcast music. These can be obtained from Phonographic Performance Limited and the Performing Rights Society. Second, security needs to be considered. The important thing about portable-tape players is that they are *portable*. ... Third, the choice of music is important. Get it wrong and the results will jar on the nerves of both patients and staff.

The author suggests as a start to try Love Themes Volume 1 and 2 by Mantovani, Reflections by the Moonlight Moods Orchestra or in the Mood for Love by Geoff Love and his Orchestra.

Umbrella organisations

The Association of Professional Music Therapists (APMT) was formed in 1976 with the purpose of fulfilling the needs of qualified music therapists in Great Britain. It acts as a protective body to music therapists already in work, to uphold clinical and ethical standards and assists in the creation of new posts. It also promotes the exchange of information between music therapists, both in Britain and abroad. There are now over 200 registered music therapists in the UK belonging to the PMT.

The British Society for Music Therapy was founded in 1958 by Juliette Alvin. Its aims include promotion of the use and development of Music Therapy. It organises conferences, workshops and meetings and is a centre of information. Its membership is open to all whose vocational activities enable them to further the objects of the Society, and there is a student membership at reduced rate for full time students.

Live Music Now is an organisation set up by Yehudi Menuhin in 1977, partly as a result of his own experiences during the war. It arranges for musicians and singers to perform for persons who would not normally have access to live music. They perform in residential care homes and in hospitals, often working with occupational therapy departments to provide workshops, providing stimulation through music.

Live Music Now set up a Welsh Branch in 1990 and the number of requests received for musical entertainers to perform for all ages in hospital and residential care homes in increasing every year.[8]

Drama

The British Association of Dramatherapists recognises six postgraduate courses for entry to its membership. In addition to the postgraduate qualification the Association requires members to complete a specified number of supervision hours in the first three years post-qualification to retain full membership.

Movement and dance

Movements such as the Shamanic Life Dance emphasise the importance of dance in initiating freedom in the individual and enabling the dancers to change the way they experience themselves and their world. A leaflet describes the dance and movement workshops as using 'the body as a gateway for creative exploration of the deeper self'.

At the present time movement and dance therapies are not included in the art therapies which are obtaining state registration.

STATE REGISTRATION

The Professions Supplementary to Medicine (Arts Therapists Board) Order of Council 1997[9] came into force on 26 March 1997. It adds the profession of arts therapists to the schedule of professions supplementary to medicine listed under the 1960 Professions Supplementary to Medicine (see Chapter 6). (In contrast chiropractors and osteopaths have obtained state registration outside the professions supplementary to medicine and through separate statutory provision (see Chapters 22 and 33).

The Order in Council has set out the framework for the new Arts Therapists Board, a total of 17 members:

- nine from the professions
- one from the Scottish Corporations
- one from the Royal College of Physicians of London

- one from the Royal College of Psychiatrists
- one expert in professional education and
- four other members.

Following the establishment of the Board, and the setting up of the appropriate register all the other provisions of the 1960 Act discussed in Chapter 6 will come into effect. Once the full provisions are in place it is a criminal offence for people falsely to claim that they are a state registered art, music or drama therapist. A therapist in art, music or drama must also be state registered in order to obtain employment within the NHS.

The Order in Council recognises the British Association of Art Therapists, the Association of Professional Music Therapists and the British Association for Dramatherapists for the purposes of consultation in making appointments to the Board.

SITUATIONS WITH LEGAL SIGNIFICANCE
Whose property?

Situation 1   Whose property?
A patient with learning disabilities was encouraged to paint, assisted by an art therapist who worked on a sessional basis for the residential care home. Materials were provided by the home. He was persuaded to take part in an exhibition and, following that, several orders were received for his paintings. Social Services have argued that the paintings belong to the home, or alternatively that the proceeds should be taken into account in assessing his means tested contribution to the fees of the home. The relatives who administer his property claim that the payments should come to them on his behalf, without any reduction for fees.

The legal situation is probably (since there is no decided case that the author is aware of) that the home is entitled to recover the cost of the materials which they provided for the patient from the proceeds of the sale, but that the work in the painting belongs to the patient. Once the income becomes part of his assets, then there is no reason why it should not be taken into account in the means testing for contributions to the fees of the home. The relatives would have a duty to show that any money they receive are used for the benefit of the patient.

In an interesting article Janet Patrick and Gary Winship[10] discuss the problems relating to disposal of creative pieces. Disposal includes:

- being given away
- sold
- destroyed (either immediately or later)
- kept and displayed
- kept and stored.

Difficulties can arise, for example when a patient committed suicide and a painting completed by the patient was still on display – should it be taken down or left up?

Or the conflicts which can arise when management requires all the paintings to be taken down.

These authors do not consider the legal dimension, including payment for the materials, rights of ownership and possession and rights of relatives. There may be a value in clarifying such issues before the creative art session begins.

Videos for sale

Situation 2   Videos for sale
As part of drama therapy, a psychiatric patient, May Brown, agreed to take part in a drama session which was videoed. No written agreement was made. The makers of the video now wish to use the video for educational purposes and May has been asked to give her consent to the video being sold. What are her rights?

May is entitled to refuse to allow the video to be sold or used outside the hospital. She has a right of confidentiality and unless there was clear agreement that, in taking part in the drama session she was giving consent to this video being used outside the hospital, she is entitled to have that confidentiality respected. The firm could, of course, offer her payment for the right to use that video but she would have the right to refuse. Had her consent been obtained before the video was made, her capacity to give consent would have had to be checked. It should be noted that, for the purposes of the Video Recordings Act 1984, the supply of videos used in training or carrying on any medical or related occupation are exempted from the provisions of that Act. This definition would probably extend to the work of a drama therapist in a health context, particularly where the patient's care is under the supervision of a registered medical practitioner.

Recorded music

Situation 3   Recorded music
Residents at a home for those with learning disabilities planned a concert to raise funds for the home. One of the acts included playing a record which the residents accompanied with singing and a drum. They raised over £1000 but have now been told that they face legal action for failure to obtain a licence.

Under the Copyright, Design and Patents Act 1988 protection is given to composers and artists. Licences should have been obtained by the producer of the show. Letters should be sent to the Phonographic Performance Limited and the Performing Rights Society to apologize for the error, which was a result of ignorance.

CONCLUSIONS

A new era has begun for art therapies. State registration should ensure that the public can be confident that registered therapists offering services are well qualified and abide by a clear Code of Professional Practice. The registered therapists should themselves benefit from the protection that this gives them. Like the other professions supplementary to medicine which are registered under the 1960 provisions, they will be involved in the major changes now being proposed following the recent consultation exercise conducted by JM Consulting Ltd under the steering group chaired by Professor Sheila McLean (see Chapter 6). Not all the varied therapies which are covered by the title to this chapter are under the umbrella of the state registered art therapies and it will be interesting to note the extent to which those not so included seek to amalgamate with those who are. Whether state registered or not, there is every sign that the contribution that these therapies can make across the whole spectrum of health care is now appreciated and their significance will grow.

Questions and Exercises

1. What are the advantages and disadvantages of state registration for art therapies?
2. Design a leaflet and consent form which explains to persons about the filming and use of a video on which they may be filmed.
3. What are the dangers in using art, drama and musical activities as a source of diagnosis?

REFERENCES

1. Department of Health 1997 Career pamphlet HSC 27 Arts therapist. DoH, London
2. Rowden R 1994 The Arts in Health Care Chapter 2 In: Wells R and Tschudin V (eds) Wells' supportive therapies in health care. Baillière Tindall, London
3. McNief S 1992 Art as Medicine: Creating a therapy of the imagination. Shambhala, London
4. Karney R The healing power of art. The Times, 26 March 1996
5. Inglis B, West R 1983 The Alternative Health Guide. Michael Joseph, London
6. Association of Professional Music Therapists Leaflet, An Introduction to Music Therapy
7. Biley F 1992 Use of music in therapeutic care. British Journal of Nursing 1(4): 178–80
8. Roy Hancock R The sound of music helps to heal. Western Mail 26 July 1997
9. SI 1997/1121
10. Patrick J, Winship G 1994 Creative therapy and the question of the disposal: What happens to created pieces? British Journal of Occupational Therapy 57(1): 20–2

20

Astrology and related disciplines

To some the idea that astrology, tarot readings, palmistry etc. could be seen as a complementary therapy defies belief. There are however several groups of people who see astrology and related disciplines as a profession whose work can assist personal fulfilment and health.

BACKGROUND

The Association of Professional Astrologers

The Association of Professional Astrologers was formed in 1989 to meet the growing demand for professional work of the highest standard. The Association has a Code of Ethics (see Box 20.1) and keeps a register of those who have the qualifications accepted by the Association. For full membership the Association requires a diploma from a body recognised by the Association plus two years post-diploma experience as a consultant. Associate membership is also available. However an alternative route to the diploma is open to those who have many years of skill in practising. In this case their application must be supported by published or presented work. This can be in the form of a book, a series of articles, or conference or seminar lecturers. This material must clearly demonstrate a level of astrological knowledge at least equal to that required for a diploma pass.

The Council of the Association consists of three officers, Chair, Secretary, and Press Officer, and four council members. The Council is elected by ballot at the annual general meeting. Any full member is eligible to stand for membership of the Council. Election is by secret ballot.

Box 20.1 Code of Ethics of the Association of Professional Astrologers

Members agree:
  1. To respect the dignity and worth of every human being and their right to self-determination. To accept a responsibility to encourage and facilitate the self-development of the client, whilst having due regard to the interests and rights of others.
  2. To preserve the confidentiality and anonymity of a client and all material relating to the client. To take great care in the publication or presentation of case-material and to maintain that anonymity unless the client otherwise agrees.
  3. To ensure that a client is made fully aware of the method of working, the duration and nature of the consultation/s, and the fees involved before any work is undertaken.
  4. To ensure that potential clients, whose needs are beyond the competence of an individual astrologer, are referred to appropriate individuals or agencies.
  5. To refrain from offering any medical, legal or financial advice to a client on astrological grounds unless the appropriate skills or qualifications have been obtained.
  6. To refrain from making public comments or predictions on the personal or emotional life of public figures or on the state of their health. Any comments on public figures should be concerned solely with the role for which they are known, and should not be made in a manner likely to bring astrology or the Association into disrepute.
  7. To maintain the highest ethical standards in all dealings with clients and to refrain from behaviour likely to bring astrology or the Association into disrepute.

Any complaint alleging a breach of the Code of Ethics must be followed by an investigation by the Council.

The British Astrological and Psychic Society

A second organisation, the British Astrological and Psychic Society (BAPS) was formed in 1976 by Russell Grant. It aims to provide a means of bringing together those actively working in, or interested in, the many different aspects of esoteric, spiritual and 'New Age' teachings such as psychic perception, astrology, palmistry, tarot, numerology and healing.

Membership is open to all those interested in learning about the different disciplines in the Society, but only those who have been a member of the Society for at least six months can become a Consultant. Consultants must also be examined with regard to their competency and professionalism. They are required to conform and be a signatory to a Code of Ethics and Conduct (see Box 20.2). The BAPS publish a national register of Consultants, many of whom are identified with several different forms of competencies. Those disciplines in which the Consultant has been vetted are shown in upper case in the Register, other disciplines (which are practised as an allied or secondary subject) are shown in lower case. Consultants can use Cons. MBAPS after their name.

The Society publishes a quarterly journal called *Mercury*. An information booklet available from the Society defines astrology, card readings, colour readings, graphology, I Ching, intuitive care reading, numerology, palmistry, psycards, psychic perception (including crystal ball), clairvoyance, aura reading, mediumship and psychic art, runes, sand reading, tarot.

The Code of Ethics and Conduct of the BAPS covers the topics shown in Box 20.2.

Box 20.2   Code of Ethics and Conduct of the BAPS

1. Stated aim to provide a service which reflects both professional and spiritual integrity.
2. Stated duty to encourage an awareness and understanding of their subjects and the spiritual reality they represent.
3. Rules relating to the fixing of fees.
4. Rules relating to the working at festivals of the Society.
5. Rules relating to the use of Cons.MBAPS.
6. Conduct as befits a professional member of the Society.
7. Rules relating to incidents of breach of Code.
8. Rules about reinstatement after removal from the Register.
9. Duty to sign a copy of the Code.

In addition to the Code of Ethics and Conduct for Consultants, the Society also has a Code of Conduct for general members. A complaints procedure enables any client or member of the Society or member of the general public to bring concerns before the Society.

LAWS RELATING TO ASTROLOGY AND SIMILAR DISCIPLINES

Fraudulent Mediums Act 1951

The provisions of this Act are set out in Box 20.3.

Box 20.3   Fraudulent Mediums Act 1951

1(1). Subject to the provisions of this section, any person who —
(a) with intent to deceive purports to act as a spiritualistic medium or to exercise any powers of telepathy, clairvoyance or other similar powers, or
(b) in purporting to act as a spiritualistic medium or to exercise such powers as aforesaid, uses any fraudulent device,
shall be guilty of an offence.
(2) A person shall not be convicted of an offence ... unless it is proved that he acted for reward; and for the purposes of this section a person shall be deemed to act for reward if any money is paid, or other valuable thing given, in respect of what he does, whether to him or to any other person.

The consent of the Director of Public Prosecutions is necessary to a prosecution being brought under the Act. The Act does not apply to anything done solely for the purpose of entertainment.

Other provisions

The criminal laws relating to obtaining a pecuniary advantage by deception and related offences and the Trade Descriptions Act are also significant laws for this group of practitioners (see Chapter 5). It is important that those practising in these fields do not offer clients more than they can accomplish and set out clearly the limitations of their work.

BAPS guidelines

The British Astrological and Psychic Society is very clear in the advice it offers to its members and the general public.[1]

In most disciplines, consultations provide two areas of information. The first is the personal information of various kinds, which covers such things as general and particular personality characteristics, strengths, weaknesses, talents, abilities, vocational tendencies, potential or actual health conditions and so forth. The second is concerned with events in the life of the client, relating to past, present and future. Certain disciplines are better at providing one kind of information than another, while some others are capable of providing both in varying degrees.

The Society emphasises the importance that

anyone seeking the help of a professional in any of these fields has some understanding of what can, and cannot, be provided through a specific discipline. In this way disappointment is avoided and value for money is obtained.

The Society also explains:

It should be understood though, that our lives are not totally pre-defined, we can and do change what will happen by the actions we take from day to day ... With the understanding of the possibility of viewing the trends and influences available, when consulting someone on the kinds of decisions that need to be made, you will be learning to take control of your future.

SITUATIONS WITH LEGAL SIGNIFICANCE

Situation 1   The lottery
Following a visit to a person advertising herself as skilled in palmistry, Jane was led to believe that she would win the lottery. With this prospect in mind, she took on considerable debts and commitments but is still waiting to achieve success. Does she have any rights against the palmist?

Civil law   There can be liability for negligent advice, but it has to be established that the advice was given in circumstances where the one person knew that there would be reliance upon that advice and as a consequence of relying upon the negligent advice loss or damage has occurred. In this situation it is extremely unlikely that any court would consider that a duty of care was owed by the palmist to the client. Even if there were such a duty, it might be considered totally unreasonable for the client to rely on any such advice in these circumstances. In any event there may be a high level of contributory negligence by the client in incurring the debts and commitments before the win was secured. It could also be argued that these debts were not the consequence of the advice. In addition how does the client establish that the advice was negligent? It could be that the palmist was following the reasonable standards of any palmist, but that the client had completely misinterpreted the comments made.

Criminal law There could be liability under the Fraudulent Mediums Act 1951 and also under the Theft Act for attempting to obtain a pecuniary advantage or property by deception. Successful prosecution would depend upon being able to prove the intent to deceive.

Situation 2   False pretences

Bob Chudd with no training or expertise in tarot, I Ching and other divinations set up a business with booths in many of the arcades of major city centres. He staffed them with school leavers to whom he gave an information leaflet on what to do. He found that he was able to make a considerable profit. People have complained to trading standards departments about these activities. Can any action be taken?

Bob Chudd would be subject to the laws relating to obtaining property by deception, the Trade Description Act (see Chapter 5) and the Fraudulent Mediums Act 1951 and regulations relating to planning permissions and bye-laws of individual councils (see Chapter 15). The fact that he has provided no training for his employees will not necessarily prove that he has committed a criminal offence, unless he has advertised to the contrary and made false claims in respect of their abilities. The Trading Standards Department of the local authority could take action if there was evidence of a criminal offence being committed (see Chapter 6).

CONCLUSIONS

The scientific basis of many of the claims made by practitioners in this field has still to be established. However it has a considerable following and regulations may be necessary to ensure that the public is protected from some dishonest practitioners.

Questions and Exercises

1. What arguments do you consider can be used to justify the inclusion of predictive disciplines in a book on complementary therapies?
2. How should the client be protected against unscrupulous people working in this field who are not associated with an organisation requiring observance of a code of conduct?
3. On what basis should insurance cover be provided for people practising in this area?

REFERENCES

1. Information Booklet and Register of Consultants. Nuffield Survey BAPS

21

Bach flower remedies

DEFINITION

Bach flower remedies are described by the Bach Centre as:

a 'natural, safe, form of healing. They restore peace of mind and help relieve negative attitudes which may be standing in the way of health and happiness.'

The Centre emphasises that

they do not treat physical disease but by bringing about a state of mind that is conducive to health and happiness, the whole system can respond positively, and one's own natural healing process then has a chance to begin.

BRIEF HISTORY

Bach flower remedies were discovered by an eminent physician, Dr Edward Bach, who dedicated his life to the healing of the sick and was determined in his quest to discover a harmless and simple means. He recognised seven major emotional states and then identified 38 negative states and formulated a Bach flower remedy for each state. In addition he devised a Rescue Remedy. The Rescue Remedy is a combination of five Bach flower remedies: rock rose, impatiens, clematis, Star of Bethlehem, and cherry plum. It is described as assisting a person to cope with every day situations such as an examination or driving test, a wedding, going to the dentist or traffic jams. The remedies are taken in water.

Dr Bach lived at Mount Vernon for the last two years of his life and the Bach Centre is now the place where the remedies are prepared. In 1933 he invited Nelsons to handle the bottling and sale of the remedies and they are still doing so.

The remedies are considered completely safe, but scientific evidence supporting their effectiveness or how they purport to work is not yet available. However practitioners and users have anecdotal evidence as to their value.

Other groups have developed flower remedies and an article by Don Dennis provides a good review of the many books covering this subject.[1]

REGISTRATION AND TRAINING

The Bach flower remedies are intended primarily for self-help. However practitioners have been trained as Bach Counsellors to provide personal advice. A list of names is available from the Centre. Workshops and seminars are provided at various venues. Practitioner training courses are provided for practitioners who have a professional practice. Applicants must be suitably qualified in their own profession. The training takes five months to complete and is arranged in three parts, the first takes place at the Centre, the second and third are by correspondence.

DEFINITIONS OF STANDARDS OF COMPETENCE

Quality standards

The control and responsibility for the production of the remedies has remained in the hands of personal assistants and successors to Dr Bach and of the Nelsons. A quality statement issued by the Dr Edward Bach Centre and the Nelsons guarantees that the preparation of Bach flowers both adheres to Dr Bach's unique instructions and also meets the highest UK and world-wide quality standards. The bottling plant is licensed and regularly inspected by the UK medicines inspectorate.

Rules on professional conduct

Practitioners recognised by the Bach Centre agree to follow a Code of ethics and practice.

LAWS RELATING TO THE THERAPY

Flower remedies could come under the provisions of the Medicines Act 1968 if claims are made about them which bring them under the definition of a medicinal product, unless they are exempt under section 12 of the Act (see Chapters 5 and 26).

The preparation and labelling of the Bach remedies is declared to be in accordance with the regulations. The label states that the dilution of the ingredients is one part in 100 000, referred to as a 5X dilution or 0.001%. Brandy is used as a preservative and is referred to as grape alcohol.

SITUATIONS WITH LEGAL SIGNIFICANCE

A rose by any other name

Situation 1   A rose by any other name
During a visit to Hong Kong, Mary saw for sale a suitcase containing all 38 of the Bach remedies and purchased it for what she considered a reasonable price. She has now discovered that she has been the subject of a fraud. Does the Centre have any right of action on her behalf?

Like so many proprietary products, it would not be surprising if fake bottles were offered of the flower remedies. Mary has a right of breach of contract, but it would be difficult for her to exercise it, unless she was to return to Hong Kong and trace the seller. The Centre would also have rights under International laws, but the cost in implementing these against the manufacturers may be extremely high and the likely success uncertain.

Situation 2   Not the correct result
A purchaser of the guide to flower remedies and the products claims that they have not been effective in her treating her friends and neighbours. Is the seller liable for her failure?

No harm has occurred so there is no potential action in negligence. There may be liability under the contract, depending on its express and implied terms, there may also be a remedy under the Sale of Goods Act, again depending on what promises were made. The purchaser would have to bring the action, since it was her contract with the seller (the doctrine of privity applies see Chapter 4). Her friends etc. would only have an action against her, if she charged for the services and it was an agreement intending to create legal relations (see Chapter 4) or if any of them could claim that she caused them harm as a result of her negligence.

CONCLUSIONS

There appears to be little research evidence supporting the clinical effectiveness of flower remedies, but many anecdotal tales are available of their working for individual clients. Perhaps if an understanding of how homeopathy works is ever discovered, this would have great implications for the use of flower remedies.

Questions and Exercises

---

1. To what extent do you consider that the purchase of all health products should come under the oversight of the Medicines Control Agency?
2. Is there any justification for including the knowledge of natural herbs and flowers as part of the basic syllabus of all medical students?

REFERENCES

1. Dennis D 1997 The New Flower Essences: A review of books from around the world. Caduceus 35

Chiropractic

DEFINITION

Chiropractic is an independent branch of medicine which specialises in mechanical disorders of joints, particularly those of the spine. The term is derived from two Greek words: 'cheir' (hand) and 'praktikos' (to use) and means treatment by hand or manipulation. It is seen as complementary to conventional medicine and not as an alternative, patients often being referred by their GPs to chiropractors for such problems as back pain and sciatica, tension headaches, neck, shoulder and arm pain and for other joint and muscle pains. Patients may thus be treated by their GPs with prescribed medications such as analgesics, non-steroidal anti-inflammatory drugs (NSAID) or muscle relaxants concurrently with treatment by a chiropractor to whom the GP has referred them.

BRIEF HISTORY

Chiropractic is one of the professions specialising in complementary therapy which has been successful in achieving state recognition and registration. Chiropractic itself was founded over a hundred years ago in the USA by a Canadian, Daniel David Palmer.

In America there has been considerable hostility to chiropractic from orthodox medicine but in September 1987 a federal judge ruled that the American Medical Association had violated anti trust rules and caused an 'unreasonable restraint of trade' by 'orchestrating a campaign to eliminate the chiropractice profession' through boycotts, denials of reimbursement or hospital privileges, and rules forbidding doctors to refer patients to chiropractors or work with them. The judge then ordered the American Medical Association to inform its members within 30 days, as well as publishing in its journal, that doctors were free to associate with chiropractors if this seemed to be in the best interests of the patient.[1]

The British Chiropractic Association (BCA) was founded in 1925 and is the largest voluntary registering body for chiropractors in the UK. The BCA was a founder member of the European Chiropractors Union which was founded in 1932.

As well as the BCA, there are three other Chiropractic Associations: The British Association for Applied Chiropractic; the McTimoney Chiropractic Association and the Scottish. The development of these is explained.

The British Chiropractic Association adopted a policy of not establishing a school of chiropractic in Europe until they were satisfied that standards comparable to the Palmer School in the USA could be achieved. This policy led to dissension within the Association and some of the Association members started to undertake informal teaching. Dr Mary Walker of the Palmer School tutored one of her patients, John McTimoney in the toggle recoil technique. John McTimoney developed this technique and founded in 1972 the Oxford McTimoney Chiropractic School. His pupils founded the McTimoney Chiropractic School to teach this method. This led to the establishment of the McTimoney Chiropractic Association.

The British Association for Applied Chiropractic was formed from the work of Hugh Corley who founded the Witney School of Chiropractic which employed the Corley method, a development of the McTimoney technique.

In preparation for the implementation of the Chiropractors Act and the state registration of chiropractors all these associations formed in 1991 the Chiropractic Registration Steering Group (CRSG) to provide a clear statement of the views of the profession on what is the currently minimum acceptable standards of safe and competent chiropractic practice in the UK. The recommendations of the CRSG on competence are discussed below.

In 1979 the British Chiropractors Association made a formal request to join the Professions Supplementary to Medicine. They were refused and despite an appeal to the Privy Council the refusal was upheld. In the House of Lords the Council of the Professions Supplementary to Medicine was severely criticised:

The Council acted in the spirit of a monopolist, the mean, narrow exclusive spirit of a medical trade union, slamming the door on specialists who might tackle some infirmities better than the general practitioners or even surgeons themselves.[2]

Ultimately the value of chiropractic has been recognised by the passing in 1994 of the Chiropractors' Act (see below).

The BMA has praised as commendable the willingness of those practising chiropractic methods to submit to research whereby patients with low back pain were allocated randomly between chiropractic and orthodox treatment.[3]

REGISTRATION AND TRAINING

The Anglo European College of Chiropractic in Bournemouth is the only college recognised by the BCA in this country as meeting the international requirements for chiropractic education. Colleges overseas which are recognised are principally in the United States, Canada and Australasia.

The four year full time degree course leading to the award of BSc in Chiropractic was approved in 1987 by the Council for National Academic Awards and following the dissolution of the CNAA the degree course is now validated through the University of Portsmouth of which the Anglo-European College of Chiropractic is an independent associate college.

The working party set up by the King's Fund and chaired by Sir Thomas Bingham (which prepared Chiropractic for state registration (see below)) recommended that the minimum standards for education and training should be the equivalent of the European Council of Chiropractic Education as at January 1992. Appendix 11 of its report[5] sets out the main areas and a summary is shown in Box 22.1.

Box 22.1   European Council on Chiropractic Education (ECCE)

Minimum educational standards:
1. Accreditation procedures
2. Chiropractic education
    - Pre-chiropractic studies
    - Chiropractic studies
    - Post-graduate studies
3. Evaluation of the chiropractic student
4. Mature students
5. Other prospective students

The working party recommended the formation of the following committees to be set up by the General Council:

- Education Committee
- Investigating Committee
- Professional Conduct Committee
- Health Committee

DEFINITIONS OF STANDARDS OF COMPETENCE

Factors leading to the Chiropractors Act

Under section 62 of the NHS and Community Care Act 1990 a committee of the Clinical Standards Advisory Group (CSAG) was set up to determine the standards of clinical care needed to deal effectively with low back pain.[4] The CSAG recommended the distinction between the vast majority of patients who have 'simple' backaches and those less commonly seen who have either nerve entrapment or serious underlying disease. The 'simple backache' patients account for the bulk of the service costs and are frequently referred inappropriately to hospital consultants, increasing waiting lists and generating chronic cases. The CSAG recommended:

- that there should be a shift of NHS resources to treatment in the community for these patients;
- that rest should be replaced by active rehabilitation;
- that there should be a discontinuation of referrals to orthopaedic or rheumatology specialists for 'simple backache' and instead patients should be given specialist attention by physiotherapy, osteopathy and chiropractic in the community;
- there should be a multi-disciplinary back pain service for those who did not respond to treatment after six months.

The Chiropractic Registration Steering Group (CRSG) invited King Edward's Hospital Fund for London, which had appointed Sir Thomas Bingham to chair a working party on osteopathy (see Chapter 33), to establish a similar working party for chiropractic. The report of this working party was published in May 1993 and formed the basis of a private member's Bill which led to the Chiropractors Act 1994 (see below).

The CRSG working party

The CRSG also set up a working party to report on current parameters for safe and competent practice in chiropractic.[6] The terms of reference were:

- To determine through a consensus process, the parameters that exist within the chiropractic profession of the UK for the safe and competent practice of chiropractic.
- To report and illustrate the parameters that constitute a competent chiropractor, whatever training that chiropractor may have received and with whichever voluntary association he or she may be registered.
- To report on competences that already exist within all three established chiropractic traditions in a manner that is representative of the profession as a whole.
- To determine the parameters in use for the safe and competent practice of certain methods of treatment that may present an increased risk to patients when performed by practitioners not formally trained in those methods, as shown by expert opinion or reputable published evidence, even though such methods of treatment may not be used by all three chiropractic traditions.

The CRSG considered standards under two broad categories: safety and competences.

Safety

The CRSG took as its starting point the definition of safety adopted by the Canadian Chiropractic Association[7]:

A judgment of the acceptability of any risk in a specific situation during the application of a specific procedure or group of procedures provided by an individual with specified and appropriate training.

The CRSG extended this definition to include safety in the environment of the chiropractor, premises, standards of hygiene etc. It also emphasised the importance of recording the underlying physical condition of the patients, recognising the importance of outcome of medical and clinical treatment and care and the significance of the patient's immediate family and wider cultural community. It acknowledged the different factors which arose when the patient was treated outside the normal consulting room and emphasised the importance of strict adherence to the relevant statutory and safety regulations.

Competences

The CRSG analysed competences under four headings:

- Assessment
- Treatment
- Advice
- Communication.

Assessment was discussed in relation to assessment before treatment, assessment in the course of treatment and the provision of specialist opinion.

Treatment was considered both in terms of the manual treatment techniques: chiropractic adjustment, mobilisation and manipulative competences and also in terms of education, exercise, nutrition and counselling which were all seen as therapeutic options in chiropractic.

Advice was seen as an integral part of any treatment programme and the objects of advice were identified. The advice could include:

- the prescription of a programme of exercises;
- advice in such areas of lifestyle, occupation, ergonomics and nutrition; and
- where a patient's condition requires treatment outside a practitioner's competence, advice to consult his or her general medical practitioner or other health care professional.

Communication with patients, other health care professionals, with legal and other regulatory bodies and the general public are also analysed.

RULES ON PROFESSIONAL CONDUCT

Members of the BCA subscribe to a Code of Ethics and Disciplinary Procedure which the BCA hoped would form the baseline for the General Chiropractic Council when it was established. In addition to the Code of Ethics the BCA had published in 1990 a Code of Publicity to the provision of Chiropractic Services. This covered the topics shown in Box 22.2.

INSURANCE COVER AND PROFESSIONAL INDEMNITY

The Chiropractors Act 1994 has an identical provision to section 37 Osteopaths Act 1993 relating to professional indemnity insurance (see Chapter 33). There is no duty for the General Council to consult the professions before making rules under this section.

Box 22.2   BCA Code of Publicity

Introduction:
  Publicity
  Interpretation and scope
  Commencement of Code

General Rules:
  Legality
  Decency
  Honesty
  Truthful presentation
  British Code of Advertising Practice
  Member to be identified

Specific Rules:
  Claims to specialisation or particular expertise
  Success rate
  Confidentiality
  Comparisons and criticisms of services
  Statements as to charges
  Physical details of publicity
  Professional announcements etc.
  Stands at exhibitions
  Joint publicity
  Members' responsibility for publicity

Unacceptable practices:
  Unsolicited direct approaches
  Inability to provide publicised services
  Unprofessional claims

Breaches of the code

LEGAL PROVISIONS

The Chiropractors Act 1994

The Chiropractors Act 1994 follows almost exactly the provisions for osteopaths set out in the Osteopaths Act 1993 which is considered in Chapter 33. The section headings are listed below.

A. *Council and Registration provisions*:

1. General Council and its committees
2. Registrar of chiropractors
3. Full registration
4. Conditional registration
5. Provisional registration
6. Registration: supplemental provision
7. Suspension of registration
8. Restoration to the register after having been struck off
9. Access to the register etc.
10. Fraud or error in relation to registration

B. *Professional education*
11. Education Committee
12. Visitors
13. The standard of proficiency
14. Recognition of qualifications
15. Recognition of qualification: supplemental
16. Withdrawal of recognition
17. Post-registration training
18. Information to be given by institutions

C. *Professional Conduct and fitness to practise*
19. The Code of Practice
20. Professional conduct and fitness to practise
21. Interim suspension powers of the Investigating committee
22. The Professional Conduct Committee
23. The Health Committee
24. Interim Suspension powers of the Professional Conduct Committee and the Health Committee
25. Revocation of interim suspension orders
26. Investigation of allegations: procedural rules
27. Legal assessors
28. Medical assessors

D. *Appeals*
29. Appeal from the Registrar
30. Appeal from the Health Committee
31. Appeal from the PCC

E. *Offences, monopoly and miscellaneous provisions*
32. Offences
33. Competition and anti-competitive practices
34. Default powers of the Privy Council
35. Rules
36. Exercise of powers of the Privy Council
37. Professional Indemnity Insurance
38. Data protection and access to personal health information
39. Supply of video recordings for use in training to be exempted supply
40. Exemption from provisions about rehabilitation of offenders
41. Financial provisions
42. Amendments to the Osteopaths Act 1993
43. Interpretation and commencement provisions.

Schedules to the Act cover the General Council, the Statutory Committees and transitional provisions.

Section 39 of the Chiropractors Act 1994 exempts video recordings made for use in the training of chiropractors and osteopaths from the Video Recordings Act 1984 under section 3(11) of that Act (see Chapter 33).

Sections relating to the Council and registration

The Act's provisions on the Council and registration are summarised in more detail in Box 22.3.

Box 22.3 General Chiropractic Council and registration

Section 1 The creation of a General Chiropractic Council consisting of chiropractors and representatives of the public.
Section 2 The General Council is responsible for the regulation, development and promotion of the whole profession and the establishment and maintenance of a statutory register of chiropractors.
Section 3 Inclusion on the register will be based on the holding of a recognised chiropractic qualification which the General Council recognises as providing the chiropractor with the necessary skills for the safe and competent practice of chiropractic.
Section 4 Transitional arrangements to protect those who were already practising chiropractic lawfully, safely and competently.

DEFINITIONS FOR PURCHASING CONTRACTS

The speed with which complementary therapies adjust to the new structure and the internal market of the NHS is likely to have a major impact upon the purchase of their services by health authorities and GP fundholders.

In response to the new NHS structure the British Chiropractic Association has published an excellent guide *Chiropractic, Back Pain and the NHS*[8] and also explicit advice in a booklet for purchasers and providers.[9] The notes give an easy guide to chiropractors on how to start a pilot year with a fundholding or another purchasing authority and how to use the guide to prepare a contract and to consult a solicitor. The booklet covers the topics set out in Box 22.4.

Box 22.4 Guide to purchasing and providers for chiropractic, back pain and the NHS

1. Role of chiropractic in the treatment of back pain;
2. Chiropractic in the NHS
3. Models for communication between chiropractors and referring GPs
4. Accessing chiropractic: 2 models for purchasing
5. 2 economic models for chiropractic in the NHS
6. Limitations of the 2 models
7. The long-term effects of chiropractic
8. Purchasing chiropractic in a pilot year
9. Other elements of quality assurance

Appendices to the booklet whose contents are listed in Box 22.4 include the epidemiology of chiropractic, process audit requirements in a chiropractic back pain service and a sample contract.

SITUATIONS WITH LEGAL SIGNIFICANCE

Retaining the patient

Situation 1   Retaining the patient
A GP refers a patient to a chiropractor who on examination discovers that the patient is suffering from a nerve root entrapment. The chiropractor is anxious to retain the work because of his financial problems and neither refers the patient back to the GP nor on to a neurologist. After several months of continuing pain, the patient seeks alternative advice and discovers the underlying reason for his pain. He is now intending to sue the chiropractor for breach of contract and for negligence.

The chiropractor in this situation has clearly failed to follow the Code of Professional Conduct. He has, presumably for financial reasons, retained the patient when professionally he should have realised the limitations of his professional expertise in relation to the patient's problems. The patient would have the right of the following actions:

• He could sue the chiropractor in negligence for causing him additional pain and suffering and failing to refer him on to a doctor or other professional at an earlier stage. This action may not be worthwhile, depending upon the amount of compensation which would be due to the patient and whether the chiropractor is properly insured.

• He could sue the chiropractor for breach of contract. In failing to use appropriate care and referring the patient on, the chiropractor could be regarded as being in breach of an implied term that he should be using all reasonable care and skill in the treatment of the patient. There may also be liability under the Supply of Goods and Services Act 1982 (see Chapter 4). It is relevant here to consider whether the patient was paying the chiropractor himself or if the reference was under the NHS.

• Refer the chiropractor to the Professional Conduct Committee of the General Council for Chiropractors.

• Seek to obtain alternative dispute resolution between himself and the chiropractor.

Negligent information

Situation 2   Negligent information
A chiropractor is asked by a patient what is the difference between an osteopath, a physiotherapist and a chiropractor. He fails to inform the patient correctly and permits him to think that they are all the same. If the patient is then informed of the correct situation by a physiotherapist would the patient have any cause of action?

Liability can exist for information which is given out negligently as it can for negligent activities. However the person suing for negligence has to prove harm. In this situation, the patient has been told wrong information by the chiropractor, but has he suffered harm? It may be that he has been going to the chiropractor for too long and inappropriately in which case he could claim loss of money or increased suffering because he was not receiving the appropriate treatment. If, however, harm cannot be established, then there would not be a successful civil court action for negligence. The chiropractor could of course be reported to the Professional Conduct Committee for Chiropractors.

Nature of services

> **Situation 3   Nature of services**
>
> A GP purchases the services of a chiropractor on a part-time basis. The chiropractor carelessly allows the patient to fall from the consulting couch. The patient fractures her pelvis and is seeking compensation. Is the GP liable?

If the GP has used the services of the chiropractor on a sessional basis, but the chiropractor remains as a self-employed professional then the GP has not become the employer of the chiropractor. The chiropractor will be personally accountable to the patient for any harm that the patient has suffered. Thus if the patient can prove that the fall was the result of the negligence of the chiropractor and the fracture is a reasonably foreseeable consequence of that negligence, then the chiropractor through insurers would be liable to pay compensation for the harm caused. The GP would not be liable, unless he was somehow directly involved in the incident (e.g. he may have provided the couch and failed to ensure that it was reasonably safe – he would then be liable as occupier of the premises). If on the other hand the GP has employed the chiropractor, then the GP would become vicariously liable for the negligent actions of the chiropractor.

Faulty diagnosis

> **Situation 4   Faulty diagnosis**
>
> A chiropractor failed to diagnose that the client was suffering from a brain tumour. After six months treatment the client died and a post mortem revealed the tumour. Would the chiropractor be accountable to the relatives for this?

The answer to this question hinges on what could reasonably be expected of a chiropractor in this situation. Would a reasonable chiropractor have diagnosed this brain tumour or sent the client back to the GP for tests to be undertaken? Was the client referred initially by a GP who had failed to diagnose the condition. What would have been the reasonable action of a GP? Even if fault can be proved in this way, those seeking compensation would also have to prove that had the diagnosis been properly made, then action could have been taken to prevent the brain tumour being fatal. This might not have been possible. In addition to possible civil litigation, the relatives could bring a complaint before the professional conduct machinery of chiropractic.

CONCLUSIONS

Chiropractors, like osteopaths, have succeeded where a lot of other complementary therapists would like to follow: they have become a state registered profession. They are probably not yet, however, seen as entirely within the sphere of orthodox medicine, and there is still a long way to go in ensuring acceptance of the benefits of this profession.

Daniel Redwood[10] states:

There is an immediate and pressing need to broaden lines of communication between the chiropractic and medical professions, both on a one-to-one basis and in small and large groups, with the goal of offering a cooperative effort to all patients. Each side must learn to recognise its own strengths and weaknesses, as well as those of the other. No one has all the answers. Although chiropractors have clear guidelines for referring to medical doctors, neither the medical profession as a whole nor its various specialty groups have developed formal guidelines for referring patients to chiropractors.

There is therefore still a considerable way to go before chiropractors can be satisfied that their full potential is realised by those who practise within the orthodox fields of health care. Further comparative research on the clinical effectiveness of chiropractic in contrast with orthodox medicine may well further its progress.

Questions and Exercises

1. A person calls himself a chiropractor before the implementation of the 1994 Act and after the implementation of the Act. What, if any, is the difference?
2. To what extent will state registration of chiropractic change the way in which chiropractors fulfil their role?
3. How can the public awareness of the significance of state registration be improved?
4. Design a research project to show the clinical effectiveness of chiropractic.

REFERENCES

1. Dunea G 1988 Letter from ... Chicago. Matters of turf. British Medical Journal 296: 277
2. Hansard Chiropractic and the NHS 21 November 1979 Column 248
3. British Medical Association 1993 Complementary Medicine: New approaches to good practice. Oxford University Press, Oxford (citing research by Meade TW *et al* Low back pain of mechanical origin: randomised comparison of chiropractic and hospital out-patient treatment. British Medical Journal 300(1990)1: 431–7
4. Clinical Standards Advisory Group 1994 Back Pain: a report of a CSAG committee on back pain. HMSO, London
5. King Edward's Hospital Fund for London 1993 Report of a Working Party on Chiropractic Chaired by Sir Thomas Bingham. King's Fund, London
6. The Chiropractic Registration Steering Group Working Party 1995 On Current Parameters for Safe and Competent Practice in Chiropractic, Chairman Professor Tony Atkinson. CRSG, Braintree

7. Clinical Guidelines for Chiropractic Practice in Canada. Supplement to the Journal of the Canadian Chiropractic Association 38(1) March 1994
8. British Chiropractic Association 1994 Chiropractic, back pain and the NHS: notes for chiropractors. BCA, Reading
9. Breen A 1994 Chiropractic, back pain and The National Health Service: A guide for purchasers and providers. CA, Reading
10. Redwood D 1996 Chiropractic, Chapter 7 In: Micozzi M (ed) Fundamentals of complementary and alternative medicine. Churchill Livingstone, New York

23

Colour and environmental therapies

DEFINITION

Colour is the energy for healing as the whole of the human body, is contracted light. When we know how each colour of the rainbow can help to balance our health we can, indeed, use this as a complementary medical treatment.[1]

BRIEF HISTORY

The influence of colour on behaviour has been recognised since the time of the Greeks. Theories relating to the link between an individual's aura and its response to specific colours each of which have their own vibration have been developed. Colour therapy has been practised in this country since the 1950s. Theo Gimbel, who founded the International Association of Colour Therapy which operates as an umbrella organisation, heads the Hygeia College of Colour Therapy, which is a registered charity (see below).

Colour products

Various organisations promote the use of colour as a therapy, selling products and consultations. Thus Aura-Soma was established in 1984 by a pharmacist, Vicky Wall. Its aim is to help people restore the natural balance needed for a healthy life and to gain an understanding of their potential and direction in the world. Aura-Soma has over 100 colour combinations and clients put a drop on a tissue to inhale, or to use for moisturising the skin. Clients select the colours, which have different meanings, such as 'challenges' and 'get up and go'. Clients can have consultations about the meanings of the colours.

Another product, Avatara Colour Therapy, has a range of 52 bottles of dual coloured liquids.

Courses are available to learn and practice colour therapy. Colour Choice uses a spectrum of 12 colours from which the client chooses three and rejects one, each choice having a specific meaning.

Hiraeth feng shui

Another therapy concerned with environment is Hiraeth Feng Shui. This therapy looks at the environment as a source of healing. Consultants give advice on how the healing energies of the home could be released and as a result relationships, health and prosperity can be improved.[2] Leaflets on Feng Sui state that

The plan of your house affects your behaviour, relationships, health and prosperity and the walls that surround you affect your breathing and therefore your vitality. The walls are the skin, giving protection and comfort. The door is the mouth – providing the nourishment, and the windows are the eyes.

Snoezelen

Another total environment therapy has been designed to alter moods by a variety of different mood enhancing equipment. One proprietary name associated with this development is that of Snoezelen (from the two Dutch words meaning 'sniff' and 'doze'). Its aim is to create an environment which makes the best use of the senses: taste, touch, smell, sight and sound. Its effects on concentration and responsiveness in people with profound multiple handicaps has been researched[3] and it has also been used as part of a strategy for the management of chronic pain.[4]

REGISTRATION AND TRAINING

The Hygeia Colour courses have been running since 1967. The curriculum of basic colour therapy training includes 75 hours of teaching over a period of 12 months. Five essays of 2–3000 words are required plus reading from a recommended book list. Research and study requires a minimum of 15 hours per week. A dissertation of 6–8000 words is followed by the advanced course of 112 hours, of which 30 hours are with supervised teaching and the rest of the time consists of practicals, interviews and written examination. A probationary year is required during which time, twelve case histories must be submitted. Successful students are awarded the Hygeia Diploma of Colour Therapy (H.DipC.Th) and are placed on the Hygeia Register of Colour Practitioners. After two years work, graduates may apply to the Institute for Complementary Medicine (see Chapter 6) for membership and to be placed on the British Register for Complementary Practitioners (BRCP). They may also become members of the International Association for Colour Therapy (IACT). A Hygeia Fellowship can be obtained by graduates on successful completion of a 25–30 000 word thesis on research into colour therapy. Successful fellows can teach colour therapy.

The Institute for Complementary Medicine is developing, in association with its affiliated members, national training standards based on NVQ criteria. It anticipates that treatment involving the use of colour will be divided into

- those offering advice on dress sense, make-up and decor (beautician)
- those using the use of colour visualisation and treatment by light at varying degrees of saturation or
- the scientific diagnostic appraisal of the cause of disease and the wavelengths required to correct the imbalance.

Definitions of standards of competence are set by the Hygeia College, which encourages its students and practitioners to develop research based practice.

RULES ON PROFESSIONAL CONDUCT AND INSURANCE

The practitioners qualified through the Hygeia College who then become members of the Institute for Complementary Medicine are required to follow the latter's Code of Conduct. In addition practitioners who are members of the International Association for Colour Therapy follow its Code of Ethics and Practice for Colour Healers and Colour Practitioners. Practitioners are required to sign the 36 clause document setting out the principles which must be followed.

The first clause of the International Association for Colour Therapy is

I will practise only those therapies for which I am registered and insured for professional indemnity and third party liability.

LAWS WHICH APPLY

Those organisations which sell colour bottles and other products are subject to the Sale of Goods legislation (see Chapter 4), the liability of the manufacturer under the *Donoghue* v. *Stephenson* principle (see Chapter 3) and the Consumer Protection Act 1987 (see Chapter 13).

SITUATIONS WITH LEGAL SIGNIFICANCE

Not fit for its purpose

Situation 1   Not fit for its purpose
James purchased 52 bottles advertised for use in colour therapy at a cost of over £350 for his fiancée. She tried them out and believed that she had had no benefit from them. Can James get his money back?

James' chance of success will depend upon any promises given by the supplier at the time he made the purchase. These promises may be set out in literature as well as stated by the seller. If the goods fail to match up with these undertakings, then there could be evidence of a breach of contract and also a breach of the terms implied into the contract by the Sale of Goods Act 1979. If bottles are sold following a consultation, then the contract may come under the Sale of Goods and Services Act 1982 (see Chapter 4).

Unfair competition

Situation 2 Unfair competition

Spencer, who is a qualified practitioner of colour therapy and has been involved in colour therapy for over ten years, has discovered that a rival competitor is undercutting him and taking his business. He is sure that his rival has not tested out the products, is not trained as a colour therapist and is making false claims. What remedies does he have?

Until there is a system of state registration for colour therapists, those who have been qualified have little protection against those who have not been through a similar training. Public education is essential to ensure that they understand the different types of training and qualification. Clearly if the rival was writing defamatory statements about him that is actionable. Spencer would have to prove that a statement was untrue, has been made to a person other than himself and would lower his reputation in the minds of right thinking people.

Epileptic fits

Situation 3 Epileptic fits

Angela paid to see a consultant about colour therapy. She was shown different colours and reacted violently to one, with a grand mal epileptic fit. She had never suffered from one before.

This situation is always a concern for the therapist when it appears that the therapy triggers a condition which the client was not aware she suffered from. It could be argued here that, if this was the very first fit, the therapist could not be held responsible, unless there were some simple tests that any reasonable therapist would have carried out to check for this particular propensity.

CONCLUSION

Like so many areas of complementary therapy, this is a growth area but more research is needed to underpin the claims which are made of its healing powers.

Questions and Exercises

1. What research project could be carried out to test the workings of colour therapy?
2. Do you consider that the law should protect a person who redecorated her house on the principles recommended by a consultant in colour and environmental therapy if the new scheme did not appear to 'work'?

REFERENCES

1. Taken from the profile of Theo Gimbel published by the Hygeia College of Colour Therapy.
2. Leaflet advertising Hiraeth Feng Sui
3. Ashby M, Lindsay WR, Pitcaithly D, Broxholme S, Geelen N 1995 Snoezelen: Its effects on concentration and responsiveness in people with profound multiple handicaps. British Journal of Occupational Therapy 58(7): 303–6
4. Schofield P 1996 Snoezelen: Its potential for people with chronic pain. Complementary Therapies in Nursing and Midwifery 2(1): 9–12

Dowsing and radionics

DEFINITIONS

Dowsing (also known as radiesthesia) and radionics are based on the theory that all matter emits radiation. This can be studied and conclusions drawn which can assist in medical diagnosis.

Using specially designed instruments, and dowsing ability or ESP, the Radionic practitioner is able to detect the causes and location at the root of any dysfunction. The energy flow can then be directed to make the necessary correction irrespective of distance between patient and practitioner.[1]

The practitioner will therefore study a wide range of matter associated with the patient including blood, hair, nail clippings. These can be studied in the absence of the patient. The dowser uses a pendulum which is swung over the material or the patient.

DOWSING

Background

The British Society of Dowsers, whilst accepting that dowsing is most commonly associated with finding water by interpreting the reactions obtained with a forked stick, states that dowsing is widely used for other purposes including medical diagnosis and healing.

The Society considers that basically anyone can dowse. A few people do find difficulty in obtaining responses whilst at the other end of the spectrum lie the very gifted dowsers. Most people can develop that art by practice and perseverance.

The British Society of Dowsers was founded in 1933 to spread information among members and the public on the use and value of dowsing in all its forms and to keep a register of practising members. The Society is a registered Charity. In 1987 it became incorporated as a company limited by guarantee. The activities of the Society are set out in Box 24.1.

The Psionic Medical Society formed of doctors and dentists make use of dowsing in their work.

Box 24.1   Activities of the British Society of Dowsers

1. To keep an active watching brief on all parliamentary developments within the UK and the EC in so far as they may affect the role and activity of the practising dowser.
2. To maintain links with international organisations concerned with dowsing and radiesthesia.
3. To foster development of local dowsing groups.
4. To publish a quarterly journal.
5. To keep a register of practising dowsers.
6. To hold public lectures, residential congresses and short courses.
7. To run a lending library.
8. To arrange for manufacture of dowsing equipment.
9. To sell books.

Registration

Membership is open to all who are interested in dowsing no matter what degree of skill they may possess.

There are no specific qualifications in order to be on the Register of members. One difficulty in proving competence is that the effect of dowsing has not been proved scientifically. Some may learn how to do it wrongly. Presumably it could be said that if a particular dowser is successful in diagnosing correctly then, competence is proved.

RADIONICS

This is the detection of disharmonics or distortion in the patient's energy patterns and the directing of corrective energy patterns by the use of various instruments.

The Radionic Association was formed in 1943 and incorporated in 1960 as a Company limited by Guarantee.

Registration and training

There are three classifications of membership of the Radionics Association:

- qualified fellows, members or licentiates
- associate members and
- Honorary Fellows or members.

The details are explained in the Association's Memorandum and Articles of Association. The School of the Radionics Association runs introductory weekend courses and a three year part-time training course.

Article 7 of the Association requires a person to satisfy the following conditions for eligibility as a member:

- over 21 years of age
- has been a licentiate for a period of not less than one year and
- has passed such oral and/or written examination or other test as is prescribed by the Council.

Article 8 enables the Council to dispense with the requirements under article 7 if the following conditions are satisfied.

- the person is at least 25 years old,
- has been an associate member for at least a year
- has been practising Radionics for a period of not less than four years immediately preceding the date of the application
- has by practical experience acquired such knowledge of the practice of Radionics in any of its branches as in the opinion of the Council qualifies him for Membership
- has satisfied such conditions as may be prescribed by Council as qualification for membership
- has proved to the Council's satisfaction that he is conversant with the rules and regulations of the Association, the ethics of Radionic practice and the law relating to Radionics
- the records kept in connection with his practice are of an adequate standard and
- his personal standing is in the opinion of the Council such as to qualify him for membership

Rules on professional conduct

Rules of Conduct are laid down in the Articles of Association of the Radionic Association, Articles 25–36. Article 37 prescribes the rules relating to discipline for any breach of the Articles. In addition as a member of the Confederation of Healing Organisations (CHO), the Radionic Association uses the Code of Conduct approved by the CHO. This Code of Conduct was adopted by the CHO from the British Complementary Medicine Association on 1 April 1993. Appendices have been added by the CHO.

Insurance cover and professional indemnity

Article 26 of the Articles of Association requires every qualified member to hold professional indemnity insurance cover, and any member can be required by Council to produce the insurance certificate. The Council can waive this requirement at its discretion for overseas members unable to obtain insurance cover at reasonable rates. The CHO emphasises that compliance with the provisions of the Code and the Appendices to the Code of Conduct added by the CHO is mandatory. Insurance cover is voided by non-compliance.

Laws relating to the therapy

In a memorandum issued by the Radionic Association the following areas of law are considered relevant to members. These are listed together with the relevant chapter number in this book.

- Law and ethics – Chapter 2
- Criminal law – Chapter 5
- Prohibited appellations and functions – Chapter 6
- Fraudulent practice – Chapter 5
- Advertising – Chapter 5
- False or misleading statements – Chapters 4 and 5
- Treatment of children – Chapter 9
- Professional negligence – Chapter 3
- The Apothecaries Act – not covered
- Oral remedies – Chapter 5 (Medicines Act) and Chapter 27
- Notifiable Diseases – Chapter 10
- Post Mortem – not covered
- Fees and Accounts – Chapter 4
- Homoeopathy – Chapter 27
- Legal advice – Chapter 2

SITUATIONS WITH LEGAL SIGNIFICANCE

Unseemly behaviour

Situation 1   Unseemly behaviour
A client reported that she saw her practitioner in Radionics coming out of a pub in a distinctly unruly manner. The acquaintance she was with recognised the therapist and mocked the client for taking part in sessions of dubious scientific validity. Does the client have any protection?

Clearly in this situation the practitioner has failed to act in the manner required by Article 35 of the Radionic Association. The client clearly believes that her own reputation has been damaged by her involvement with the practitioner. She has the right to complain to the Association and would be required to give evidence on the way in which the member has failed to comply with the Articles of the Association. In its commentary on the Articles relating to Conduct, the Radionic Association states that whilst

a member's private life is for the most part outside the jurisdiction of the Association … Prima facie evidence of drunkenness, for example, might indicate habits which were a danger to a member's patients and discreditable to the profession of Radionics and might thus give rise to an enquiry.

Misdiagnosis

Situation 2   Misdiagnosis
A parent took her daughter of 8 years to a dowser. The child had been complaining of headaches and the dowser suggested that the child probably needed to wear spectacles. When the parent saw the optometrist, she was advised that urgent medical attention was required because there were signs of a tumour.

Whether or not the dowser would be held responsible for failing to detect the brain tumour, depends upon what promises were made by the dowser as to her abilities and the reasonableness of the parents in relying upon dowsing for a diagnosis of their child's headaches. The parents may be considered to be at fault in failing to obtain orthodox medical advice. If she were to die, manslaughter charges could be brought against the parents and also the dowser on the grounds that she was aiding and abetting parents in their failure to take reasonable care of their child.

Further, the Code of Professional Ethics of the Radionics Association make it clear, under Article 31, that a practitioner is not to perform functions of a registered medical practitioner:

administer general or local anaesthetic, perform an operation, prescribe medicines classified as dangerous drugs or make an internal physical examination.

Overcharging

> **Situation 3**   Overcharging
>
> A member of the Radionic Association developed a considerable reputation for his work in diagnosing ailments. Such was the demand for his services that he was able to charge £200 for a half hour session. Other members of the Radionic Association have complained to the Association that he is bringing the name of the Association into disrepute.

It could be argued on behalf of the member complained about that he is in fact bringing renown to the Association, since in other professions high fees are seen as a symbol of success and eminence. As far as the Association is concerned the Council only fixes the maximum fees of licentiates since these persons are newly qualified and relatively inexperienced. Fellows and Members are therefore able to make whatever fee arrangements they like with their patients. Possibly members may have more justification in attempting to bring disciplinary proceedings if no fees or very little was charged, thus preventing others from making a reasonable charge.

Fraud or true belief?

> **Case**   Fraud or true belief?
>
> In 1960 a person who had brought an instrument designed by George de la Warr sued him because he found that it did not work. The judge held that there was no fraud, since the defendant honestly believed it to work.

Had the contract contained an express term guaranteeing the effectiveness of the box, then the plaintiff may have won a case on breach of contract or under the previous Sale of Goods Act (see Chapter 4).

CONCLUSIONS

Unless clear scientific evidence is forthcoming to support the clinical effectiveness of this field of complementary therapies, it is unlikely to play a major part alongside orthodox medicine. Individual experiences of success will however continue to attract clients.

Questions and Exercises

1. Do you consider that dowsing and radionics could achieve state registration? What would be the advantages to the general public and to the practitioners if state registration were required?
2. In what circumstances do you consider that a practitioner in dowsing or radionics should be liable for failing to diagnose a serious medical condition?
3. In what ways do you consider that it would be possible to improve the research basis of dowsing and radionics?

REFERENCES

1. Booklet on Members of the Confederation of Healing Organisations. November 1996 CHO

25

Healing

DEFINITION

Healing has been defined as

the beneficial effect which healers in the Confederation of Healing Organisation (CHO) terms are believed to have on patients when, motivated by their own beliefs and following their normal practices, they administer healing in contact through the hands or at a distance by thought (or prayer) transference or by radionic instrument.[1]

The simple definition is 'to make well'.

A more complex definition is provided by the College of Healing in its Appendix III to the BCMA Code of Conduct.

To the extent that it occurs, healing is the transference of harmonising paraphysical energies. What energies are transferred depend upon the needs, beliefs, capabilities and procedures of the persons involved. Every living being is maintained by these energies which may be transferred in the presence of those concerned or at a distance.

Healing may be one individual to another or between groups and individuals or it may be self-induced.

Healing as a form of complementary or alternative therapy takes several different forms: Therapeutic touch, spiritualism, faith healing, reiki, crystal healing or simply healing. All forms postulate the existence of an energy force which can be used to 'heal' the client. In some therapies, this is linked with a particular religious faith. All forms are briefly discussed in this chapter.

Healing has been described by a practitioner as

A gentle and non-intrusive method of restoring balance, harmony, strength and well-being. It is a therapy that seeks to understand the conscious or subconscious pattern behind 'symptoms' be they physical, emotional or mental. Then through a careful process of unblocking, realigning and energising it seeks to alleviate the causes. The healing process is a subtle transference of universal energy that aims to re-establish the natural flow and balance within the client, replenishing their energy system.[2]

The concept of healing is not necessarily linked with a particular religion or philosophy and many practitioners may use healing in association with other forms of therapy such as crystal, massage or allergy therapy.

HEALING AND ITS SCIENTIFIC BASIS

Some might be appalled that any attempt at scientific principles should be applied to their faith or work of healing: by its very nature a religious or ethical belief is not susceptible to being proved according to the scientific principles of testing hypotheses. Thus a book such as *Here and Now*[3] gives accounts of 'stories' of individuals who have benefited from the workings of the Holy Spirit by means of Gestalt Therapy.

Some books such as Helen Graham's *The Magic Shop*[4] emphasise that

the art of healing throughout all ages and parts of the world is rooted in magic ... magic may be properly thought of as practical or applied mysticism.

Graham has however shown that many of the claims relating to meditation and its effect in inducing relaxation are supported by research.[5]

Research into the effects of healing on patients with chronic conditions is being conducted by seven GPs in Devon and publication of the results is awaited. It has recently been announced that the first Professor of Complementary Medicine in the world, Professor Ernst based at Exeter University, is receiving a grant of £45 000 donated by the Wellcome Trust to carry out research into healing. He is planning to conduct a controlled experiment to ascertain whether spiritual healers actually do achieve results. The placebo effect will be avoided by placing the healer behind a curtain, so that the patient will not know whether or not the healer is there and by using actors to imitate healers. It is hoped that the results will be published within a year.[6]

REGULATION OF THE HEALING PROFESSIONS

In spite of the difficulties of establishing the scientific basis of healing, it is important that patients are able to trust the integrity of those organisations and therapists who purport to provide healing services. The CHO thus provides an important service in protecting the patient.

Confederation of Healing Organisations

The CHO is an umbrella group for various organisations with a total membership of 11 000. Those within the organisation at the time of writing are listed in Box 25.1.

Box 25.1   Organisations in the CHO (1997)

- Association of Professional Healers
- Association for Therapeutic Healers
- The British Alliance of Healing Associations
- The College of Healing
- The CPS (College of Psychic Studies)
- Fellowship of Erasmus
- Greater World Spiritual Healing Fellowship
- The Healing Foundation of the R.T. Trust
- Maitreya School of Healing
- The National Federation of Spiritual Healers
- The Radionic Association
- Rainbow Healing Association
- Spiritualist Association of Great Britain
- Sufi Healing Order of Great Britain
- The White Eagle Lodge
- World Federation of Healing

There are probably no more than 7000 healers altogether in CHO; many join more than one organisation. It has supported the fundamental requirements for the protection of the patient laid down by the Junior Health Minister in 1986 requiring each member organisation to have the following:

- A mandatory Code of Conduct
- A disciplinary (and complaints) procedure to enforce the Code
- Minimum standards for entry into membership and training
- Public liability insurance cover for each healer, comparable to a GP's
- A facility for checking membership (e.g. a Register).

In addition the CHO has added to the requirements registration of the member associations with the Charity Commissioners and insisted that healing should take place as complementary to orthodox medicine, not as an alternative.

The CHO has done much to expand the availability of healing within the NHS and is also encouraging the use of research in healing.

The Code of Conduct

The CHO's Code of Conduct was originally written in the early 1980s in consultation with the Royal Colleges, the BMA and the GMC. It was used by the BCMA in the preparation of its Code which is now used by all its member organisations (see Chapter 6). The CHO now uses the BCMA Code with CHO appendices on matters relevant to healers. These include:

- healing and the law
- additional principles for healers
- treatment of animals (agreed with the Royal College of Veterinary Surgeons)
- the definition of healing
- notifiable diseases
- an equal opportunities policy.

The CHO emphasises that healers must not claim to cure, and they are forbidden to take responsibility for a medical diagnosis.

Training and education

The Vice Chairman of the CHO's training committee is responsible for co-ordinating competence based training in the National Federation of Spiritual Healers. The Chairman of the CHO's training committee Richard Booth, is development manager of the College of Healing (see below).

The CHO specifies minimum standards for entry, training, and includes two years supervised probation. Before acceptance as full healers, probationers must have their supervisor's recommendation and generate at least four certificates from patients.

The CHO aspires to create an NVQ in healing. To this end it has run a pilot study on competence based training at three levels and applied to develop National Occupational Standards in healing on the way to the qualification itself. Details are set out in a published booklet.[7]

Insurance

Professional indemnity cover is mandatory and the CHO has organised insurance for its members with an extremely low premium. This reflects the fact that the therapy is extremely low risk, especially since it is not invasive, does not require contact and can be done at a distance. It covers risks relating to injuries on the premises, being sued for healing activities undertaken on a voluntary basis. It also covers clients alleging sexual impropriety by any healer, but here cover will only provide defence up to the point of a court determining that a healer is guilty. The policy will not cover deliberate acts or any criminal acts, but will pay the costs of any successfully defended case. There are very few claims: in 16 years the CHO states that there has only been one successful claim as a result of a collapsing portable couch.

Member organisations

Of the member organisations, regulation details are given of only two, the College of Healing and the National Federation of Spiritual Healers, as an illustration of how the self-regulatory mechanism operates. Space does not permit a detailed account of all the members of the CHO listed in Box 25.1.

College of Healing

The College of Healing was formed as the result of a group of healers and doctors coming together in 1983. It has the aims shown in Box 25.2. It teaches in a non-denominational way. It is a member of the Confederation of Healing Organisations.

The College of Healing offers courses at different levels:

- Level 1 Introductory course in Healing
- Level 2 Foundation course in Healing

Box 25.2 Aims of the College of Healing

- To provide education, training and research
- To educate and inform the public and healthcare professionals about the nature of healing
- To train individuals in healing and self-development
- To train professional healers to teach healing
- To provide continuing professional development
- To research the nature and successes of healing
- To develop new and different healing techniques.

- Level 3 Basic Practitioner course in Healing
- Professional diploma course in Healing
- Post-graduate development course

The College of Healing has as one of its main aims (see Box 25.1) to research the nature and successes of healing.

As a member organisation of the British Complementary Medicine Association (BCMA) it has adopted the Code of Practice of that organisation for its own members (see Chapter 6 for details). In addition it has devised an appendix solely for members of the CHO's associations. It emphasises that compliance with the Code and the appendix is mandatory. Insurance cover is voided by non-compliance.

The appendix covers the topics shown in Box 25.3.

Box 25.3 Content of appendix to Code of Conduct for CHO

- The Healer must keep within the law
- The Healer must not offer clairvoyant reading during a healing session
- Healers sometimes say or do certain things because they are impressed to do so – they must apply reason and common sense to such impressions
- Healing must only be given in response to an invitation from the patient or their representative
- To avoid offending some patients healers must not raise the question of their religious beliefs unless this is invited by the patient
- When a healer is giving healing privately to a person of the opposite sex it is advisable for the healer to request the presence of a third party whose bona fides the healer and patient can accept

---

A second appendix to the BCMA Code of Conduct for CHO members is concerned with the treatment of animals. The Royal College of Veterinary Surgeons has recognised as ethically acceptable healing within the terms of this appendix. This requires healers to ensure that an animal has been examined by a veterinary surgeon before being treated with healing.

National Federation of Spiritual Healers

One of the largest member organisations of the CHO is the National Federation of Spiritual Healers. This has, as at July 1997, over 2000 probationers and almost

3500 full healer members. Full members have to satisfy certain criteria in including evidence of four successful healings. It is a charitable organisation formed for the achievement of the principles and objectives as defined in the articles of association. Article 2 states that

The object of the Federation is to serve the public good by the promotion of the study and practice of the art and science of spiritual healing.

Its current president is a general practitioner. At present major changes are taking place in the review of the Code of Practice and the Constitution.

Certain centres of healing are affiliated to the National Federation of Spiritual Healers. It is non-denominational. All members of the NFSH, healers and probationers, operating in the UK are automatically covered by the independent insurance policy upon their becoming members of NFSH. This policy only covers members when they are carrying out spiritual healing in accordance with the Code of Conduct. It does not cover the practice of other therapies. The Federation has recently arranged insurance cover with Bervale Mead which covers healing equipment, buildings and contents as well as healing activities.

Article 3 requires members of the Federation to acknowledge the principle that the paramount consideration in all healing activity is the welfare of the patient and healers should act in accordance with the Oath of Hippocrates.

LINKS WITH THE NHS

The GMC[8] permits a doctor to suggest or agree to a patient seeking help from a healer provided the doctor continues to give and to remain responsible for whatever medical treatment is considered necessary. (For further information on the attitude of the GMC to complementary therapy see Chapter 6.) The NFSH state that 1500 hospitals have agreed to the National Consumer Council Guide to Patients Rights[9] and this states that patients in some NHS hospitals can request healing providing the doctor treating the patient is told. The NFSH requests that any instances of refusal to refer a patient should be reported to it.

The input of healing into the NHS is increasing with over 70 GPs using the services of healers for their patients.

SPECIALIST FORMS OF HEALING

Therapeutic touch

Definition

Therapeutic Touch (TT) has been described as

a healing art (complementary therapy) that has been developed by a nurse (Dr Dolores Kreiger, Professor Emeritus New York University) for nurses. It is based on the nursing theory of Rogers' Science of Unitary Human Beings (SUHB) and is the most widely researched (by US nurses) of all the complementary therapies used by nurses.[10]

It is linked with other hand-mediated healing modalities, i.e. healing touch, polarity, reiki, jin shin, jyutsu, external qigong, touch for health, reflexology, acupressure and shiatsu massage.

Background

The theory underlying the principles of therapeutic touch can be found in Eastern Philosophies, which see humans and the environment as being inseparable and co-extensive with the universe. In 1964 Martha Rogers published her book *Science of Unitary Human Beings* which provided a radical vision of nursing, far removed from the medical model. The elements of the Science of Unitary Human Beings are[11]:

- Human beings are energy fields
- Humans and the environment are continually, simultaneously and mutually exchanging energy with each other
- Universal order is a force innate to all energy fields.

In the application of these theories to nursing, the role of the nurse is seen as being the observing and repatterning of the energy fields of their patients, therefore promoting relaxation and pain relief. This involves the following phases: centering, assessment, clearing, intervention or balancing and evaluation.[12]

It has achieved considerable acceptance within nursing and is seen as part of mainstream nursing practice in the US. In this sense it could be questioned whether it is properly included in a book on complementary therapy. According to J Sayre-Adams no harmful effects of therapeutic touch have yet been demonstrated when done by practitioners who have been trained by Krieger and her students and who follow the guidelines as set up by the governing bodies of TT.

Research shows that patients will respond differently to Therapeutic Touch;[13] there is considerable unpredictability in the effect on the patient. This clearly makes research into its clinical effectiveness difficult. A pilot study by Sian Vaughan[14] did not support earlier findings that the effect of TT was to lower diastolic blood pressure; nor was there an increase in relaxation response compared to the placebo group; however there did appear to be benefits in terms of pain relief. She recommends that more research of a qualitative nature be carried out.

Hand-mediated Energetic healing (HMEH)

Hand-mediated Energetic healing (HMEH) is discussed by Victoria E Slater[15] who states that

Physiologic and psychoneuroimmunologic responses do not easily explain HMEH, because the recipient is often not physically touched. Quantum and electromagnetic theories seem to offer the best explanations for HMEH, but they are hard to understand and usually are not taught to students of the health care sciences. While anecdotal reports abound of salutary effects, relatively few research studies of HMEH have been published. The results of these studies appear mixed at first, until one takes a closer look. For people experiencing real distress, HMEH has been shown to offer effective relief.

Spiritualism

Background

The seven principles of spiritualism are shown in Box 25.4.

Box 25.4 Seven principles of spiritualism
1. The Fatherhood of God 2. The Brotherhood of Man 3. The Communion of Spirits and the Ministry of Angels 4. The Continuous Existence of the Human Soul 5. Personal Responsibility 6. Compensation and Retribution 7. Eternal Progress open to every human soul

In contrast to healing *per se* members of the National Spiritualist Church hold healing sessions as part of their religious beliefs in a fulfilment of Christ's exhortation 'heal the sick'. There are two spiritualist associations in the CHO: the Spiritualist Association of Great Britain (SAGB) and the Greater World Christian Spiritualist Association.

The Spiritual National Union (SNU) which, with the Guild of Spiritualist Healers, had been a founder member of the CHO is no longer affiliated to the CHO. It joined the Guild of Spiritualist Healers in 1994 and the National Executive Committee of the SNU instituted a new Standing Committee, to be known as the Spiritualist Healing Committee with special responsibility for healing throughout the Union.

Registration and training

The SNU is an organisation limited by guarantee which is a registered charity and has a training programme which can lead to SNU Approved Healer status. Training is given under supervision in a variety of healing methods: absent healing, contact healing and magnetic healing. There is a required 100 week training period. Following completion of the basic course, students must provide two references from patients who have received healing and must also undertake a practical assessment. SNU approved healers can then work towards gaining a Certificate or Diploma of Recognition in Spiritualist Healing.

Rules on professional conduct

Its Code of Conduct is obligatory and any insurance cover only applies when healers are giving healing according to the Code of Conduct. It is regularly updated. The Code of Conduct recognises that some healing may take place in the altered state of consciousness i.e. trance. When this occurs, it requires healers to obey specific criteria (including conducting healing on a private appointment basis not publicly) and to ensure that a third party is present at all times during the healing session. All trance healers must be registered as such with the healing committee for information purposes only.

Reiki

Background

The word Reiki is Japanese and means 'Universal Life Force Energy'. It originates in Tibet and was used by lamas in the monasteries. Its modern usage results from the work of Dr Mikao Usui in the late 1800s. As a therapy it has been defined as

an interactive approach where healing is transferred from healer to client. The aim is to restore balance in the client's energy field. A range of techniques may be used during healing, such as visualization and the laying on of hands.[16]

Its benefits are described as including: stress reduction, increase of confidence and self-esteem, overcoming fears and anxieties, increasing energy levels, relieving aching muscles, exploring problem areas, amplifying the soul purpose, increasing self-worth and improving relationships.[17]

Registration and training

It is taught in three Degrees (levels):

- the first degree (which can take place over a weekend) covers the use of hands to channel Reiki energy
- the second degree covers the mental/emotional balancing distant healing practices
- the third degree covers the understanding necessary to teach others.

Two organisations are involved in the training of Reiki: the Reiki Association which is part of an international Reiki community and follows the Usui method; and the Reiki Kyokai, set up by two members of the Reiki Association, which has its own standards, training and guidelines for finding a therapist. Both associations insist that initiates should wait between courses in order to integrate what has been taught.[18] The Reiki Association is concerned at the number of bogus Reiki practitioners and is increasingly concerned with the need to improve on its self-regulation. At present it is possible for a person to claim to be Reiki trained after only a weekend of training.

Crystal healing

The Affiliation for Crystal Healing Organisations (ACHO) is an umbrella group for such associations as The International College of Crystal Healing, The School of White Crystal Healing and the Cornwall School of Crystal Healing. The ACHO sets guidelines and standards for its members. Some of its members are themselves members of the British Complementary Medicine Association and use its Code of Ethics and practice.

The course content for crystal healing would include such topics as: crystal healing techniques, choosing caring for and cleansing crystals, tuning and dedicating crystals, planetary healing with crystals, crystals and colour, use of a crystal pendulum, crystal gridwork and sacred geometry.

THE LAW AND HEALING

In theory of course, healing whether by therapeutic touch, spiritualism, reiki, crystals within or outside the context of a specific religious belief, should give rise to no legal issues since, by its very nature, it is non-invasive and even touching is not essential (healing can take place from a distance and out of sight of the individual).

Missed diagnoses

However problems can still arise if a patient, in reliance on a healer, fails to obtain orthodox medical advice and as a consequence a serious underlying condition is not identified and treated in time. The healer might disclaim any responsibility for such a failure arguing that they do not purport to diagnose any condition and therefore they should not be held responsible. It has already been stated that the CHO insists that members do not diagnose medical conditions. Any member of an organisation coming under the CHO who is in breach of the Code could face disciplinary proceedings for such activities.

The religious context

The Church of Scientology case

The Church of Scientology claimed a dramatic victory recently when an appeals court in France held that the Church was a genuine religion, not a cult, and reduced sentences on members of the Church who had been convicted on charges ranging from manslaughter to fraud following the suicide of one of its members. The prosecution had argued that the Church was a sect that aimed at defrauding gullible individuals. The defence argued that it was a religion with the legal right to ask members for money. Patrick Vic had committed suicide hours after he had asked his wife for a loan of Ffr30 000 to pay for a Scientology purification course. Lawyers for the prosecution accused the Church of exploiting the good faith and credulity of its victims for commercial profit by pseudo-scientific and semi-medical practices to the detriment of their financial interests, while exposing them to certain medico-psychological risks.

The decision of the Court was praised by the Reverend Heber Jentzsch, head of the Church in Los Angeles[1] as:

A dream come true for my Church and minority religions. The court has returned to the French tradition of liberty and equality.

Cures and shrines

Where healing is undertaken as part of a religious creed, regulation of the activity becomes extremely fraught. In a democratic country it could be argued that people should be entitled to take part in activities which they believe might lead to a cure or amelioration of their condition. Thus thousands of believers flock each year to shrines such as Lourdes to be healed. There are no laws to prevent such visits. Adult mentally competent persons are entitled to seek to obtain succour from where ever they wish. When there is fanaticism for a particular cult and the members are mentally competent adults it is difficult to control any organisation, even if ultimately it leads to a mass suicide. (There are however laws to prevent fraudulent misrepresentation and false advertising and these are covered in Chapters 4 and 5.)

Children

Children are in a different category. If parents reject orthodox medicine, insisting instead in taking their diseased child to a shrine, then social services could argue that the best interests of the child are not being looked after and they could seek an order under the Children Act 1989.

Case Child dying of diabetes[20]

The parents, instead of ensuring that their daughter received insulin for her diabetes, tried to treat her with a homeopathic remedy and the girl died, they were both found guilty of failing to take reasonable care of her and the father was imprisoned.[20]

In other words, whilst the law would permit parents to take a sick child to a shrine, a healer or some other source of assistance, this must be complementary to the treatments available from orthodox medicine, not as an alternative to them. Unless, of course, the practitioners of orthodox medicine have said that there is nothing further that they can do to help the child.

Charitable status

In a recent case the High Court held that faith healing is charitable.[21] Gwendolen le Cren Clarke died leaving her residuary estate to two persons with whom she had been involved in a small religious and healing movement which was centred on her home. They were directed to use 'the same ... to further the spiritual work now carried on by us together ... for so long as the law permits'. The residuary estate was worth about £150 000. The judge held that these words created a trust and it had to be decided if the trust was for charitable purposes. Private religious meetings were not charitable, since they were confined to religious services for a closed group. It was argued that in this situation the sessions were open to the public. The judge held that spiritual work in the form of faith healing was charitable. Any private work of the group was ancillary or subsidiary to the public faith healing part of the group's work. The gift was therefore a charitable gift.

SITUATIONS WITH LEGAL SIGNIFICANCE
No success

Situation 1 No success

A client paid £500 to visit a healer. Unknown to the healer the client had just been diagnosed as having cancer of the pancreas. Following the session the client deteriorated and died within a few weeks. The wife is now reclaiming the £500 from the healer.

If it can be established that the healer took the £500 on the understanding that the client would be cured of all illnesses, then it could be said that there was a breach of contract by the healer. However on the facts the client did not tell the healer that he was suffering from cancer, so the healer could argue that curing this was not part of the agreement between them. If the healer is a member of an organisation within the CHO, then it should have been made clear to the patient that the healer could not make a medical diagnosis.

The payment and receipt of the money puts the relationship of the healer and patient within the scope of the law relating to the sale and supply of goods and services (see Chapter 4). The wife's success in recovering the money, will depend to a large extent on establishing what was promised in exchange for that sum. If, on the other hand, the healer argues that the money was a gift, then it would have to be shown that it did not result from any fraudulent misrepresentation or any deception to obtain pecuniary advantage since this could result in a prosecution under the Theft Act. The burden of course would be on the prosecution to establish the deception beyond all reasonable doubt.

It should also be pointed out that most healers do not charge a fee, but may accept an offer to defray expenses. Some full-time healers may charge moderate fees.

Unexplained trauma

> **Situation 2**   Unexplained trauma
>
> Avril visited a healer, having heard that he would be able to support her following her bereavement. The healer impressed Avril with his understanding of her situation and advised her to utilise the energies which she possessed to recover her peace of mind. Since visiting the healer, Avril has found herself to be in a very depressed condition unable to work and carry on with any social life. Her doctor sees her as being in a state of post traumatic stress disorder. Avril blames the healer for this state.

Avril may be able to show that the healer was in breach of the duty of care which he owed to her. However she may have difficulty in establishing that the harm from which she is suffering is caused by any breach of duty by the healer, rather than being the effect of her bereavement. Chapter 3 covers the law relating to negligence and reference should be made to the difficulties relating to causation.

If Avril can show the duty of care, the breach of the duty of care, and the fact that this caused the PTSD from which she is suffering, she may well have a claim against the healer. In addition healers who are members of an organisation under the CHO could face disciplinary proceedings if they fail to comply with the Code and give false hopes to a patient.

A poodle

Healers who belong to member organisations of the Confederation of Healing Organisations will be bound to observe the BCMA's Code of Conduct and the appendices to this framed by the CHO. Appendix 2 relates to the healing of animals

---

Situation 3 A poodle

Dennis had been concerned that his poodle was off his food, loosing weight and generally out of condition. He learnt that healers were also prepared to treat animals and took the poodle to a well-known local healer. The healer laid his hands upon the poodle and reassured Dennis that its appetite would soon return. Unfortunately his prediction did not materialise. When Dennis eventually took the poodle to the vet he was told that the poodle had an inoperative cancer but had he brought him in earlier, then there would have been a chance that surgery would have been successful. The poodle was put down.

---

and paragraph 4 makes it clear that it is a requirement that 'before treating an animal, the healer must seek assurance from the owner that the animal has been examined by a veterinary surgeon'. Here the healer has clearly not done this. Had he done so, the vet might have diagnosed the cancer in time to cure the animal. As a consequence the owner may have a claim against the healer, who, since he has failed to comply with the Code of Conduct, may find that his insurance cover is now void. He would thus be personally liable for any compensation. Unfortunately this may mean that Dennis is unable to secure from the healer compensation for the loss of his dog. It depends on the healer's personal resources.

An element of contributory negligence may be present, since it could be claimed that any reasonable animal owner, should himself have gone to the vet prior to seeking assistance from the healer. How much compensation would be deducted on account of this contributory negligence would depend upon the detailed facts of the case (see Chapter 3 on contributory negligence).

The healer will also face disciplinary proceedings for failing to obey the Code.

CONCLUSIONS

It is clear that applying the Bolam test of competence and reasonable practice to therapists in this field will always be difficult, and, because of the essentially intuitive, subjective nature of the therapy, probably entirely inappropriate.

Healing, under whatever philosophy or school of thought will also probably never be amenable to the scientific standards of proof and causation that practitioners of orthodox medicine seek before being prepared to accept any claims. The results of current research projects into healing will be extremely interesting in this respect.[22]

In the meantime there will always be attempts to explain by normal scientific processes the miracles or cures which are evidenced in the writings on this topic. For example an explanation of the healing properties of attendance at a shrine is given by Dr Stuttaford.[23] He states that

psoriasis is improved by exposure to sunlight or change of mood. The effect of both of these factors provides a possible, logical explanation for some of the miraculous cures of leprosy which have followed a pilgrimage. The combination of exposure to sun while walking to a shrine, coupled with the sense of relief derived from worshipping, whether at Walsingham or Lourdes, in those who have previously been tormented by their anxieties could well have accounted for the occasional cure.

The cured client might feel that the explanation is not important.

Recent years have seen major developments in the recognition of healing and its acceptance by orthodox medicine within the NHS. Much credit must be given to the work of the CHO in establishing standards of conduct and practice.

Questions and Exercises

1. Draft a pamphlet setting out the work of a healer to be given to clients.
2. What promises do you consider that a healer could validly make as part of a contract for services?
3. What are the arguments for and against a healer requesting gifts rather than payment from clients?
4. In what ways, if any, do you consider persons should be protected from the work of healers who do not belong to a recognised association?

REFERENCES

1. Confederation of Healing Organisations (CHO) Appendix III to the code of conduct of the BCMA CHO, Berkhampstead
2. Clare Dakin, 3 Burra Close, Sandford on Thames, Oxon. OX4 4YE (personal communication to author)
3. Davidson I 1991 Here and Now: An approach to Christian Healing through Gestalt. Darton Longman and Todd, London
4. Graham H 1992 The Magic Shop: An imaginative guide to self-healing. Rider, London
5. Graham H 1990 Time, Energy, and the Psychology of Healing. Jessica Kingsley, London
6. Ahuja A Charity puts spiritual healers to the test. The Times 17 June 1997, p 8
7. Confederation of Healing Organisations 1997 Competence based qualification in healing/radionics. CHO, Berkhampstead
8. GMC letter MRD/PW of 1 November 1977 and 6 March 1978 quoted in the Members Code of Conduct of the NFSH. (see now the Duties of a doctor: Guidance from the GMC, booklet on Good Medical Practice para. 28. (no date)
9. National Consumer Council, Guide for NHS patients and doctors 'Patients' Rights'. HMSO (no date given). (see also now the Patient's Charter).
10. Didsbury Touch Therapeutic Touch, leaflet (no date)
11. Sayre-Adams J 1933 Therapeutic touch – principles and practice. Complementary Therapies in Medicine 1: 96–99
12. Sayre-Adams J 1994 Therapeutic touch – A nursing function. Nursing Standard 8(17): 25–28
13. Sayre-Adams J 1993 Therapeutic touch – principles and practice. Complementary Therapies in Medicine 1: 96–99
14. Vaughan S 1995 The gentle touch. Journal of Clinical Nursing 4: 359–68
15. Slater VE In: chapter 9 Marc M 1996 (ed) Fundamentals of complementary and alternative medicine. Churchill Livingstone, New York
16. Rankin-Box R 1995 The nurses' handbook of complementary therapies. Churchill Livingstone, New York
17. Leaflet on Reiki by Carrie Ebdon Reiki Master and Teacher, Cardiff
18. Bonita L 1997 Reiki, the healing power of the universe. Caduceus issue No 35 Spring 1997
19. Mcintyre B Scientology is not a cult, says court. The Times 30 July 1997
20. News report. The Times 6 November 1993; and editorial A right to life: parents cannot condemn their children to die. The Times 8 November 1993.
21. Funnel and another v. Stewart and others The Times Law Report 9 December 1995
22. For further information into on-going research contact the CHO and the RCCM
23. Stuttaford T The pain and shame of psoriasis. The Times 17 July 1997, p 16

26

Herbal medicine

DEFINITION

Herbalism is the use of plants in healing. Its stated aims are at stimulating the body's own natural healing abilities by rebalancing and cleansing it. It should also be noted, however, that plants and herbs can have direct medicinal and/or toxic effects, e.g. aspirin (originally obtained from willowbark), quinine, digitalis (from foxgloves) and opium derivatives.

BACKGROUND

Brief history

Herbalism is probably the oldest known therapy. The earliest known records of medicinal herbs are from northern China, carbon-dated at 3000 BC and include myrrh and frankincense.

Hippocrates (460–360 BC) separated medicine from superstition and mysticism and established a school of healing, combining herbal remedies, diet and hydrotherapy.

In 1653 Nicholas Culpeper published his book *Complete Herbal*.

Herbalism aims to establish the root cause of any ailment, thus an infection may result from a weakness due to faulty diet. Herbal remedies will bring the body to health, reducing the risk of re-infection.

Traditional Chinese Medicine (TCM)

There is evidence that Chinese medicine was practised over 2000 years BC. Its philosophy and the terms yin and yang are discussed in Chapter 16 on acupuncture. Illness is seen as an imbalance of qi within the body, caused by external or internal factors or factors which are neither. Diagnosis is based on four skills:

- inspection
- listening and smelling
- inquiry
- palpation.

Treatment includes:
- acupuncture
- moxibustion (see Chapter 16)
- cupping and bleeding
- massage and the manipulation of qi by exercise
- breathing
- herbal medicine and dietetics.[1]

A register is kept of practitioners in Chinese herbal medicine.

Chinese traditional medicine does not lend itself to the criteria laid down by modern Western scientific methods, i.e. randomized, placebo controlled, and double blinded clinical trials. However the Office of Alternative Medicine in the USA has funded studies on a range of different TCM treatments linked with specific medical conditions e.g. osteoarthritis and acupuncture, menopausal hot flushes and chinese herbs.

Ayurvedic medicine

This is a therapy which is derived from Indian medicine dating back to 1200–800 BC.[2] According to Ayurveda the cosmos is composed of five basic elements: earth, fire, water and space. Certain forces cause these to interact, giving rise to all that exists. In human beings these five elements occur as the three doshas (forces) that, along with the seven dhatus (tissues) and three malas (waste products), make up the human body. When in equilibrium the three doshas maintain health, but when an imbalance occurs among them, they defile the normal functioning of the body, leading to the manifestation of disease. Restoring a person to health entails the complete process of diagnosis and therapeutics which take into account both mental and physical components integrated with the social and physical worlds. After diagnosis treatment involves purification using oils and enemas and alleviation therapy which utilises food such as honey, butter or ghee, sesame or castor oil and natural medicines.

It was reported that Sir James Goldsmith consulted Prakasch, a practitioner of Ayurvedic medicine, after he had been told that there was no more that conventional medicine could do to cure his cancer. Seven days before he died he refused to take conventional pain killers because he believed that they would counteract the effects of the Ayurvedic treatment.[3]

Current research

Claims by herbalists are being authenticated through scientific research and there is thus a growing body of data from randomised controlled trials on the efficacy of certain herbal remedies.

Use in pregnancy and postnatally

Helen Stapleton gives a brief history of herbalism and suggests that herbs are a safe and accessible way of treating disorders of pregnancy.[5] She emphasises that 'if there are no signs of improvement within 7–10 days, their use should be discontinued and qualified help sought'. Her suggestions include raspberry leaf tea which has a tightening and toning effect on pelvic structures, so women may continue to drink it for 6–8 weeks postnatally. **NB the excessive astringency of raspberry leaf tea contraindicates its use in the first and early second trimesters.** Chamomile, meadowsweet, spearmint, and ginger or aniseed can help alleviate nausea:

For persistent cases of nausea, a visit to a qualified herbalist to obtain more specific herbs, such as wild yam or gentian roots, may be necessary.

She states that heartburn, anaemia, urogenital infections, stress, fatigue and moods, varicose veins, constipation, haemorrhoids and perineal healing and breast problems can all be relieved by herbs.

Ingestion of garlic by breast feeding mothers significantly improves suckling time.

Derma trust

On the 6 November 1995, dermatologists at the Royal Free Hospital launched an appeal in the House of Lords to fund research into Chinese herbal medicine. The research will not only investigate the use of herbs in the treatment of skin diseases but, because of their proven immunosuppressant powers, their effect on diseases including psoriasis, rheumatoid arthritis and inflammatory bowel disease. The Charity which has been set up is called Dermatrust.[4]

Controlling bodies

The National Institute of Medical Herbalists (NIMH) which describes itself as 'a professional body of practitioners of phytotherapy' has set standards and training for herbalists. It was established in 1864 with two main aims: the safeguarding of the profession and the training of new members.

The Ayurvedic Medical Association keeps a list of practitioners and the Ayurvedic Company of Great Britain Ltd can be contacted by those wishing to visit its practitioners.

REGISTRATION AND TRAINING

Accreditation of courses

The Accreditation Board of the National Institute of Medical Herbalists requires the information set out in Box 26.1 to start the accreditation process for approval of courses. It is the only professional body of herbal practitioners, not only in England but in most of Europe.

Box 26.1 Information required for course accreditation

1. The philosophy of the institution with a clear statement of involvement in the teaching of herbal medicine
2. The entrance requirements for students and whether credit for prior training and/or experiential learning is given
3. The annual intake of students
4. The breakdown of the financial structure of the institution
5. Length of course, qualification obtained and any external validation
6. Content of the course and core skills
7. Methods of assessment and hours of course
8. Recommended texts
9. Resources available
10. Clinical training and number of hours
11. Involvement of students in course content and assessment
12. Student support mechanisms

Initially the training carried out by the National Institute of Medical Herbalists itself was the responsibility of its department of education, which in 1975 changed its name to the School of Herbal Medicine. The School became independent in 1982 and subsequently came under the aegis of the College of Phytotherapy.

Now known as the School of Phytotherapy and based in Sussex it runs a four year degree course as well as tutorial courses (leading to a Diploma in Herbal Medicine), a one year course (leading to a Certificate in herbal studies, which does not constitute a licence to practise professionally) and specially structured courses (leading to a Diploma in Herbal Medicine) for professionals such as GPs and osteopaths who already have substantial clinical experience.

A four year honours degree course was introduced at Middlesex University in 1995. Dr Ting Ming Li a clinical geneticist at the Royal London Hospital Whitechapel has established an Institute of Chinese Medicine in Chandos Place London. He has initiated on the NHS a pilot study giving GPs an introductory course on Chinese Medicine at the Royal London.

Definitions of competence

The Accreditation Board of the National Institute of Medical Herbalists defines the core skills of a medical herbalist as shown in Box 26.2.

Rules on professional conduct and insurance

Members of the National Institute of Medical Herbalists have to obey a Code of Practice and Ethics and membership provides professional indemnity insurance.

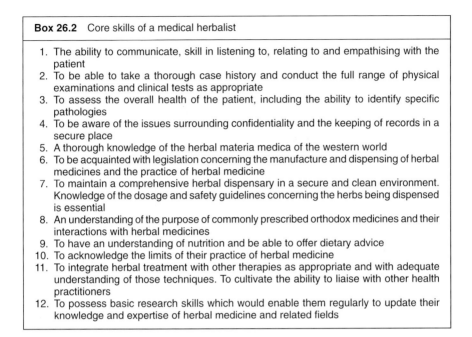

Box 26.2   Core skills of a medical herbalist

1. The ability to communicate, skill in listening to, relating to and empathising with the patient
2. To be able to take a thorough case history and conduct the full range of physical examinations and clinical tests as appropriate
3. To assess the overall health of the patient, including the ability to identify specific pathologies
4. To be aware of the issues surrounding confidentiality and the keeping of records in a secure place
5. A thorough knowledge of the herbal materia medica of the western world
6. To be acquainted with legislation concerning the manufacture and dispensing of herbal medicines and the practice of herbal medicine
7. To maintain a comprehensive herbal dispensary in a secure and clean environment. Knowledge of the dosage and safety guidelines concerning the herbs being dispensed is essential
8. An understanding of the purpose of commonly prescribed orthodox medicines and their interactions with herbal medicines
9. To have an understanding of nutrition and be able to offer dietary advice
10. To acknowledge the limits of their practice of herbal medicine
11. To integrate herbal treatment with other therapies as appropriate and with adequate understanding of those techniques. To cultivate the ability to liaise with other health practitioners
12. To possess basic research skills which would enable them regularly to update their knowledge and expertise of herbal medicine and related fields

LAWS RELATING TO THE THERAPY

The Herbalist's Charter

The Medical Act 1512 made it an offence to practise physic or surgery unless the practitioner was a university graduate or had been licensed by the bishop of the diocese in which he lived. Because of the unpopularity of this Act, an amending Act was passed in 1542 which became known as 'the Herbalist's Charter'.

The preamble to the Act noted that, since making the earlier Act,

the Company and felowship of Surgeons of London, minding only their own Lucres, and nothing the Profit or Ease of the Diseases or Patient have sued, troubled and vexed divers honest Persons, as well Men as Women, whom God hath endued with the Knowledge of Nature, Kind and Operation of certain Herbs, Roots and Waters.

It also noted that

it is now well known, that the Surgeons admitted will do no Cure to any Person, but where they shall know to be rewarded with a greater Sum or Reward than the Cure extendeth unto...

This Act made it lawful for anyone who

having Knowledge and Experience of the Nature of Herbs, Roots and Waters, or of the Operation of the same, by Speculation or Practice, within any Part of the Realm of England or within any other the King's Dominions, to practise, use and minister in and to any outward Sore, Uncome, Wound, Apostemations, outward Swelling or Disease, any Herb or Herbs, Ointments, Baths, Pultess and Emplaisters, according to their Cunning, Experience and Knowledge in any of the Diseases, Sores and Maladies beforesaid, and all other like to the time, or Drinks for the Stone, Strangury or Agues, without Suit, Vexation, Trouble, Penalty, or Loss of their Goods.

Since this time, the focus of any restraint over practice of herbalism has been through control of the product rather than of the practitioner.

The Medicines Act 1968

Baroness Trumpington, Parliamentary Under Secretary of State, speaking in 1987[6] described the impact of the Medicines Act 1968 on alternative medicines.

All medicines – conventional and alternative – that were on the market when the Medicines Act 1968 came into force in 1971 were given licences as of right. Nothing was done at that time to check them for safety, quality and efficacy – the basic requirements for a Medicines Act licence. The intention was that over the following years this could be done by the DHSS as the Medicines Act Licensing Authority. Of the 39 000 medicines on the market in 1971, about 15 000 remain to be reviewed. Many of the original 39 000 were withdrawn, usually voluntarily by the manufacturer because they had outlived their usefulness.

Effort in reviewing these old medicines has concentrated on the more powerful conventional medicines and only in the past year have we started to look at alternatives…

Over the next few years we expect to review some 700 herbal products. The DHSS will be looking for no more than an appropriate level of proof of efficacy, manufacturers will need to satisfy the DHSS as licensing authority that the products are absolutely safe and that the quality of manufacture is completely satisfactory. … By this means I expect most herbal products to remain on the market but with unsubstantiated claims removed. As a result, on completion of the review consumers will be able to choose from the herbal remedies on sale with increased confidence about their safety and their effectiveness for the conditions given on the packet label. In this way the review will increase the freedom of the consumer to exercise an informed choice.

The present situation is that the Medicines Control Agency has classified some herbal products as medicines which therefore come under the Medicines Act 1968 (see Chapters 6 and 27). Toxic materials come under the Control of Substances Hazardous to Health Regulations (see Chapter 13). The vast majority of herbal products, however, are not licensed and do not require a licence for their production and sale.

Licensing policy for herbal medicines

The attempt by the Medicine Control Agency in 1994 to introduce licensing for every herbal remedy met with such uproar that the project was abandoned. There are, however, still calls for such a scheme in view of the fact that herbal products are not entirely harmless.

Peter A G M de Smet[7] suggests that in view of the

herbal wave sweeping over society … the time seems ripe for a licensing policy that promotes the safety and quality of herbal medicine-like products without imposing an unbearable conventional burden on their manufacturers.

He recommends that special herbal licensing offers

opportunities before marketing to screen the declared constituents, demand proof of product quality, restrict the level of potentially hazardous constituents, and enforce warnings about correct and safe use. In addition the possibility exists to oblige licence holders to report suspected adverse reactions. The presence of a licence number on the label would make the regulatory efforts visible to retailers, consumers, health care providers and inspectors and would facilitate post marketing surveillance and, if necessary, recalls.

There has been recent media concern over the promotion of vitamins. Birmingham University is starting research on the effect of vitamin supplements on stress and intellect in people under 60.[8] The research is headed by Professor Doug Carroll with a £200 000 grant from Roche.[9] (see also Chapter 5 and the Medicines Act)

SITUATIONS WITH LEGAL SIGNIFICANCE

Whilst many people consider herbal medicines safe, since they are 'natural', the National Poisons Unit at Guy's Hospital has received 5500 inquiries about side effects of alternative medicines, herbal preparations and food supplements in recent years.[10]

Kidney damage

Case   Kidney damage[11]
30 Belgian women suffered from severe kidney damage after taking a slimming remedy based on Chinese Herb medicine.

In the case above the mistake was thought to arise from the fact that three plants in Chinese herb medicine have the same name.

Missed diagnosis

Situation 1   Missed diagnosis
A registered midwife who had also had a training in herbal medicine, obtained the consent of a mother to use herbal remedies during the pregnancy. She made use of raspberry leaf tea, in the post-natal care. This has a tightening and toning effect on pelvic structures. The mother complained of pain, similar to the contractions. The midwife assured her that these indicated the womb tightening and returning to its pre-pregnancy state. The mother was encouraged to continue to drink the raspberry tea. It subsequently transpired that the pains were the result of an inflamed gall bladder and an operation was necessary. The mother blames the midwife for missing these symptoms as a result of which she suffered severe and undiagnosed pain and is threatening to complain to the UKCC.

The midwife/herbalist would appear to have acted outside her competence and as a result of that her client suffered unnecessary pain. There would certainly appear to be grounds for an investigation by the Preliminary Investigating Committee of the UKCC, who would decide whether professional conduct proceedings were justified. The success of any civil litigation would depend upon the mother proving that the midwife failed to follow the reasonable standard of a midwife. This might prove easier than establishing the reasonable standard of a herbalist. If the midwife was an employee the employer would be vicariously liable for the harm.

Raspberry leaf tea contraindicated

Situation 2   Raspberry leaf tea contraindicated

A midwife without herbalist training mentioned to a client early in her first trimester that she had read about the use of raspberry leaf tea in connection with pregnancy and suggested that her client should try it. Unbeknown to either, raspberry leaf tea is contraindicated for the early stages and the client miscarried. The client is seeking compensation.

The midwife here almost certainly acted outside her competency and in breach of the UKCC guidelines. She could therefore be subject to professional conduct proceedings. She has also probably acted in breach of her duty of care to the client in advising the administration of any medicinal substance without due knowledge of its potential effects. She and, through the principle of vicarious liability, her employers could be liable to pay compensation if it can be proved on the balance of probabilities that the miscarriage was due to the ingestion of raspberry leaf tea. There would be little or no contributory negligence to reduce the claim as it is reasonable for the client to trust the health professional on such matters. (See generally Chapter 3).

Sleepless nights

Situation 3   Sleepless nights

Parents were at their wits end following the birth of their first baby, who appeared not to require sleep other than in ten minute bouts. The general practitioner told them that it was only a phase, and eventually the baby would sleep. The health visitor suggested that they took it in turns to sleep but made no other suggestions. A friend suggested that they should visit a health shop.
   The shop assistant was extremely helpful and gave them a herbal product which she assured them would benefit the baby. They used it for several nights running without any immediate effect. They increased the dose and also gave the baby a medicine that they had purchased from the chemists to assist sleeping.
   Unfortunately the baby died. Subsequently they learnt that the herbal product was not recommended for any child under 10 years. The parents are angry and want to prevent any other child dying in this way.

Post mortem evidence and the inquest should answer the question as to why the baby died. If it is established that it was the result of the herbal product and its possible interaction with the other medical product, then it is possible that criminal proceedings for manslaughter could be brought against the persons responsible.

These include:

- the parents
- the shop assistant
- the manufacturers of both products.

Criminal liability will depend upon the facts and establishing that both the objective ingredients (*actus reus*) failing to inform or giving the wrong information and the mental element (*mens rea*) carelessness amounting to recklessness are present (see Chapter 5). Civil liability on the part of the manufacturers would be possible under the principles of the case of *Donague* v. *Stevenson* (see Chapter 3) if adequate warnings were not given on the packaging or if the product was defective as a result of negligence on the part of the manufacturer. The Consumer Protection Act, 1987, may also apply (see Chapter 13).

Liability excluded

Situation 4   Liability excluded
A therapist trained in allergy therapy also gave advice to clients about the use of herbal products, although she was not qualified in herbal medicine. One client has complained that her eczema, which had started improving, is now worse than ever and is blaming one of the herbs which had been recommended. The therapist has checked with her insurance and has discovered that it does not provide cover for liability associated with any activity not disclosed in the application form. She had not specifically mentioned that she gave advice on herbs.

It may be extremely difficult for the client to prove that her aggravated eczema is the result of herbs or of any advice given by the therapist. Unfortunately for the therapist, if the insurance cover excludes advice on herbs, she may not obtain any assistance in defending any litigation were the client able to establish breach of the duty of care and harm arising from that breach to enable it to be brought. She would therefore have to pay for the costs of defending herself out of her own resources, subject to any entitlement to legal aid.

CONCLUSION

It was estimated in 1992 by Mintel, the market analysts that sales of herbal and homeopathic remedies and aromatherapy oils have reached a total of £62.7 million of which herbal medicines account for £32 million and the total is rising.[12] There is no reason why this popularity should not increase and there would appear to be sound arguments, in view of the possible toxicity of the herbal products, for the tighter controls advocated by De Smet (above) to be introduced. As well as controlling the products, there would also appear to be strong arguments in favour of controlling the use of the professional title to ensure that nobody can call themselves a herbalist, unless they have been qualified on an accredited course.

Questions and Exercises

1. To what extent do you consider herbal preparations should be on open sale to the public without being subject to tight controls on marketing, labelling and promotion?
2. What are the advantages and disadvantages of state registration for herbalists?
3. Do the regulations on the Control of Substances Hazardous to Health apply to herbs? (refer to Chapter 13 for the regulations).

REFERENCES

1. Kevin V 1996 China's Traditional Medicine In: Micozzi M (ed) Fundamentals of Complementary and Alternative Medicine. Churchill Livingstone, New York
2. Zysk KG 1996 Tradition Ayurveda In: Micozzi M Fundamentals of Complementary and Alternative Medicine. Churchill Livingstone, New York
3. Ridley Y Healer blamed for Goldsmith's agony. The Sunday Times 3 August 1997
4. Stuttaford T Lords hear case for herbal medicine. The Times 6 November 1995, p 6
5. Stapleton H 1984 Herbal medicines for disorders of pregnancy. Modern Midwife 5(4): 18–22
6. Trumpington 1987 Alternative medicine and therapies and the DHSS. Journal of the Royal Society of Medicine 80: 336–8
7. de Smet PAGM 1995 Should herbal medicine-like products be licensed as medicines? British Medical Journal 310: 1023
8. Stuttaford T Don't hold your breath in the vitamin dispute. The Times 22 July 1997
9. Ahuja A Critic of vitamins industry to test magic bullet pills. The Times 21 July 1997
10. Laurance J Great cures, or mumbo jumbo? The Times 5 July 1995, p 20
11. Hawkes N old Chinese cure or killer? The Times 1 February 1994
12. Laurance J Great cures, or mumbo jumbo? The Times 5 July 1995, p 20

27

Homeopathy

DEFINITION

Homeopathy is literally the therapy of treating like with like. The Society of Homeopaths defines it as

An effective and scientific system of healing which assists the natural tendency of the body to heal itself. It recognises that all symptoms of ill health are expressions of disharmony within the whole person and that it is the patient who needs treatment not the disease.

BACKGROUND

Homeopathy is known to have been practised by the Ancient Greeks and Hippocrates stated that there were two ways of treating ill health, the way of opposites and the way of similars.

Its modern development dates from the work of Samuel Hahnemann, a Leipzig physician in the 18th century, who discovered that the same medicines which caused the patient's ill health could be used in minute doses to treat the condition. Since his discoveries the practice of homeopathy has developed in popularity. It became extremely popular in the United States at the end of the 19th century, when 15% of the doctors were homeopaths. After a drop in popularity, homeopathy is now widely practised both by lay persons and professionals who also practise in orthodox medicine.

Fundamental principles

There are three fundamental principles underlying homeopathy:

- the law of similars
- the single remedy
- the minimum dose.

The law of similars The homeopath seeks a remedy which is known to produce a similar picture to that of the patient's condition. The prescribed similar remedy then stimulates and assists the patient's own natural healing efforts.

The single remedy An attempt is made to treat the patient's complex condition by one single remedy. The effect of this is observed and evaluated before a further prescription is considered.

The minimum dose Only a minute dose is given, in the form of a specially prepared potency. The potency and number of doses is determined by the homeopath according to the needs of individual patients.

Homeopathic effect

The Society gives as an example of homeopathy the treatment of insomnia. Traditional medicine might involve giving to the patient large doses of medicine to create artificial sleep. The homeopath, in contrast, would give to the patient a minute dose of a substance which in large doses causes sleeplessness in a healthy person. This will enable the patient to sleep naturally and because of the minute dosage no side effects or addiction will result. In order to determine which is the most appropriate homeopathic substance suitable to the patient, a lengthy interview takes place to determine all the symptoms, emotional and mental as well as physical, that the patient is experiencing and to understand the patient's history.

How homeopathy actually works has never been convincingly scientifically demonstrated. A French scientist, Jacques Benveniste, put forward a theory in the 1980s that water in some way acts like a magnetic medium, retaining a memory of things that it has been in contact with. He was the subject of a critical examination led by the editor of Nature. The theory could explain why even very dilute mixtures could be potent. Dr Fisher, consultant physician at the Royal London Homeopathic Hospital, is quoted as saying that

There is starting to be physical evidence from Nuclear Magnetic Resonance which says that water treated in this way, diluted, and shaken is different from ordinary water. No body knows exactly what the difference means, but there is a consistent difference.[1]

Research

Research into the scientific bases of homeopathy is extensive and a study was published in 1991 in the British Medical Journal by medical school professors, who were asked by the Dutch Government to review the existing research.[2]

Controlling bodies

There are two distinct organisations for homeopaths:

- one which requires practitioners to have a medical or veterinary qualification, the Faculty of Homeopathy
- one which enables those who do not have a medical training to secure a qualification in homeopathy, the Society of Homeopaths.

In addition the British Homeopathic Association exists to develop and promote homeopathy. Membership is available to members of the public interested in the development of homeopathy on payment of a subscription. However prospective members must sign that they will not use the membership of the British Homeopathic Association for any professional purpose whatsoever.

LINKS WITH ORTHODOX MEDICINE

When homeopathy was introduced into this country in the 19th century it had a considerable take up from orthodox doctors. The Faculty of Homeopathy was established in 1848 to train doctors in homeopathy. Five schools of homeopathy were established: London, Liverpool, Bristol, Glasgow and Tunbridge Wells and have received state support.

In 1977 a homeopathic clinic was planned at the newly built Royal Liverpool Hospital to replace an earlier facility which was closed down. There was opposition from Medical Consultants, and discussion in the House of Commons. Tom Ellis MP stated that

For sheer blind prejudice and bigotry, crass ignorance and highly questionable ethical behaviour, it would be hard to find a better example, even from the minutes of the Wapping Bargees' Mutual Benefit Society, let alone a body of professional men.[3]

The Liverpool Clinic was opened.

In 1979 attempts to close the Royal London Homeopathic Hospital by the Area Health Authority failed.

Examples of homeopathy in midwifery

An article[5] discusses the benefits of homeopathy in midwifery at all stages of the pregnancy and points out that there is no evidence that it has caused side effects in pregnancy or labour, interfered with the action of orthodox drugs, created an overdose, or built up in the body, become toxic or addictive. Case histories which the author describes include mothers suffering from haemorrhoids, occipito-posterior labour, postpartum haemorrhage and a baby with evening colic. All patients were successfully treated with a homeopathic remedy.

UKCC Advice to its registered practitioners

In 1992 the UKCC advised its practitioners[6] on the use of homeopathic medicines as shown in Box 27.1.

Box 27.1   Advice of UKCC

Paragraph 38 Homeopathic and herbal medicines are subject to the licensing provisions of the Medicines Act 1968, although those on the market when that Act became operative (which means most of those now available) received product licences without any evaluation of their efficacy, safety or quality. Practitioners should, therefore, make themselves generally aware of common substances used in their particular area of practice. It is necessary to respect the right of individuals to administer to themselves, or to request a practitioner to assist in the administration of substances in these categories. If, when faced with a patient or client whose desire to receive medicines of this kind appears to create potential difficulties, or if it is felt that the substances might either be an inappropriate response to the presenting symptoms or likely to negate or enhance the effect of prescribed medicines, the practitioner, acting in the interests of the patient or client, should consider contacting the relevant registered medical practitioner, but must also be mindful of the need not to override the patient's rights.

Similar advice to that contained in Box 27.1 is given by the UKCC in its advisory document *The Midwife's Code of Conduct*[6] clause 34 and clause 35, relating to the wishes of the mother, is shown in Box 27.2.

Box 27.2   UKCC Midwife's Code of Conduct

Clause 35 When a mother wishes to receive medicines of this [i.e. homeopathic or herbal] kind and you believe that the substances might either be an inappropriate response to the presenting symptoms or likely to negate or enhance the effect of prescribed medicines, you have a duty to discuss this fully with the mother. The midwife, acting in the best interests of the mother and in her full knowledge, should consider contacting the relevant expert practitioner to seek advice, but must also be mindful of the need not to override the woman's rights.

GPs and vets as homeopaths

The Faculty of Homeopathy is an academic institution, which was established by Act of Parliament, the Faculty of Homeopathy Act 1950, based at the Royal London Homeopathic Hospital, Great Ormond Street, London. It is responsible for the teaching and examination of doctors and veterinary surgeons, all of whom must be registered practitioners, in homeopathic medicine. It can award the membership qualification MFHom and VetMFHom and the fellowship qualification FFHom and VetFFHom.

Society of Homeopaths guidelines

The Society of Homeopaths recommends that a client should maintain his or her relationship with the GP who will arrange any tests or X-Rays. It states[4]

Homeopathy has an alternative philosophy but by working in this way with your GP the two systems of health care can provide complementary services.

Definitions for purchasing contracts

Some health authorities have negotiated contracts for the purchase of homeopathy for their patients. However it was reported on 22 May 1997[7] that Lambeth, Southwark and Lewisham health authority, which had been sending 800 patients a year at a cost of £250 000 to the Royal Homeopathic Hospital Holborn, has decided to stop referring patients because it does not believe the treatment is effective. In future patients of non-fundholding GPs in the area will only be able to access homeopathy through the NHS in exceptional circumstances. The health authority stated that, after studying the evidence, it had found that no good scientific effect is produced by homeopathic treatment. It would continue to purchase other forms of complementary medicine such as acupuncture, osteopathy and chiropractic treatment for up to six weeks, because there was evidence that this could be beneficial.

Not surprisingly this announcement met with a strong reaction from the Royal Homeopathic Hospital and the spokesman stated

Ten years ago we might have struggled to prove that homeopathy was effective but there is now so much evidence to show that it does work that it should be unarguable.

A letter in the Times on the 27 May 1997 from the Director of Research to the Royal London Homeopathic Hospital, Peter Fisher, stated

It is not true to say that homeopathy is unsupported by scientific evidence: independent reviews of the clinical-trial evidence consistently support its efficacy. The most recent review, conducted by an expert group supported by the European Commission identified 184 clinical trials of homeopathy and came to a clearly positive conclusion.

Meanwhile patients and their GPs are voting with their feet; sales of homeopathic medicines are rising at 15% annually, and GP fundholder referrals to this hospital rose 27% last year. NHS purchasing should be based on evidence and patient demand, not, as seems to be the case here, on a 'we don't understand how it works, therefore it doesn't work' argument.

REGISTRATION AND TRAINING

The Faculty of Homeopathy

The Faculty does not keep a register, so in that sense homeopathy is not a state registered profession but the Act of Parliament does give to the Faculty limited disciplinary powers. The Faculty is therefore permitted to expel members or fellows and to strip them of their qualifications should they be deemed to have brought the Faculty into disrepute through inappropriate actions or malpractice. The Faculty also provides training for other state registered health professionals including dentists, pharmacists, midwives, health visitors and nurses. All homeopathic practitioners are advised by the Faculty to liaise with the general practitioners of their patients.

The Society of Homeopaths

The Society of Homeopaths is the professional body for homeopaths practising in the Hahnemannian tradition. Its aims are set out in Box 27.3.

Box 27.3 Aims of the Society of Homeopaths

1. To develop and maintain high standards for the practice of homeopathy.
2. To develop and maintain for public use a Register of homeopaths who practise to the standards required by the Society and abide by the Society's Code of Ethics.
3. To protect the public's freedom to have homeopathic treatment now and in the future.
4. To promote public awareness of homeopathy and to encourage its responsible use in the home.
5. To promote and support the establishment of education and training in homeopathy.

The Society of Homeopaths keeps a register of Homeopaths. Persons are only included on the Register after they have been examined by the Registration Committee of the Society of Homeopaths in relation to the criteria set out in Box 27.4.

Box 27.4 Admission criteria for the Society of Homeopaths

1. They practise according to the principles and practice established by Samuel Hahnemann, the founder of homeopathy.
2. They have a proper understanding and knowledge of homeopathic materia medica and repertory.
3. They have been adequately trained in the essential medical sciences and skills and have had suitable clinical training and experience.
4. They agree to abide by the Society's Code of Ethics.

Practitioners who satisfy the criteria set out in Box 27.4 are issued with a Certificate of Registration and may use the initials RSHom. Those who have been made fellows use the initials FSHom.

Definitions of standards of competence

These are set by the Society and the Faculty.

Rules on professional misconduct

Any complaint about one of the members registered with the Society of Homeopaths can be pursued through the Professional Conduct Director of the Society. The Faculty's disciplinary powers are referred to above.

LAWS WHICH APPLY

Medicines Act 1968 – sections 12 and 56

Refer to Baroness Trumpington's description of the effect of the Medicines Act 1968 in Chapter 26 on herbal medicine.

In relation to homeopathic medicines she said[8]:

I foresee problems when applying the Medicines Act to homeopathic remedies. The Act is built around the concept that a particular medicine has a particular purpose or set of purposes. Consequently a medicine's effectiveness can be judged against the extent to which that purpose is achieved. In accordance with homeopathic philosophy, a practitioner might treat the same condition in two patients with entirely different medicines. He might treat two different conditions in two patients with the same medicine. His decision in each case would depend on his analysis of the whole patient. I am not qualified to debate the validity of this approach but it does present a difficulty when the Medicines Act licences of right for homeopathic remedies come to be reviewed – which would certainly not be for several years – or when new licences for homeopathics are applied for.

She then discussed the possibility of introducing a modified form of licensing for homeopathics which deals only with the safety and quality of the ingredients and the acceptability of the method of manufacture. The question of efficacy would be left to the professionals and the patient would look to the prescribing doctor or to the pharmacist for advice.

EC Directives

Council Directive 92/73/EEC widens the scope of Directives 65/65/EEC and 75/319/EEC.

The aims of the directive

The 1992 Directive recognised that:

1. Homeopathic medicine is officially recognised in certain member states but is only tolerated in other Member states.
2. Even if homeopathic medicinal products are not always officially recognised, they are nevertheless prescribed and used in all member states.
3. It is desirable in the first instance to provide users of these medicinal products with a very clear indication of their homeopathic character and with sufficient guarantees of their quality and safety.
4. The rules relating to the manufacture, control and inspection of homeopathic medicinal products must be harmonised to permit the circulation throughout the Community of medicinal products which are safe and of good quality.
5. Having regard to the particular characteristics of these medicinal products (such as the very low level of active principles they contain and the difficulty of applying to them the convention statistical methods relating to clinical trials) it is desirable to provide a special, simplified registration procedure for those traditional homeopathic medicinal products which are placed on the market without therapeutic indications in a pharmaceutical form and dosage which do not present a risk for the patient.
6. On the other hand the usual rules governing the authorisation to market medicinal products should be applied to homeopathic medicinal products placed on the market with therapeutic indications or in a form which may present risks which

must be balanced against the desired therapeutic effect. Those Member states which have a homeopathic tradition should be able to apply particular rules for the evaluation of the results of tests and trials intended to establish the safety and efficacy of these medicinal products provided that they notify them to the Commission.

Implementation in the UK

A Department of Health press release on 24 January 1994 relating to the registration of homeopathic products, described the Medicines (Homeopathic Medicinal Products for Human Use) Regulations 1994 SI 1994/105 as a new scheme to cover products for oral or external use in humans with no therapeutic indications and which are of good quality and sufficiently diluted to guarantee safety.

Market authorisation

Medicines for Human Use (Marketing Authorisations etc.) Regs 1994 SI No 3144 made it an offence to place a medicinal product on the market without marketing authorisation, which was granted by the Medicine Control Agency. These Regulations implement for the UK, a range of EEC Council Directives. The Regulations also set down a procedure for the consideration of an application, revocation and suspension of marketing authorisation and the suspension of the use of marketing or medicinal products. There are also provisions on the labelling of medicinal products.

In a recent case[9], it was held that, where there was a challenge by way of judicial review over the decision of the Medical Control Agency in relation to the classification of a product as medicinal, it was not for the High Court to make the classification, but for the High Court to review the decision on the usual principles of judicial review (i.e. the principles of natural justice). The Medicines Control Agency had decided that melatonin, a product marketed by Pharma Nord Ltd, was a medicinal product.

Regulations relating to homeopathic products

The Medicines (Advisory Board on the Registration of Homeopathic Products) Order 1995, SI 1995/309, made fresh provision for the establishment of the Advisory Board on the Registration of Homeopathic Products, clarifying the purposes for which the Board is established i.e. to give advice with respect to the safety and quality of any homeopathic medicinal product which meets the specified conditions set out in the Order and any homeopathic medicinal product which satisfies the conditions set out in the EEC Council Directive 92/74 and to which any relevant provision of the Medicines Act 1968 applies.

Medicines (Homeopathic Medicinal Products for Human Use) Amendment Regulations 1996 came into force 1 April 1996, SI 1996/482. These Regulations amend the Medicines (Homeopathic Medicinal Products for Human Use) Regulations 1994, SI 1994/105 which relate to the simplified registration procedure for the marketing of homeopathic medicinal products for human use. New provisions are made for fees payable in respect of applications for certificates of registration under Part III of the Regulations, prescribing fees for certificates of registration ranging from £100 to £650 determined by the number of homeopathic stocks used in the preparation of homeopathic medicinal products and by criteria relating to whether the licensing authority has previously assessed stocks and formulations identical to those proposed.

SITUATIONS WITH LEGAL SIGNIFICANCE

Failure to take a full history

Situation 1   Failure to take a full history

A Homeopath fails to take a full account of the history of a client and therefore does not discover that the client may be pregnant. He recommends a remedy which is inappropriate because it has an abortive effect. The client seeks to recover compensation.

The likelihood of the client succeeding in this situation will depend upon her being able to prove that any reasonable homeopath would have asked her about the pregnancy and would not have advised a remedy which could have brought about a miscarriage. In addition, however, and this may be difficult, she would have to prove that it was because she took this remedy that she miscarried, i.e. that the breach of duty by the homeopath caused the harm. In his defence the homeopath may be able to show that there was contributory negligence by the client in failing to inform him of the possibility of a pregnancy. There may also be a dispute over the facts as to what questions she was asked, whether she answered the questions fully and honestly, or whether she withheld information from him. If the homeopath is also a registered medical practitioner, then he would be judged according to the Bolam test as to what would have been reasonable practice by a doctor as well as what a reasonable homeopath would have done.

Failure to warn

Situation 2   Failure to warn

Following a consultation with a homeopath a client was told that he would be sent certain tablets to cure a problem relating to sinusitis. The client was not told to give up drinking coffee, menthol and peppermint during the time he was taking the tablets. After several return visits to the homeopath the client was advised that the tablets were probably ineffective because the coffee he continued to drink had a counteractive effect. He has now asked for the return of all his fees and the cost of the remedies.

In this situation the client is unlikely to be able to sue for negligence since it appears that he has not suffered harm. This in any event is very difficult to establish with homeopathic remedies since the level of toxicity is minute. However he could probably sue for breach of contract since the information of which drinks and foods to avoid whilst taking the remedies would appear to be vital information and the homeopath could be regarded as failing in his contractual duty to give necessary information to the client.

Allergic response

Situation 3   Allergic response
Following a homeopathic consultation, a client was given a preparation for pain relief. The homeopath had failed to check whether the client suffered from any allergies and was therefore not aware that this client was allergic to lactose. Lactose was used as the tablet base for the remedy and the client suffered a severe reaction from which he died. His family are now suing the homeopath.

There is a high probability that the family would succeed in their action against the homeopath if they can prove that death was caused by the lactose. Most would probably agree that any homeopath following a reasonable standard of care would have ascertained any information about allergies. Nor would it be possible for a homeopath who did not belong to the Society to argue that he was entitled to practise at a lower standard of care than those who had Society membership.

Care of a child

Case   Care of a child[19] (see also Chapter 25)
Parents refused to have a diabetic child treated by conventional medicine, believing entirely in the efficacy of homeopathic treatment. As a consequence the child died.

In this case both parents were found guilty of failing to take reasonable care of their daughter and the father was imprisoned. It could also be possible for criminal proceedings for manslaughter against the parents, and also the homeopath, to be brought. The success of a prosecution against a homeopath in such circumstances will depend upon the advice which he gave the parents and his own knowledge of the child's condition (see Chapter 5).

Side effects

Situation 4   Side effects
A client alleged that he had suffered the side effects from homeopathic medication. He had been given a homeopathic preparation based on ammonium compound and arsenic. The homeopath stated that it was impossible that any homeopathic substances could have caused side effects because only a minute amount of the active ingredient was used in homeopathic preparations.

If the client brings an action for negligence, it will be essential to establish the extent to which the homeopathic preparation could have caused any side effects, and whether a reasonable homeopath should have been aware of this possibility and taken action to ensure that the client was informed of this.

Loss of sight

Situation 5   Loss of sight
A patient refused to take steroid treatment for temporal arteritis and insisted on homeopathic treatment. The Homeopath failed to refer the patient to the appropriate specialist when the patient's problem deteriorated. As a result the patient lost the vision in one eye.

In a situation where the patient is refusing to consider any other investigation or specialist, the therapist would have a responsibility to ensure that the patient was competent to make such a decision and had all the necessary information. Where the homeopath was also a registered medical practitioner he would have to satisfy the Bolam test in ensuring that the patient was advised to agree to a referral to the appropriate specialist.

Brain damage

Situation 6   Brain damage
A homeopath who was also a registered medical practitioner failed to diagnose a brain tumour in a five year old child. Only homeopathic treatment was given as a result the child suffered from brain damage.

Like Case 1 this tragic outcome could result in both civil and criminal proceedings. If the parents were unaware of the need to obtain orthodox medical treatment and diagnostic tests such as X-Rays, then they may not be to blame. However the doctor's failure to arrange for the appropriate tests could lead to successful prosecution and civil action depending on what facts can be proved and the extent, if any, that the doctor was grossly negligent and reckless in relating to the health of the child.

CONCLUSIONS

In spite of its history and the establishment of the Faculty of Homeopathy in 1950, homeopathy has still not lost its identity as a complementary therapy rather than being seen as part of orthodox medicine. This is surprising in view of figures such as those produced by Swayne.[11] He showed that of a total of 7218 consultations carried out by members of the Faculty 88% were part of the NHS.

The clinical effectiveness initiative, the pressure on funding and increasing comparative research may, however, pave the way for greater use of homeopathic remedies. For example there is evidence that in France the annual cost for the Social Security System for homeopathic physician is 15% less than that of a conventional physician and the price of the average homeopathic medicine is one third that of standard drugs.[12]

The authors suggest that outcomes research will prove to be the most important area of homeopathic research over the next five years using such indicators as overall health status, patient satisfaction, days missed from school or work, and the cost of treatment.

There is now increasing evidence of the use of homeopathic remedies being used by veterinary surgeons. Since animals are unlikely to be affected by the placebo effect, results such as those shown by Day on the use of homeopathy in treating mastitis in cows[13] are extremely important. If homeopathic remedies can hold their own in comparative research trials, then there is every possibility of their becoming an integral part of the NHS.

Perhaps the 21st century will be the one in which the scientific basis for the effectiveness of homeopathy is understood thus opening up a new arena for exploration.

Whilst the safety of homeopathic remedies are stressed by many writers evidence is emerging from Medical Defence Societies that there are complaints and litigation in relation to missed diagnoses and failing to continue with necessary orthodox medicine. As the popularity of homeopathy grows, so may the number of criticisms.

Questions and Exercises

1. A patient has been receiving homeopathic treatment for several months and has found that she had benefited from it. She learns that her health authority has now decided not to contract for such treatments and as her GP is not a fundholder there is no way in which she can receive this treatment under the NHS. She is not able to pay for the treatment privately and does not wish to change her non-fundholding GP. Does she have any rights?
2. What action can a homeopathic practitioner take when he discovers that a neighbour is setting up a practice in various complementary therapies, including homeopathy, without being a member of any recognised homeopathic association?
3. A patient with severe eczema attends a homeopath and is advised to take a specific preparation which is based on sulphur. The patient fails to keep to the set dose and the eczema becomes inflamed and irritated. He claims that the homeopath was at fault in recommending that particular product. Will he succeed?

REFERENCES

1. Brown M Look for the perfect match. The Times 5 July 1997
2. Kleijen J, Knipschild P, Riet G 1991 Clinical trials of homeopathy. British Medical Journal 302(6772): 516
3. House of Commons Adjournment Debate 7 April 1977, quoted in Fulder S 1988 The Handbook of Complementary Medicine. Coronet,
4. Society of Homeopaths Leaflet. Homeopathy Simply Explained

5. Cummings B 1994 Using homeopathy in midwifery practice. Modern Midwife 4(11): 17–20
6. UKCC 1992 Standards for the Administration of Medicines. UKCC, London
7. Murray I Health Authority halts homeopathy. The Times 22 May 1997
8. Trumpington 1987 Alternative medicine and therapies and the DHSS. Journal of the Royal Society of Medicine 80: 336–8
9. R v. Medicines Control Agency, ex parte Pharma Nord Ltd. The Times 29 July 1997
10. News report. The Times 6 November 1993; and editorial A right to life: parents cannot condemn their children to die. The Times 8 November 1993.
11. Swayne JMD 1989 Survey of the use of homeopathic medicine in the UK health system. Journal of the Royal College of General Practitioners 39: 503–6
12. Jacobs J, Moskowitz R 1996 Homeopathy, chapter 5 In: Micozzi M (ed) Fundamentals of complementary and alternative medicine. Churchill Livingstone, New York
13. Day C 1988 Clinical trials in bovine mastitis. British Homeopathic Journal 75: 11–14

28

Hypnotherapy

DEFINITION

Hypnotherapy is the use of hypnosis (i.e. placing a person in a trance like state) to enhance that person's sense of health and well-being.[1]

BACKGROUND

Hypnosis involves creating a state of mind in which normal methods of thinking are temporarily suspended and experiences of an unusual nature may take place. Hypnotherapy uses hypnosis to effect therapeutic change. Hypnosis to anaesthetise a patient during an operation has been used for nearly 100 years in the West and probably longer in China.[2] However, like so many other complementary therapies, hypnosis was dismissed for many years as a deception but is now widely accepted by psychiatrists and clinical psychologists as an invaluable therapeutic tool, particularly in the United States.[3]

Anton Mesmer an Austrian (1734–1815) discovered a technique to induce convulsions and a loss of mental and physical control in his patients. Hence the term 'mesmerism'. He attributed the success to some form of fluid which was being redistributed by the force of magnetic poles.

In the 1830s hypnotist John Elliotson, a distinguished professor with an unorthodox manner and a fascination with the paranormal, offended the medical establishment by a demonstration of mesmerism (as hypnotism was then called) in front of lay audiences that included Charles Dickens. Elliotson is quoted as saying that 'in a mesmeric trance state, wounds give no pain'. Elliotson's work was denounced as unscientific by the *Lancet* and he had to resign from University College London.[4] Elliotson's work however was followed by James Esdaile.

In India in the 19th century, a Scottish surgeon, Dr James Esdaile, carried out more than 300 major yet apparently painless operations on hypnotised patients, ranging from limb amputations to the removal of scrotal tumours. A medical committee chaired by the deputy governor of Bengal subsequently endorsed Dr James Esdaile's unorthodox use of hypnosis, which he advocated as a far more effective and safer anaesthetic than chloroform.[5]

James Braid (1795–1860) an English physician, sought to remedy mesmerism's tainted reputation by postulating that its effects were due to a mental force, not a mysterious fluid.[6] He changed its name to hypnosis, after the Greek God for sleep. Braid suggested that Mesmer's subjects had been in a trance state which could be induced by watching a swinging pendulum or staring at a distant point or light. He called this state neurohypnotism.

Dr Milton H Erickson, an American psychiatrist, defined hypnosis as a state in which subjects experience a heightened awareness, concentrating their attention on thoughts, beliefs, memories and so on that are beyond normal waking awareness. His approach was widely practised in the second half of the 20th century in the United States.[7]

The BMA subcommittee in 1955 published a report recommending that the subject of hypnosis be taught to all medical undergraduates in Britain, and that trainee psychiatrists, anaesthetists and obstetricians be trained in its clinical use. Nevertheless, a survey carried out in 1978[8] found that such teaching was virtually unheard of in medical and dental schools.

Case 1 No anaesthetic
The report of the first patient to undergo a vasectomy without an anaesthetic was published in April 1994.[9][10] Andy Bryant had the operation, normally performed under local anaesthetic, with the help of a hypnotist at the Marie Stopes clinic in London.

Mandy Langford, a hypno-therapist and former chair of the British Complementary Medicine Association stated that

The technique was widely used to counter pain, especially in dentistry and for chronic back problems. Hypnotism doesn't stop the pain but it enables a person to manage and control their levels of pain. It is about taking the attention away from here and now and focusing it on something more enjoyable.

Dr Stuttaford, the columnist of the *Times*, quoted Dr Craft, a consultant psychiatrist at the Charter Nightingale Hospital in London, as saying that hypnosis helps patients who have a wide variety of phobias, from claustrophobia to a fear of flying, and also those who have anxieties. It is also valuable in treating people who have intractable pain.

Hypnosis is useful in selected cases. I am, however, careful not to use it with psychotic patients. It seems that hypnosis sometimes enhances paranoia and all too often I can become part of the delusion.[11]

REGULATION

There is no single system of nationally accredited courses in hypnosis. The Institute of Complementary Medicine maintains a register of hypnotists affiliated to professional organisations.

There is nothing, however, to prevent any person setting him or herself up as a hypnotist and offering services. It is estimated that there are over 4000 hypnotherapists in this country and there are numerous organisations representing them. There is not however one single umbrella organisation which links them. Hypnotherapy is one of the eight sections recognised by the United Kingdom Council for Psychotherapy (UKCP) (see Chapter 35). Five organisations are registered under that section including the National Register of Hypnotherapists and Psychotherapists.

Hypnotherapy by the medically qualified

Because of the dangers of causing harm two organisations regulating hypnosis in Britain (the British Society for Experimental and Clinical Hypnosis and the British Society of Medical and Dental Hypnosis) only allow qualified physicians, dentists or psychologists to be members. These organisations will provide lists of members.

A Hypnosis Unit opened at University College London in 1993. Its intake includes dentists, psychiatrists, psychologists, anaesthetists, general practitioners and paediatricians. The Head of the Unit, Dr Oakely, is reported[12] as saying

Hypnosis is not a therapy in its own right. It can only be effective in the context of another medical or psychological treatment.

Definitions of standards of competence

A project is being funded by the Department of Education and Employment for the Development of National Occupational Standards for Complementary Therapies. Hypnotherapy is one of several therapies in the project which is under the aegis of the Care Sector Consortium which is the Occupational Standards Council for Health and Social Care in the UK.

In the absence of a single controlling body on hypnotherapy there could be considerable debate over what were accepted standards of practice, except in the most extreme situations. There would probably be different standards of care between those hypnotists who are also registered as dental or mental practitioners and those who have no other professional health training. Most hypnotists would probably agree with the list given by Denise Rankin-Box of areas of therapeutic potential for hypnosis in nursing (shown in Box 28.1) and with her list of contraindications (shown in Box 28.2).

Rules on professional misconduct

All those who are members of an organisation registered with the UKCP are obliged to obey ethical guidelines on professional practice. In addition organisations have their individual Codes of Practice which can lead to practitioners being removed from the register of members.

Box 28.1 Therapeutic potential in nursing

- Relaxation
- Acute and chronic pain management
- Childbirth – management of labour pain
- Stress management
- Control of certain phobias – needle phobia during, for example, renal dialysis, chemotherapy, diabetes management
- Post-amputation phantom pain management
- Relief of nausea during pregnancy, drug treatment, post operatively
- insomnia
- hypertension
- irritable bowel syndrome

In casualty simple trance techniques may be used to relax or 'numb' an area requiring suturing – this can be effective in both children and adults.

Self-hypnosis can be taught to clients for pain control in labour, acute anxiety attacks, insomnia, relaxation etc.

Box 28.2 Contraindications for use

Whilst hypnosis can be extremely valuable it is important that the therapist is competent to deal with the particular problems.

Avoid long-standing psychological problems which may require professional counselling/treatment.

Occasionally clients may feel lightheaded when coming out of a deep trance state and it is important to know how to manage this and any abreactions that may occur.

However those treated by persons not members of a recognised association are vulnerable. For example, Dr Whorwell in a letter to the editor of the *British Medical Journal*[13] points out that

Anybody can set up as a therapist, even to the extent of concocting bogus qualifications from a fictitious training institution. The time has come to impose strict controls over the provision of hypnotherapy, particularly as it is a powerful phenomenon which cannot be allowed to get into the hands of unscrupulous people. A single register, easily accessible to the public is needed, from which practitioners can be erased for transgressions. The criteria for inclusion on the register should be well defined. Having a list of recognised qualifications or colleges would be pointless as a potential patient would find it almost impossible to ascertain which were bona fide, in addition, there would be no opportunity to impose sanctions.

He does not however insist that hypnotherapists should have a medical qualification.

Insurance cover and professional indemnity

Those organisations who are members of the UKCP are obliged to have professional indemnity insurance cover.

LEGAL PROVISIONS

> **Case 2** First successful action
>
> In 1948 a successful legal case was brought against a stage hypnotist for assault and professional negligence.

The Hypnotism Act 1952

In 1952 Leo Abse successfully introduced a private members Bill into Parliament which resulted in an Act being passed to regulate the demonstration of hypnotic phenomena for purposes of public entertainment. Its basic provisions are shown in Box 28.3.

> **Box 28.3** Hypnotism Act 1952
>
> **1. Control of demonstrations of hypnotism at places licensed for public entertainment**.
> [The licensing powers of local authorities] shall include the power to attach conditions regulating or prohibiting the giving of an exhibition, demonstration or performance of hypnotism on any person at the place to which the licence relates.
>
> **2. Control of demonstrations of hypnotism at other places.**
> (1) No person shall give an exhibition, demonstration or performance of hypnotism on any living person at or in connection with an entertainment to which the public are admitted, whether on payment or otherwise, at any place in relation to which such a licence as is mentioned in section one of this Act is not in force unless the controlling authority have authorised that exhibition, demonstration or performance.
> 2(1) (A) The foregoing subsection shall not apply to an exhibition, demonstration or performance of hypnotism that takes place in the course of a performance of a play (within the meaning of the Theatres Act 1968) given either at premises in respect of which a licence under that Act is in force or under the authority of any such letters patent as are mentioned in section 17(1) of that Act.
> 2(2) Any authorisation under this section may be made subject to any conditions.
> 2(3) [Contravention of this section or conditions imposed is an offence].
>
> **3. Prohibition on hypnotising persons under eighteen**.
> A person who gives an exhibition, demonstration or performance of hypnotism on a person who had not attained the age of eighteen years at or in connection with an entertainment to which the public are admitted, whether or payment or otherwise, shall, unless he had reasonable cause to believe that that person had attained that age, be liable on summary conviction...
>
> **4. Entry of premises**.
> Any police constable may enter any premises where any entertainment is held if he has reasonable cause to believe that any act is being or may be done in contravention of this Act.
>
> **5. Saving for scientific purposes**.
> *Nothing in this Act shall prevent the exhibition, demonstration or performance of hypnotism (otherwise than at or in connection with an entertainment) for scientific or research purposes or for the treatment of mental or physical disease.* [author's emphasis]
>
> **6. Definition of hypnotism**.
> ...includes hypnotism, mesmerism and any similar act or process which produces or is intended to produce in any person any form of induced sleep or trance in which the susceptibility of the mind of that person to suggestion or direction is increased or intended to be increased but does not include hypnotism, mesmerism or any such similar act or process which is self-induced.

Advice was given to Local Authorities in 1989 to attach conditions to licences, including checking whether the hypnotist has been refused a licence in the past. Volunteers should not be made to behave in an 'indecent, offensive or harmful manner' or to consume harmful substances and all hypnotic suggestions must be removed from the minds of subjects including the audience. The guidance recommended that no inducement should be offered to members of the public to take part.

Continued concerns

Colin Pickthall MP for Lancashire West told the House of Commons on 14 December 1994 that because the Act excluded Hypnotism for medical and scientific research a hypnotist had gone ahead with performance in a public house after having been refused a licence on the grounds that the Act did not require permission for research and he claimed that his show was private research. Colin Pickthall emphasised in the House of Commons that

It is possible for someone to learn quickly how to hypnotise people and within a day to be doing so on stage, even though that person does not understand and possibly does not even care about the consequences of what he is doing. It is those cowboys that we are most worried about.

In December 1994 it was reported[14] that the government was to review the law governing stage hypnosis after a series of complaints over acts in pubs and clubs and growing fears about safety. Campaigners for a change in the law want a central register of hypnotists, a code of conduct and compulsory liability insurance. Others are demanding an outright ban.

Circular No 39 of the Home Office issued in 1996 set out guidance to local authorities for the granting of licences for the performance of stage hypnotism. An Annex to the circular provides model conditions to be attached to the licence. This model covers the following areas:

- consent to the licence
- form of application
- publicity
- insurance
- physical arrangements
- treatment of audience and subjects
- prohibited actions
- authorised access (to constable, or member of licensing or fire authority)

Rules relating to the performance of stage hypnotism will also be covered by the general rules applying to public entertainments licences for music and dancing.

Recent cases

Case 3 Regression
It was reported[15] that following a hypnotist's show Christopher Gates who had been put into regression, felt unwell. He was referred to a psychiatric unit for four weeks. Nine months later his condition has deteriorated severely and he now thinks of himself as eight years old and behaves like an eight year old. He must be accompanied by an adult at all times.

Case 4   Death following hypnotism

Sharon Tabarn aged 24 died five hours after being hypnotised in a nightclub[16] She died from a fit hours after being told to emerge from a hypnotic trance as if a 10 000-volt electric shock had passed through her chair. The inquest recorded a verdict of accidental death and an expert witness declared that there was no connection between the hypnosis and any physical side effects.

Her mother founded the Campaign against Stage Hypnotism. Following this campaign, it was reported on August 7 1996[17] that in the light of a report by a panel of psychologists, and psychiatrists highlighting the risks of stage hypnosis, the Home Office has sent a guidance paper to Local Councils who could consult a blacklist of stage hypnotists whose acts had provoked complaints, before issuing licences. These proposals are described as an attempt to keep controls to a minimum and reflect the level of risk. Any action which would be likely to cause harm, anxiety or distress would be banned. Stage hypnotists would also be prohibited from trying to treat any medical condition. Margaret Harper, the campaigner whose daughter died said she would have preferred to see a total ban. She considered the proposals still favoured the performers. She also was concerned at who would be monitoring the proposals.

Subsequently it was announced that a solicitor representing families who claim to be victims of stage hypnosis has lodged an application with the Attorney General for a fresh inquest after a verdict of death by natural causes on Sharon Tabarn.[18]

Case 5   Suicide attempts

The solicitor in case 4 also represented Lynne Howarth who sued Philip Green a hypnotist for causing psychiatric damage and leading her to attempt suicide twice. Mrs Howarth was asked to pretend that she would be brought out of her trance by a 10 000 volt shock. She is claiming damages for mental suffering and loss of earnings after her husband took six months off work to look after her. She stated that for six months she did not go out of the house and tried to commit suicide. 'I became very abusive towards my children. I just wasn't myself. It makes me very angry that these people can get away with this.' On March 20 1997[19] judgment was entered in her favour at Blackburn County Court because the hypnotist had failed to file a defence. However the amount of compensation is still to be settled.

SITUATIONS WITH LEGAL SIGNIFICANCE
Liability for failure?

Situation 1   Liability for failure?

A hypnotist agrees with a patient that he will assist the patient to stop smoking. After a series of sessions, the patient is smoking more than ever and the hypnotist confesses that there is nothing more that he can do. The patient threatens to sue the hypnotist for breach of contract and negligence in causing him to become an even heavier smoker. Will he succeed?

In this situation, the likelihood of the patient succeeding in his legal action will depend upon the following factors:

- What terms have been agreed as part of the contract for services?
- What is the standard of care which the hypnotist owed to the patient and was he in breach of this standard?

If the hypnotist undertook to end the patient's smoking habit, then he is clearly in breach of contract. If, which is more likely, he undertook to assist him to give up but warned him that he could not guarantee the result, then an action for breach of contract is unlikely to succeed (see Chapter 4 for further details on breach of contract).

The fact that the patient has become an even heavier smoker may not have been caused by the actions of the hypnotist and therefore compensation may not be recoverable for that. The burden is on the patient to prove what was the reasonable standard of care expected of a hypnotist and how the defendant fell below this. Expert witnesses would have to show in what ways the defendant failed to measure up to any such standard. In addition the patient would have to show that the fact that he is now a heavier smoker was a reasonably foreseeable result of the alleged breach of duty.

Evidence that the hypnotist gave a warning that the therapy might not succeed will make it more difficult for the patient to win the case both in contract and in negligence.

Sexual abuse

Situation 2   Sexual abuse
A hypnotherapist agrees to hypnotise a woman to help her reduce weight. She now claims that during the session whilst she was in a trance he abused her sexually. What rights does she have?

Clearly an offence has been committed, but the prosecution will have to prove guilt beyond all reasonable doubt (see Chapter 5 on the criminal law). The difficulty for the patient is that it is her word against that of the hypnotist unless other patients come forward with similar allegations. The problem of sexual abuse by therapists is well documented[20] and Julia Stone and others quote a letter in the *British Medical Journal* where PJ Whorwell cites a case of a hypnotherapist who used hypnosis to abuse female patients and urges greater regulation of such therapies.[21]

If a criminal act has been proved it is open to the victim to claim compensation from the Criminal Injuries Compensation Board (the CICB). The compensation scheme has been subject to recent review under the Criminal Injuries Compensation Act 1995.

CONCLUSION

As the popularity of hypnosis expands as a therapeutic tool, so we are likely to see an increase in the number of legal actions and pressure on the professions to increase self-regulation, especially for those who are not registered as medical practitioners or dentists.

It is essential that those who use hypnotism develop standard forms for making contracts with patients and explain the limitations of hypnotherapy. There is a danger that the reputation of hypnotists will be tarnished by the excessive promises and the abuse of its powers by a few.

There would appear to be considerable advantage in state regulation to limit the use of the word 'hypnotherapist' to those with the appropriate accredited training in order that the general public can be protected.

Questions and Exercises

1. Do you consider that there should be a law to regulate religious worship where some forms of hypnotism may be used incidentally?
2. Can a distinction be drawn between hypnotism as a stage performance and hypnotherapy for therapeutic purposes?
3. What would be the advantages of national accreditation of courses in hypnotism.

REFERENCES

1. Rankin-Box D 1995 Hypnosis, chapter 15 In: Rankin-Box D (ed) The nurses' handbook of complementary therapies. Churchill Livingstone, New York
2. Stuttaford T Local Anaesthetic is more reliable. The Times 23 April 1994
3. Watkins A D 1996 Contemporary context of complementary and alternative medicine, chapter 4 In: Micozzi M (ed) Fundamentals of complementary and alternative medicine. Churchill Livingstone, New York
4. Greenhalgh T People laugh if I tell them how hypnosis helped. The Times 2 November 1995
5. Robertson I The strange power of suggestion. The Times 10 February 1994
6. Kaptchuk TJ 1996 Historical context of the concept of vitalism in complementary and alternative medicine, chapter 3 In: Micozzi M (ed) Fundamentals of complementary and alternative medicine. Churchill Livingstone, New York
7. Stanway A 1987 The Natural Family Doctor. Gaia Books, London
8. Robertson I The strange power of suggestion. The Times 10 February 1994
9. Laurance J Vasectomy patient says pain is all in the mind. The Times April 23 1994
10. Editorial, Patients, awake! The Times 23 April 1994
11. Stuttaford T Psychiatrists wake up to the healing power of hypnotism. The Times 5 April 1996
12. Greenhalgh T People laugh if I tell them how hypnosis helped. The Times 2 November 1995
13. Whorwell PJ 1993 Letter to the editor. British Medical Journal 307: 326
14. Ford R, Curphey M Minister orders legal review of stage hypnosis. The Times 14 December 1994, p 8
15. Ford R, Curphey M Minister orders legal review of stage hypnosis. The Times 14 December 1994, p 8
16. Ford R, Curphey M Minister orders legal review of stage hypnosis. The Times 14 December 1994, p 8
17. Tendler S Hypnosis acts face stricter controls. The Times 7 August 1996

18. Fresco A Call for curbs on stage hypnotists. The Times 23 September 1996
19. Fresco A Woman wins first judgment against stage hypnotist. The Times 20 March 1997
20. Stone J, Matthews J 1996 Complementary medicine and the law. Oxford University Press, Oxford
21. Whorwell PJ 1993 Letter to the editor. British Medical Journal 307: 327

29

Iridology

DEFINITION

Iridology is the use of the iris of the eye to diagnose weaknesses in the body, on the assumption that the iris can indicate the state of the internal organs. Many practitioners are also naturopaths (see Chapter 31).

BACKGROUND

Iridology owes its existence to the experiences of a 19th century Prussian surgeon, Ignatz von Peczely, who discovered that when an owl was hurt a streak appeared across its eye. He subsequently examined patients' eyes to see if there was any link with their presenting symptoms. He prepared a map of the eye, showing the regions and their links with parts of the body. His work was developed by Dr Bernard Jensen in the USA in the 1950s. The left iris relates to the left side of the body, the right iris to the right side.

REGISTRATION AND TRAINING

The Guild of Naturopathic Iridologists runs a course following which practitioners can become members on its register. They are required to be qualified in another therapy.

The International Association of Clinical Iridologists keeps a register of those who have graduated from the UK College of Iris Analysis.

Both organisations define standards of competence and lay down rules on professional misconduct.

However as in the other non-state registered therapies, anyone can set up in practice and call themselves an iridologist.

SITUATIONS WITH LEGAL SIGNIFICANCE
Too obscure

Situation   Too obscure
A person at a health fair saw a stall advertising the art of iridology. Not having heard about it, she asked for a session and it was agreed that she would have a consultation the next day. The iridologist advised her that she was fundamentally in very good health, but could try and reduce the stress in her life. The client has now discovered that she has severe diabetes, and in fact is losing her vision. She also discovers that the iridologist did not belong to any recognised organisation.

Although diabetes can manifest itself in changes in the retina it is extremely debateable as to whether the client would be able to sue the iridologist (who studies the iris) successfully for negligence in failing to diagnose diabetes.

Clearly the practitioner would owe a duty of care to the client, but the nature of that duty would be difficult to identify. If there is clear research that establishes that the iris is a reliable form of diagnosis and that diabetes should have shown up and been identified by the iridologist, then it could be said that there has been a breach of the duty of care. If no such proposition could be made, then the client will fail. In addition the client would still have to establish that she has suffered harm from the diagnosis being made later rather than earlier.

In addition there may be an element of contributory negligence by the client. It could be argued that any reasonable person would seek orthodox medical care to diagnose any condition such as diabetes – just as one does not go to a jeweller if one wants ear piercing done to the standard of a surgeon (see the case of *Phillips* v. *Whitely* discussed in Chapter 3). However such a statement undermines the practice of any complementary therapy which is not based on clear scientific evidence of effectiveness.

CONCLUSIONS
The exercise of diagnosis is perhaps one of the most important skills in orthodox medicine, since once a condition has been correctly identified then, if there is a recognised treatment, it is relatively straightforward to apply the treatment. If clients are to rely upon diagnosis through the iris, it is essential that they can trust those who are offering the service. Since it is so easy to offer services to the public in this field without being a member of a recognised organisation, it might be thought that this is a field where some form of state control over the use of the title is essential.

Questions and Exercises

1. Many practitioners of complementary therapy become trained in more than one. Why do you think that this is, and which combinations do you think go best together?
2. Do you agree with the statement that the skill of diagnosis is one of the most important elements in the duty of care?

30

Kinesiology

DEFINITION

Kinesiology is the application of the science of muscle testing to detect allergies or imbalance in the body.

BACKGROUND

History

Applied kinesiology was created in 1965 through the efforts of Dr George Goodheart, a respected chiropractor. He discovered that the kinesiological tests used to determine relative muscle strength and tone over the range of movement of the joints could also give qualitative information about the functions of body organs – the liver, kidneys, small intestines etc. He developed a relatively complete diagnosis and treatment system.

Theoretical basis

Its theoretical basis rests on the assumption that muscle weakness is the result of the functional state of the nervous system (or energy channels), expressed in the muscle–nerve connections (motor neurone facilitation). The organs express their function via nerves to specific muscle groups.[1] As well as detecting incorrect joint function, spinal lesions, muscle weakness, organic dysfunction and psychological effects on the function of the body as a whole, it is also used to detect nutritional needs and allergy responses (see Chapter 32 on nutritional therapies). The theory, like Chinese Medicine, is based on the view that the energy channels in the body can be blocked thereby causing dysfunction (see Chapter 16 on acupuncture).

Controlling body

The Kinesiology Federation (KF) is an umbrella organisation for practitioners involved in a variety of applications: acupressure points, nutritional supplementation, flower essences, emotional work and gentle bodywork. It has established interim arrangements for the recognition of professional practitioner members prior to the establishment of National Occupational Standards in Kinesiology.

REGISTRATION AND TRAINING

Guidelines have been prepared for training courses to obtain recognition by the Kinesiology Federation. Three main categories of courses may be submitted for approval:

- Professional courses consisting of at least 10 credits of kinesiology taken to an advanced level including the KF foundation level syllabus (a credit is the equivalent of 30 notional hours of work)
- Shorter courses suitable for lay people and/or existing kinesiology practitioners wishing to add to their skills
- Programmes containing totally new material and skills.

The KF criteria for recognition of approved systems of kinesiology are shown in Box 30.1.

Box 30.1   KF criteria for approved systems of kinesiology

The System must:
1. Use manual muscle testing as a means of assessment
2. Contain procedures encompassing the structural, chemical, psychological/emotional and subtle energy aspects of a person's functioning
3. Employ a systematic framework of enquiry primarily through muscle testing to:
   - identify any disorganisation which may adversely affect the accuracy of the muscle testing
   - identity dysfunction/imbalance within the person's system
   - determine and carry out appropriate techniques to redress any dysfunction/imbalance
   - validate the effectiveness of techniques employed through changed muscle response

---

There is a register held by the Kinesiology Federation for practitioners who have met the current standard.

Assessment includes anatomy, physiology and nutrition as well as interpersonal skills and practice management. Membership of the Kinesiology Federation also requires an average of at least 15 hours per year of postgraduate training.

RULES ON PROFESSIONAL MISCONDUCT

The KF has adopted the Code of Conduct and the Guidance to Practitioners of the

BCMA with an addendum for its own members. Its addendum emphasises the duty to act in the best interests of the client, the duty of confidentiality, and that members must not make diagnostic statements unless the member is a GP practitioner. Where members believe a client problem is outside their professional knowledge and expertise they must refer the client to an appropriately qualified practitioner.

Members must keep to the Code of Conduct. Any complaint regarding unethical behaviour or professional misconduct will be examined by the Therapy Council whose jurisdiction is final.

INSURANCE COVER

It is a requirement that all members of KF must be insured. It recommends that Bridge insurance policy issued by Balens Insurance, which covers members for use of the various therapies using kinesiology principles.

SITUATIONS WITH LEGAL SIGNIFICANCE
Varicose veins

Situation 1   Varicose veins

A practitioner of gentle massage and member of the KF failed to take account of the fact that the client had very severe varicose veins. During the massage, the veins started to haemorrhage. The client is now suing the practitioner and the KF.

In this situation, the practitioner is clearly at fault, if it can be established that any responsible practitioner following the reasonable standard of care would not have used massage on legs with varicose veins. Thus if a breach of the duty of care can be shown and it is a result of that breach that harm, i.e. the haemorrhaging, has occurred, then the practitioner will be liable.

What about the claim against the KF? This could only be maintained if it can be shown that:

1. The KF owed a duty of care to the individual client treated by a practitioner trained on one of the courses which it had approved.
2. The KF was in breach of this duty by failing to use all reasonable care in the approval of the course.
3. It was a reasonably foreseeable result of this breach that the haemorraghing occurred.

It is not clear that any of these three elements could be proved against the KF. Obviously much will depend on the specific circumstances of the actual situation.

Failure to diagnose

Situation 2 Failure to diagnose
A client underwent several sessions of treatment and advice from a practitioner of kinesiology paying out in total several hundred pounds. He has now been identified as suffering from a malignant tumour, which the practitioner had not identified. He is now prepared to sue the practitioner both for negligence in failing to identify the tumour and also for breach of contract for the recovery of his money.

The likely success of the action for negligence will depend upon the standard of care which can be expected from a kinesiologist and whether it could be reasonably expected that a tumour in a particular site could be diagnosed. Even if the client could show, with expert evidence, that a reasonable practitioner should have diagnosed the tumour, it is still essential that he shows that additional harm has been caused because of this failure to diagnose e.g. that had the tumour been diagnosed earlier treatment would have been more successful.

As far as the breach of contract case is concerned the practitioner would have to show that one of the express or implied terms of the contract was to the effect that the practitioner would identify any underlying disease and there was a failure to fulfil this. If the contract merely stipulated that a certain number of sessions would be carried out without identifying any specific benefits, then the client is unlikely to be able to recover his fees.

It should be emphasised that the Kinesiology Federation does not expect members to make diagnoses or hold themselves out as being able to diagnose. Members are expected to work alongside orthodox medical practitioners and clients should confirm that they are seeking orthodox medical advice.

CONCLUSION

More research is essential in this field in order to establish the clinical effectiveness of both the theory and its application to a wide range of therapies. If claims made by its practitioners can be substantiated, referrals within the NHS are likely to increase.

Questions and Exercises.

1. To what extent do you consider that an organisation with the responsibility of approving training courses, should owe a duty of care to the ultimate client of practitioners who pursue the course?
2. If a therapy is not supported by positive research findings showing that it is successful, how can a reasonable standard of care be identified?
3. Do you consider that a practitioner of applied kinesiology has a duty to notify clients that research evidence does not support the use of muscle testing as a form of diagnosis?

REFERENCES

1. Fulder S 1988 The handbook of complementary medicine. Oxford University Press, Oxford

31

Naturopathy

DEFINITION

Naturopathy is defined by the Commission of Naturopathic Medicine set up in 1989 as

a system of primary care medicine which seeks to facilitate and promote the body's inherent physiological self-healing mechanisms.

Like acupuncture, herbal medicine, homeopathy, chiropractic and osteopathy it holds itself to be a complete system of healing. It is based on a philosophy described as follows by Milton Power.

The Philosophy of Nature Cure holds that the constant effort or impulse of the life force in the human body is towards self-cleaning, self-repairing and positive health; that even acute disease is a manifestation of this self-curative force. Ill health and disease can therefore be eradicated only by removing all obstructions and by raising the tone of the body so that this natural inherent reconstructive self-purifying activity can do its own work safely and fully.[1]

Chronic diseases are seen in many cases as the results of mistaken efforts to 'cure', alter or suppress these acute ailments or natural healing crises by means of poisonous drugs, wrong feeding, inoculation, vaccination, hypnotism, or needless surgical intervention.

HISTORY AND UNDERLYING PRINCIPLES

The Nature Cure Movement began in Europe in the 19th century. Vincent Priessnitz is described as the 'Father of Nature Cure'. He was born in Grafenburg and saw healing power in water applied both internally and externally. Nature Cures developed over Austria and Germany. In the middle of the 19th century similar developments took place in the USA with James Caleb Jackson who, having been cured by a disciple of Priessnitz, established the Jackson Sanatorium in New York. Another American pioneer was Dr Russel T Thrall who founded the Hygieotherapeutic

College in New York. Dr H Lindlahr worked on the coordination of all the different aspects of naturopathic treatments into one science. His theory was that 'every acute disease is a healing effort of Nature'. He founded the Lindlahr Sanatorium in Chicago. In England a Hydropathic establishment was built by John Smedley in Matlock in Derbyshire in 1853.

Bernarr Macfadden, a health culturist and writer well known in America, opened a publishing office in London. He opened a health sanatorium on the sea front at Brighton in 1909. After its closure as a result of the First World War, he opened a health home at Orchard Leigh in the Chilterns. A graduate of his, Stanely Lief, took charge at Orchard Leigh and was a significant figure in the spreading of Nature Cure in Great Britain.

The Pitcairn-Knowles family established the Riposo Nature Cure Hydro near Hastings in 1913. James Thomson, who had trained in Dr Lindlahr's Chicago Sanatorium opened a practice in Edinburgh and started the first training college in Britain, the Edinburgh School of Natural Therapeutics in 1919 which ran a four year course.

Milton Powell who worked at the Brighton Sanatorium established a practice in a small Nature Cure Health Home in Northampton. He urged the foundation of a Nature Cure Association with the aims of:

- Providing a Register of Naturopaths.
- Providing moral and legal support to Nature Cure Practitioners.
- Establishing, maintaining or recognising approved Nature Cure training schools.
- Standing firmly for the principle of freedom of choice as applied to every individual seeking advice and treatment.
- Spreading by every suitable means and among all sections of the public, the ideas, principles and methods of Nature Cure.

As a result of his efforts, The Nature Cure Association of Great Britain and Ireland (NCA) was founded in 1920. In 1925 it became a non-profit making company limited by guarantee. An ethical committee was established to prepare a Code of Professional Conduct and an Educational Council set professional and technical standards of proficiency and working towards the regulation of Nature Cure Training Schools and the establishment of a Register for approved applicants.

Stanley Lief, who had qualified at Bernarr Macfadden's training college in the USA became the proprietor of Orchard Leigh and later transferred to Champneys in Tring in 1925. Lief also founded the magazine *Health for All* and the British College of Naturopathy and Osteopathy in Hampstead.

1945 saw the amalgamation of the Nature Cure Association of Great Britain and Ireland and the British Association of Naturopaths to form the British Naturopathic Association. The Guild of Naturopathy and Osteopathy was formed in 1949. In 1961 the British Naturopathic Association changed its title to the British Naturopathic and Osteopathic Association.

Joseph E Pizzorno Jr[2], states that

Naturopathic medicine is more than a system of health care; it is a way of life. Although the term naturopathy was coined in the late nineteenth century, its philosophical roots can be traced back to Hippocrates and the folk medicines of all peoples of the earth. It is a distinct system of medicine that stresses health maintenance, disease prevention, patient education and patient responsibility – in contrast to the currently dominant system that emphasizes treatment of disease.

He concludes:

Naturopathic medicine as well as the entire concept of natural medicine, might appear to be an unscientific fad that will soon pass away. To the informed, it is clear that naturopathic medicine is at the forefront of the future of medicine. The scientific tools now exist to assess and appreciate many aspects of natural medicine. It is now common for conventional medical organisations that in the past have spoken out strongly against naturopathic medicine to endorse naturopathic techniques as lifestyle modification, stress reduction, exercise, consuming a high fibre diet rich in whole foods and other dietary measures, supplementary nutrients, toxin reduction and many others.

This illustrates the paradigm shift that is occurring in medicine. What was once disregarded is now becoming more generally accepted as effective. In fact, in many instances, the naturopathic alternative offers significant benefit with standard medical practices. In the future, the concepts, philosophies and practices of naturopathy should become accepted.

A Commission on Naturopathic Medicine was set up in 1989 by the British Naturopathic and Osteopathic Association to establish a statement of basic naturopathic philosophy and policy. The Commission defined naturopathy and identified the fundamental principles in a way which could embrace all shades of practise. It also considered the following topics:

- education and research
- the role of the naturopath in health care
- the role of the naturopath in society.

The Commission identified the therapies shown in Box 31.1 as of primary importance in the naturopathic treatment of disease. It also recognised that other therapies may be considered to be naturopathic in principle and therefore complementary to the methods listed in Box 31.1. These complementary therapies include: osteopathy, chiropractic, relaxation techniques, herbalism, electrotherapy, nutritional biochemistry and homeopathy.

Box 31.1   Therapies of primary importance in the naturopathic treatment of disease

1. Nutrition and dietetics
2. Fasting
3. Structural adjustments
4. Hydrotherapy
5. Healthy life style
6. Education

The main conclusions of the Commission were accepted by the British Naturopathic and Osteopathic Association and the General Council and Register of Naturopaths in October 1990.

CONTROLLING BODY AND REGISTRATION

The British Naturopathic and Osteopathic Association in 1992 was amalgamated with the Osteopathic Association of Great Britain and restarted as the British Naturopathic Association.

An official register of members compiled by the General Council of Naturopaths is published each year and is available in public libraries. The letters MRN are used to designate a Registered Naturopath. Since December 1952 the Register has only been available to graduates of the British College of Naturopathy and Osteopathy and graduates of the British Naturopathic and Osteopathic Association's postgraduate course in Naturopathic Medicine. The Council retains a discretion in respect of suitably qualified applicants.

There are other registers of Naturopaths outside the General Council.

TRAINING

The General Council and Register of Naturopaths insist upon a sound basic education, thorough training and satisfactory examination results. The British College is the only recognised college of naturopathy and osteopathy in Western Europe which has been approved for certain major county awards to cover the cost of training. The Manifesto of the General Council emphasises the importance of practitioners being taught to recognise both their scope and limitations as naturopaths.

RULES ON PROFESSIONAL MISCONDUCT, CONTROL AND DISCIPLINE

The General Council and Register of Naturopaths (GCRN) was founded in 1967 for the benefit and protection of the public to set out and monitor standards of clinical training in naturopathy, and to maintain and enforce a strict Code of Professional Conduct for registered naturopaths. It publishes a handbook which covers the topics listed in Box 31.2.

Box 31.2 Handbook of the GCRN

1. The Registered Naturopath and the law
2. Relationships with Patients
3. Relationships with Medical Practitioners and Surgeons
4. Relationships within the profession
5. Relationships with other health care professions
6. Scope and standards of practice
7. The Management and Control of Practices
8. Promoting the Individual and the Profession
9. Guidelines for Advertising
10. Professional Misconduct
11. Disciplinary Procedures.

Proscribed conduct for a professional on the Register is

any conduct of a member in contravention of the Code of Ethics of the Register for the time being in force, or any other conduct which brings or is likely to bring the Register into disrepute.

This definition is wide enough to enable the Professional Ethics Subcommittee, to take into account in its adjudication conventional standards of morality, comparable to the definition of professional misconduct for the UKCC as conduct unworthy of a nurse, midwife or health visitor.

INSURANCE COVER AND PROFESSIONAL INDEMNITY

The GCRN requires practising members to hold professional indemnity insurance cover as a condition of membership. Criteria are laid down by the Council which must be met by any acceptable indemnity cover. These include:

- cover for legal liability for payment of damages in a wide range of situations
- cover not less than the minimum specified by the Council
- cover not only for the assured but also in respect of anyone else who may become the partner, employee, volunteer or other specified associate in respect of claims arising from work undertaken on behalf of the member
- public liability including health and safety at work.

Insurance is provided on a group basis for the assured to cover damages arising out of any bodily injury, mental injury, illness, disease or death of any patient caused by any malpractice which is defined as

any negligent act error or omission committed by the Assured in or about the conduct of the Assured's occupation or business as stated in the Proposal or Renewal Declaration Form, or Good Samaritan Acts.

PURCHASING CONTRACTS

The GCRN states in its handbook:

Most private health insurance companies require that a policy holder should be referred to a Registered Naturopath by his general practitioner, and occasionally by a consultant, in order for benefit for Naturopathic treatment to become payable.

SITUATIONS WITH LEGAL SIGNIFICANCE
Professional boundaries

Situation 1   Professional boundaries
A patient is referred to a naturopath by a general practitioner who believes that the chronic condition suffered by the patient would be ameliorated by naturopathy. The patient subsequently meets an osteopath who makes it clear that in his view, the referral was incorrect.

Situation 1 sets out one of the most difficult problems for those who practise orthodox medicine, to know the correct professional to whom any referral should be made. It may often be difficult for general practitioners to select which specialty in orthodox medicine is appropriate even when they have a basic understanding from their training of these areas. It is even more difficult when they are ignorant of the potential of certain complementary therapies and their sphere of limitation. (Some might consider that in fact they have no limitations but are holistic and comprehensive in their contribution to human health and well-being.)

If it can be proved that there is an inappropriate referral which is negligent, then, if harm can also be established the patient may be able to claim compensation if no reasonable general practitioner would have made that referral. Alternatively, the referral might have been reasonable, but the practitioner to whom the referral was made should have realised, after the initial meeting with the patient, that she did not have the necessary skills to assist the patient and should therefore have advised the patient accordingly as the next situation illustrates.

An additional issue, of course, is that the referral and the consequential treatment were entirely appropriate but that the osteopath was making a defamatory statement.

Outside the competence

Situation 2   Outside the competence
A naturopath ignores a chronic disease of rheumatism and fails to obtain pain relief for the patient who commits suicide.

In situation 2 the naturopath should have been aware of the seriousness of the patient's suffering and should have monitored his condition to ascertain if he was able to assist the patient or if another practitioner, of a different therapy, should be brought in. The naturopath has assumed a duty of care to the patient. If he has failed to follow the reasonable standard expected of a reasonable body of competent naturopaths in not referring the patient on, and if this failure caused the patient's pain to go unrelieved and therefore to lead to the suicide, then the naturopath could be held accountable for that death. The relatives could act on behalf of the estate under the Law Reform (Miscellaneous Provisions) Act 1934 but compensation is limited to £7500. If they can show dependency upon the deceased, then they may have personal claims for that loss under the Fatal Accidents Acts. In addition, if they can prove that one or other has suffered post traumatic stress syndrome, beyond that of normal bereavement, as a result of the events, then there may be a claim for their own suffering (see Chapter 3).

The handbook of professional practice issued by the GCRN emphasises the importance of good contact between its members and general practitioners, surgeons, osteopaths and dentists. Its recommendations are shown in Box 31.3.

Box 31.3   Cross-referral procedures recommended by the GCRN
When a patient has been referred, either formally or informally, the Registered Naturopath should write a formal letter giving details of the case history, the clinical examination, his findings and the proposed treatment.

Similar communication should take place following the discharge by the naturopath. If there has been no referral then it is essential to obtain the patient's consent to this communication.

Elimination diet

Situation 3 Elimination diet
Following consultation with a naturopath a client was advised to go onto an elimination diet to clear the body of toxins. Unknown to the therapist the client was in a pre-diabetic state and as a result of the reduction in blood sugars went into a coma. Her family are prepared to sue the naturopath.

As in situation 2, the success of any litigation will depend upon establishing that the naturopath failed to follow a reasonable standard of care and that this failure led to the harm which has occurred. Expert advice would be necessary from senior members of a recognised organisation of naturopaths. Again should the client die the relatives could claim for the death under the Law Reform (Miscellaneous Provisions) Act, 1934. If there are dependents, they may have the right to recover compensation resulting from the death in respect of their dependency under the Fatal Accidents Acts.

CONCLUSION

The naturopathic profession is growing rapidly; its therapeutic and diagnostic skills are becoming more sophisticated; licensing is being established in new states of the USA; and public interest is strong. Key to the profession's future is becoming an integral part of the health care system and this will depend upon research into clinical effectiveness.

Questions and Exercises

1. Design a pamphlet for the general public explaining the role of the naturopath and distinguishing it from related professions.
2. Design a research project to show that naturopathy has beneficial effects compared with orthodox medicine.
3. Since any person can set up as a naturopath, what advice would you give to a person who has qualified on an approved course to protect their practice and image.

REFERENCES

1. British Naturopathic Association 1996 The British Naturopathic Association: The first fifty years 1996
2. Pizzorno JE Jr 1996 Naturopathic Medicine, chapter 12 In: Micozzi M (ed) Fundamentals of complementary and alternative medicine. Churchill Livingstone, New York

Nutritional therapies

DEFINITION

Nutritional therapies is an umbrella term describing a number of different therapies which are concerned with the exploration of 'all possible avenues whereby a patient's nutrition can be manipulated to obtain maximum health promotion'.[1] The therapies focus on the effects of certain foods on the individual's health and well-being.

BRIEF HISTORY AND CONTROLLING BODIES

There is evidence that concern with different properties of foods existed centuries ago. Thus garlic was used in Ancient Egypt, Babylonia and Greece as a cure for many disorders. There are accounts of cabbage being used by Hippocrates for cardiac problems. Recent concerns centre on vitamins, cholesterol levels and high fibre diet.

Dietitians obtained state registration under the Professions Supplementary to Medicine Act 1960. Their training therefore comes under the financial support of the Department of Health and takes place in colleges and universities accredited through recognised validation schemes.

Outside of the state registered dietitians, a variety of organisations have grown up. Thus for example the Institute of Allergy Therapy was founded to provide guidance to individuals on health eating. It uses kinesiology methods (see Chapter 30) to identify foods and other products which affect the strength of the body and indicate a possible allergy. It does not provide a qualification in itself but provides an additional training for those who already have a qualification in an area of complementary therapy and grounding physiology and anatomy. Any unacceptable practice by members is met by preventing them having access to the homoeopathic supplies which are necessary for their practice. In the ten years that the Institute has been running, there has only been one such example where an individual has been excluded from the register.

The Institute for Complementary Medicine has a division devoted to nutritional therapies (see Chapter 6). In other therapies such as naturopathy (see Chapter 31) nutrition is an essential aspect of the therapy and its philosophy.

The Society for the Promotion of Nutritional Therapy has a register of more than 400 qualified practitioners and is involved in educational activities and in unifying the profession.

REGISTRATION, MISCONDUCT AND INSURANCE

The Institute of Allergy Therapy is an Associate of the Kinesiology Federation, which is a member of the British Complementary Medicine Association (BCMA). Members would therefore be required to follow the Code of Conduct and Guidance to Practitioners of the BCMA (see Chapter 6).

The BCMA rules would apply in relation to misconduct and complaints which if upheld against members could lead to their being struck off the membership list.

Membership of the Institute provides professional indemnity insurance cover. All members of the Institute of Allergy Therapy carry appropriate practice insurance either in a scheme covering their original therapy or in the Institute's scheme.

LAWS RELATING TO THE THERAPY

Any nutritionists who produce their own products for sale would be subject to the laws relating to the sale of foods. Any products which are defined as medicinal products would come under the Medicines Act and the Medicines Control Agency (see Chapters 26 and 27 on herbal medicine and homeopathy and Chapter 5 on the criminal law).

There is increasing concern that manufacturers of food supplements are making claims in relation to the health giving properties of their products which could bring these products under the definition of medicinal product for the purposes of the Medicines Act 1968. This is considered in Chapter 5.

SITUATIONS WITH LEGAL SIGNIFICANCE
An unlikely allergy

Situation 1   An unlikely allergy

A practitioner of allergy therapy told the client following muscle testing that she was allergic to all forms of dairy products, red meats, wheat, coffee and tea but no other allergy was detected. The client commenced a very strict diet but, in order to keep up a supply of protein, ate vast quantities of nuts. She then suffered a severe allergic reaction and was rushed to hospital, being placed on life support. Her family are threatening to sue the practitioner.

The family suing on behalf of the client would have to show that the harm occurred as a result of the breach of duty owed by the practitioner to the client and that the practitioner had not followed the reasonable standard of care in the advice she gave.

Expert evidence would be required as to what is reasonable. Difficulties could arise in view of the fact that some of the claims made by allergy therapists have not been substantiated by research.[2] On this basis it could be argued that any advice given by the allergy therapist on the basis of muscle testing is ill-founded and therefore subject to legal action. In contrast many practitioners in this field attest to miraculous results from identifying foods to avoid. At present on the evidence of clinical effectiveness data, it would be difficult to establish clear standards of advice and practice.

Whose recommendation?

Situation 2   Whose recommendation?
Following a session of allergy therapy, based on kinesiology principles, a client was advised to take certain preparations to reduce her candida level. She was told that these would be forwarded to her from a firm. She paid the therapist and within 10 days received the preparation. She has subsequently become extremely ill, with ME type symptoms. She is blaming the pills sent to her. What action can she take?

More information would be required about her previous medical history and her present illness, the nature of the pills, the advice given to her by the therapist and any diet which she has been following. It could be that when this information was obtained, there would be no chance of a successful legal action, since her present illness was not the result of anything that the therapist advised and that the pills had no toxic effect i.e. she would have had her illness anyway. To show negligence by the therapist the client would have to show a failure by the therapist to follow the reasonable standard of care and that this failure itself caused her present illness.

Alternatively, if she could show that the pills were in some way defective, she may have a right of action against the supplier under the Consumer Protection Act 1987 (see Chapter 13). In such actions, the consumer only has to show a defect in the product and the harm which has resulted, the consumer does not have to identify negligence by the supplier.

Who is the supplier? It would be the firm sending the product to her, if this is identifiable from the packaging. If this cannot be identified, then the therapist would have to pass on the information as to who was the supplier to the client or be deemed to be the supplier herself.

Is there a contract between the client and the firm who supplied the pills? This does not have to be established for the purposes of the Consumer Protection Act nor for the law of negligence (see Chapter 3 and the case of *Donoghue* v. *Stevenson*) but, to establish a claim in the law of contract, the contracting party would have to be identified. One could argue that if the client made the cheque out to the therapist, the contract is between the therapist and the client. If on the other hand the client made the cheque payable to the firm, then the therapist was acting as agent of the firm in sending the order on to the firm.

CONCLUSIONS

The field of nutritional therapy is a growth area, fuelled by recent government health promotion campaigns and healthy eating strategies. More research is needed, not only in relation to the effects of specific foods or high or low cholesterol foods and vitamins etc., but also into the clinical effectiveness of kinesiology as applied to the diagnosis of food allergies.

Questions and Exercises

1. Design a leaflet for the initial interview for a client receiving nutritional advice which points out warnings and essential information which must be given to the therapist.
2. An allergy therapist sets up a consulting room in her own house. A client becomes fixated on her and she receives harassing phone calls from him and is sure that he is constantly hanging around her house watching for her. What action can she take? (see chapter 5)
3. Dietitians who are qualified under the Council of Professions Supplementary to Medicine are state registered health professionals (see chapter 6). To what extent do you consider that all those who are giving nutritional advice should be state registered?

REFERENCES

1. Society for the Promotion of Nutritional Therapy quoted by Trevelyan J and Booth B 1994 Complementary Medicine for Nurses, Midwives and Health Visitors. Macmillan, London
2. Kennedy JJ, et al 1988 Applied Kinesiology: unreliable for assessing nutritional status. Journal of the American Diet Association 88: 698–704

33

Osteopathy

DEFINITION

Osteopathy is the manipulation of joints and spinal vertebrae directed towards resolving mechanicial problems of the body.

BRIEF HISTORY AND CONTROLLING BODY

Osteopathy originated with the work of Dr Andrew Still in Kirksville, Missouri in the USA in the 19th century. In 1874 he treated a child suffering from dysentery by easing tension in the contracted back muscles and restoring movement to the joints of the spine.

The Natural Therapeutic and Osteopathic Society is a professional body set up in 1948 and renamed in 1977. It has acted as a regulating and registering body for qualified osteopathic practitioners. It ensures that all osteopaths so registered are fully insured for professional indemnity and public liability risks. All members are governed by the Constitution and Code of Ethics of the Society.

Recent developments

Following the recommendations of the then Minister of Health osteopaths established the General Council and Register of Osteopaths in 1936 as an independent governing and registering body. In 1957 the osteopaths asked those involved in drafting the Professions Supplementary to Medicine Regulations whether they intended to include osteopathy and were told that osteopathy was not considered as a profession supplementary to medicine.

In 1976 some osteopaths tried again. A private members Bill to set up a state register for osteopaths was introduced by Joyce Butler MP. The Secretary of State for Health and Social Security felt that state registration was premature.

In 1985 there was a House of Lords debate on registration.[1] The Act of 1993 is discussed in full below.

On February 1 1996 the first General Osteopathic Council (GOsC) was appointed by the Department of Health. Under the Osteopathy Act 1993 the 24 members of the Council have responsibilities for regulating the osteopathic profession and for its promotion and development. The GOsC is the first self-regulating, statutory Council within the arena of health care to be established for over 30 years. It will regulate the profession along similar lines to the General Medical Council and General Dental Councils. GOsC members will develop the structures necessary for the regulation of professional conduct, education and training of osteopaths, opening a statutory register for osteopaths during 1997. Once the Osteopaths Act is fully in force, only those practitioners admitted to the register will, by law, be allowed to call themselves 'osteopaths' and to practise as such. Further details are available from the Osteopathic Information Service.[2]

State registration is now available to those who meet the educational requirements laid down.

REGULATORY MATTERS

Definitions of standards of competence

Competence is based on the theoretical and practical experience gained through an accredited course. Expert evidence from those in senior positions within the Osteopaths' organisation would be available to determine the reasonable standard of care in any given situation.

Rules on professional misconduct

These are set out under the Act (see below). There is statutory provision for a Code of Conduct (see below) and failure to follow this could be evidence of misconduct.

Insurance cover and professional indemnity

Section 37 of the 1993 Act enables the General Council to make rules to provide for proper insurance cover. The exact wording is set out in Box 33.1.

Concern was expressed in the House of Commons that section 37 did not actually require the General Council to establish a scheme of professional indemnity insurance. However it accepted that responsibility for making the appropriate decision should be left to the General Council.

Definitions for purchasing contracts

Referrals to osteopaths within the NHS are increasing, but these tend to be on an individual basis.

Box 33.1   Section 37 – professional indemnity insurance

(1) the General Council may by rules make provision requiring —
(a) registered osteopaths who are practising as osteopaths, or
(b) prescribed categories of registered osteopaths who are practising as osteopaths, to secure that they are properly insured against liability to, or in relation to their patients.

(2) The rules may, in particular —
(a) prescribe risks, or descriptions of risk, with respect to which insurance is required;
(b) prescribe the amount of insurance that is required either generally or with respect to prescribed risks;
(c) make such provision as the General Council considers appropriate for the purpose of securing, so far as is reasonably practicable, that the requirements of the rules are complied with;
(d) make provision with respect to failure to comply with their requirements (including provision for treating any failure as constituting unacceptable professional conduct).

LAW RELATING TO THE THERAPY

The Osteopaths Act 1993

The main provisions of this Act are as follows:

A. Council and Registration provisions:

1. General Council and its committees
2. Registrar of Osteopaths
3. Full registration
4. Conditional registration
5. Provisional registration
6. Registration (supplemental provisions)
7. Suspension of registration
8. Restoration to the register of osteopaths who have been struck off
9. Access to the register etc.
10. Fraud or error in relation to registration

B. Professional education:

11. Education Committee
12. Visitors
13. The standard of proficiency
14. Recognition of qualifications
15. Recognition of qualification (supplemental)
16. Withdrawal of recognition
17. Post-registration training
18. Information to be given by institutions

C. Professional Conduct and fitness to practise:

19. The Code of Practice
20. Professional conduct and fitness to practise
21. Interim suspension powers of the Investigating Committee

22. Consideration of allegations by the Professional Conduct Committee
23. Consideration of allegations by the Health Committee
24. Interim Suspension powers of the Professional Conduct Committee and the Health Committee
25. Revocation of interim suspension orders
26. Investigation of allegations (procedural rules)
27. Legal assessors
28. Medical assessors

D. Appeals against the decision of:

29. The Registrar
30. The Health Committee
31. The Professional Conduct Committee

E. Offences, monopoly and miscellaneous provisions:

32. Offences
33. Competition and anti-competitive practices
34. Default powers of the Privy Council
35. Rules
36. Exercise of powers of the Privy Council
37. Professional indemnity insurance
38. Data protection and access to personal health information
39. Exemption from provisions about rehabilitation of offenders
40. Financial provision
41. Interpretation
42. Title and commencement

Schedules to the Act cover the General Council, the Statutory Committees and transitional provisions.

Amendments to the Act

Schedule 2 of the Chiropractors Act 1994 made certain amendments to the Osteopaths Act 1993:

- section 9 (access to the Register etc.) is amended in relation to the publication of the Register
- section 13 is amended in relation to the standard of proficiency
- section 18 is amended in relation to information to be given to institutions and replacing the General Council by the Education Committee
- section 20 is amended to require the General Council to make rules for the procedures to be followed by the Investigating Committee
- section 22 has added to it details on the condition of practice order to specify a period for it to have effect and/or a test of competence.

There are other changes to section 27 (legal assessors) and section 28 (medical assessors) to add the Registrar to the list of people who can be given advice. Minor changes are made to sections 30 and 31 (appeals against the Health Committee and Professional Conduct Committee) and the powers of the General Council. The definition of registered address is amended.

Section 3(10) of the Video Recordings Act 1984 exempted from the provisions of that Act the supply of videos used in training or carrying on any medical or related occupation, and this exemption was extended to chiropractors and osteopaths by section 39 of the Chiropractors Act 1994.

Coming into force

The provisions relating to the General Osteopathic Council and its functions and those of the Privy Council came into force on 14 January 1997.[3]

Some organisations of osteopaths not included within the umbrella organisation will find that following the implementation of the Act it becomes illegal for them to use that title, since the Act makes it an offence for a person to use the term osteopath if that person is not registered under the provisions of the Act.

CRANIOSACRAL THERAPY

One specialist area of osteopathy which has not been integrated within the Osteopathy Registration is the use of craniosacral therapy. In this therapy emphasis is placed upon the cranial concept. This is defined by the Craniosacral Therapy Association[4] as follows:

The 'Cranial Concept' is a grand concept of the human system, which acknowledges its deepest roots and highest potentials. In this concept, we, as human beings, are seen to be an expression of life itself. Life takes shape and form. This movement of life into form creates the infrastructure of pulsation which becomes the human body. Life is movement and pulsation; expansion and contraction. These movements are the manifestation of the basic energies of life. Dr Sutherland called these basic energies the 'Breath of Life'. The main intention of life in this field is to allow this Life Breath to express itself more fully in the human system. The process and relationships which express this in the body is sometimes called 'The Involuntary Mechanism' and its physical relationships are called the Primary Respiratory Mechanism or System. The Primary Respiratory System is composed of the anatomical and physiological elements of the core of the body...

The term 'Craniosacral System' recognises this implicit truth [i.e. of the body being an integrated whole and patterns of resistance which arise in one area of the body will have repercussions for other parts]. The more the system has to express patterns of resistance and restriction in its craniosacral dynamics, the more resistant it becomes to its own inherent life energies and the more prone it becomes to tissue congestion and break-down and the more likely it is that pathology will result.

Five inter-related aspects are identified in the Primary Respiratory System:

- the inherent fluctuation of cerebrospinal fluid
- the inherent motility of the brain and spinal cord
- the mobility of the cranial sutures
- the reciprocal tension membrane system
- the involuntary movement of the sacrum between the ilia

A basic premise in Craniosacral Therapy is that if the dynamics of these relationships become resistant and restricted, then the system is more prone to disorganisation, chaos, disease and pathology. It is the role of the Practitioner to relate to these dynamics with comprehension, skill and sensitivity. It is the intention of the work to assist the system to release fulcrums and patterns of resistance and to help the system express its vitality and healing potency with greater strength and integrity.

The standards of Practitioner Competencies identifies the areas shown in Box 33.2 as requirements of competence.

Box 33.2 Competencies in craniosacral therapy

1. The mobility of the cranial sutures (eight competencies)
2. The reciprocal tension membrane system (three competencies)
3. The involuntary motion of the sacrum between the ilia (three competencies)
4. Craniosacral motion dynamics
5. Whole body dynamics and the craniosacral system
6. The viscera, organs and organ system
7. Trauma, shock, and tissue memory
8. Communication and process skills
9. Skills in relationship to infants, adults, and the birth process
10. Anatomy, physiology and pathology
11. Practice management:
    - clinical environment
    - establishing a professional relationship
    - case histories
    - record keeping
    - communicating with other health professionals
    - financial records
    - time management
    - managing one's own professional life
    - legal aspects of practice

The Code of Ethics and Practice of the Craniosacral Therapy Association sets out the principles necessary to establish and maintain standards for the practice of Craniosacral Therapy and to inform and protect members of the public seeking Craniosacral treatment. It covers such areas as:

- Duties
- Obligations
- Conduct
- Adjudication
- The Rules and objects of the Association (including grades of membership)
- Subscriptions
- Council of the Association
- Accounts and funds of the Association
- The Annual General Meeting.

The Disciplinary and Complaints Procedure enables the following disciplinary action to be taken:

- A warning with a probationary period
- Suspension of membership
- Expulsion from the association

SITUATIONS WITH LEGAL SIGNIFICANCE

Concern was expressed in a letter to the BMJ[5] by E Ernst about who prescribes osteopathic treatment.

Will an osteopath be able to treat on the NHS a patient with back pain who happens to have a spinal therapeutic approach but which an osteopath is much more likely to misdiagnose than a doctor? ... I would be happier if there were more scientifically sound data suggesting that osteopathy (or other complementary remedies) was clinically effective. The most authoritative meta-analysis on the matter to date concluded that 'data are insufficient concerning the efficacy of spinal manipulation for chronic low-back pain'.[6]

Misdiagnosis

Situation 1 Misdiagnosis
An osteopath who is newly qualified, failed to appreciate that the pain suffered by a client was caused by a dislocated ulna. The client did not therefore receive the appropriate treatment, and has been told that he is likely to have a permanent disability. Does he have any right of action?

In this situation the following questions must be answered:

- Was the patient referred to the osteopath following diagnosis by a GP or other doctor?
- Did the osteopath follow a reasonable standard of care in treating the client?
- Can it clearly be established that the disability followed the failure to diagnose by the osteopath, or would it have occurred anyway?

It may be that negligence could be established against the GP who should never have referred the patient to the osteopath.

The fact that the osteopath is newly qualified, is no defence if he has failed to follow the standard of care which any reasonable osteopath would have provided.

What is the difference?

Situation 2 What is the difference?
Following an unsuccessful operation by a neurosurgeon, a patient was advised that there was nothing further which could be done for her bad back. She obtained pain killers from her GP and suggested to him that there may be benefit in seeking the help of a specialist. The GP was uncertain about the respective spheres of activity of osteopaths, chiropractors, craniosacral therapists or physiotherapists but as a GP fundholder was prepared to purchase the service. He suggested that the patient should make enquiries as to what she thought would help her.

Situation 2 appears to be a case where the GP is absolving himself of responsibility for the care the patient should be receiving. However, as the popularity of different therapies expands, it is possible that patients can obtain much information themselves about the various treatments provided by individual therapies. It is true that many GPs may not have the knowledge to make an appropriate referral.

Ultimately the GP could be held responsible if the referral is totally inappropriate, but there may be some contributory negligence by the patient.

Expert witness

Situation 3 Expert witness
A client who was injured in a manual handling incident at work was seeking compensation from his employer. His solicitor approached an osteopath to advise him on the prognosis and the amount of compensation which the client should obtain. The osteopath provided a report which suggested that the client's condition was not serious and there was considerable hysterical overlay. Does the court have to see this report?

The report provided by the expert would be privileged from disclosure under the doctrine known as professional legal privilege (see Chapters 10 and 14), since it was obtained in course of preparing for litigation. As the law stands at present, the solicitors would not have to make this report available to the other side and there would be nothing to prevent them from seeking a report from another osteopath which was more favourable to the client. Osteopaths and others acting as expert witnesses are advised to obtain payment for such reports before they are submitted, especially where the solicitors may wish to make no use of them.

It is important to stress that practitioners called as expert witnesses should give a detached, independent opinion, not affected by the party (plaintiff or defendant) which has requested the opinion. This is considered in detail in Chapter 14. The recommendations for improvements to the civil proceedings made by Lord Woolf, which include the use of court appointed experts, are mentioned in Chapter 3.

Prolonged pain

Situation 4 Prolonged pain
A client complained of pain after excessive spinal manipulation by an osteopath. She has been referred to a pain clinic but has now been told that there is nothing further that the clinic can do. The client has been considering litigation and has been told of another client who claims that he suffered worsening pain after the mismanagement of a prolapsed intravertebral disc by the same osteopath.

Any liability of the osteopath to the first client will depend upon establishing that the osteopath was at fault in the manipulation which was carried out and also in showing that it was this excessive manipulation which has caused the excessive pain.

Expert witnesses would be required on both issues. The evidential value of the second client's statement will be of little weight and each client would have to bring their own case against the osteopath.

CONCLUSIONS

Now that osteopathy has obtained state registration it will be interesting to study the effects of this in the uptake of osteopathy services within the NHS and the extent to which orthodox doctors are prepared to refer patients and accept its contribution to patient care. In addition it will be significant to see how those osteopath groups which were not included in the registration provisions have fared. The workings of the state registration machinery will also be watched closely by other groups who are intent on obtaining this status. Evidence from medical defence organisations shows that even when practised by a registered medical practitioner, osteopathy can cause harm. The possibility, therefore, of increasing litigation in this field is clear.

Questions and Exercises

1. A GP suggests that a patient should see an osteopath for his treatment. To what extent do you consider that the GP should remain responsible for the care which the osteopath provides?
2. Since osteopathy is now state registered, do you consider that a patient should have direct access to the services of an osteopath rather than going through a GP?
3. To what extent do you consider that the Osteopaths Act could be the model for other complementary therapies? And if so which?
4. Is a client who seeks treatment from an osteopath privately in a different legal position from one who is referred through a GP? (see Chapter 4 on contract law).

REFERENCES

1. Editorial 1985 Lords debate alternatives: no action until BMA report. Journal of Alternative Medicine 3(4): 2
2. Osteopathic Information Service PO Box 2074 Reading Berkshire RG1 4YR (Tel 01734 512051)
3. The Osteopaths Act 1993 (Commencement No 1 and Transitional Provision) Order 1997 SI 1997/34
4. Craniosacral therapy association Standards of Practitioner Competencies (undated)
5. Ernst E 1993 Letter to the editor. British Medical Journal 307: 326
6. Shekelle PG, Adams AH, Chassin MR, Hurtwitz EL, Brook RH 1992 Spinal manipulation for chronic back pain. Annals of International Medicine 117: 590–8

Physiology and massage therapy

BACKGROUND

There are several different professional groups which are included within the umbrella term of physiologists. They include: physical/manipulative therapists, remedial masseurs, osteopaths, and chiropodists.

Controlling bodies

The London and Counties Society of Physiologists (LCSP) includes the above practitioners on its register as well as health and beauty therapists and body masseurs. The LCSP itself was founded in 1919 and is the oldest and largest organisation of private practitioners of remedial massage and manipulative therapy in the country.

The British Massage Therapy Council was set up in 1992 and provides a list of organisations and training schools and individual practitioners.

The Massage Therapy Institute of Great Britain based in London keeps a register of approved practitioners.

The ideal therapeutic system

The LCSP aims to meet the demand of the public by means of advanced and proven remedial massage and manipulative therapeutic methods. It quotes the debate in the House of Lords in February 1985 when Lord Colwyn described the requirements of the ideal therapeutic system (see Box 34.1) and states that the aim of the Society encompasses these requirements.

Box 34.1 Requirements of the ideal therapeutic system

1. Treatments should be effective
2. There should be very few, if any, side-effects
3. The patient's well-being should be enhanced
4. The quality of life should be ensured
5. Treatment should be reasonably inexpensive
6. Treatment should be readily available
7. The patient should have his trouble explained to him, and the methods being used to assuage it

---

Aims of the LCSP

1. To provide an organisation, international in scope and activity, for persons engaged in the scientific study of physiology; but, in particular, for those persons engaged in the professions of Remedial Massage, Manipulative Therapy (including the practice of Osteopathy and Chiropractic), Physical and allied therapies, Chiropody, and Health and Beauty Therapy, prescribing a standard of professional ability, proficiency and experience essential to the election of Members, thereby conferring a recognised and approved status by virtue of membership.

2. To conduct examinations in the theory and practice of the therapies mentioned in 1 above, and to grant certificates of proficiency dependent on the results thereof. And further, to promote and support facilities for the education of persons in such therapies.

3. To establish, promote and enforce a Code of Conduct and Ethics to safeguard the integrity of members' professional status.

4. To print, publish, buy or support books or literature or any publication for circulation to Members, insofar as such may be of interest to Members in their professional activities, and which may tend to promote the objects of the Society.

5. To purchase, have, hold and dispose of any building for use as a training establishment or lecture or demonstration rooms or clinics; or any other property, real or personal, for the advancement of the objects of the Society.

6. To do all such other things as are conducive to the attainments of the objects for which the Society is formed as may be determined from time to time by the Council of the Society.

REGISTRATION AND TRAINING

Physiotherapists who have completed successfully a course of training recognised by the Physiotherapy Board on behalf of the Council of Professions Supplementary to Medicine become state registered. The current debate over changes to this system of registration is discussed in Chapter 6.

Eligibility for membership of the LCSP requires that the practitioner is predominantly engaged in the profession of physical therapy, (which embraces osteopathy, chiropractic, manipulative therapy, electro-therapy, remedial massage and allied therapies; health and beauty therapy; or chiropody) or that the applicant is a *bona fide* student undergoing training in one or more of these therapies. It conducts examinations and/or interviews for membership but does not function as a training organisation nor qualifying body as such. It accredits colleges and courses for the purpose of the recognition of its courses as leading to membership of the Society.

The LCSP regards the Northern Institute of Massage (founded in 1924) located at Blackpool as its official training establishment. In addition it approves training in remedial massage provided through certain other schools in the UK as meeting the criteria for membership of the Society.

The LCSP publishes a Register of Practitioner Members which is distributed to libraries and other centres. It accepts on to the register members from its associate training college The Northern Institute, and also graduates from elsewhere who meet the standards it sets.

The British Massage Therapy Council is developing a register for approved members and a training scheme which has NVQ status.

The Association of Physical and Natural Therapists (APNT) requires its members to observe both its own Code of Ethics and also the Code of Ethics of the BCMA. Its administrator reports that whilst every member has public liability and professional indemnity insurance, there are no examples of claims in respect of professional misconduct or negligence.

In spite of these developments in self-regulation, any person can set up in practice and offer massage and other health and beauty services.

REGULATORY MATTERS

Rules on professional misconduct

The LCSP

The LCSP requires that its members adhere to a Code of Ethics and professional conduct. Members in particular are required to work as far as possible in close liaison with the medical profession. The Council of the Society exerts firm disciplinary control over the activities of its membership and acts firmly, promptly and resolutely in cases where it is felt that a member has infringed the Society's Code of Conduct. Disciplinary action could involve suspension or termination of membership, with a subsequent loss of professional indemnity insurance cover for the member.

The APNT rules

The rules set out by the Association of Physical and Natural Therapists are shown in Box 34.2.

The Code of Ethics of the APNT expands on and explains further these rules.

Insurance cover and professional indemnity

The LCSP takes out a master policy arranged through underwriters at Lloyds to provide extensive insurance cover for each practising member of the Society insofar

---

Box 34.2   Code of Ethics of the APNT

   1. Members shall at all times conduct themselves in an honourable manner in their relationship with their patients, the public, and with other members of the Association.
   2. No member may advertise, allow his or her name to be advertised in any way, or be involved in any publicity, except in the form laid down by the Association.
   3. Members are permitted to engage in the teaching of any therapy in which they are qualified (as recognised by the Association) provided that:

• teaching is in the form of a workshop only;
• no certification is issued other than a certificate of attendance; and
• if a member wishes to teach a formal course leading to a certification of proficiency or a diploma such courses must be approved by the Association.

   4. Members of the Association may belong to other organisations or associations provided that they accept their dual membership does not give them immunity from this Code of Ethics.
   5. Infringement of the Ethical Code renders members liable to disciplinary action with subsequent loss of privileges and benefits of the Association.

---

as claims arising in respect of professional indemnity (malpractice); public liability and products liability.

The members of the APNT also have full public liability and professional indemnity insurance cover through their membership.

SITUATIONS WITH LEGAL SIGNIFICANCE

Title

The LCSP has laid down clear rules to prevent any misguidance of the public in the use of the term Doctor:

The use of the title 'Doctor' by any practitioner associated with any of the healing arts might generally be considered to imply that the holder possesses a medical doctorate approved by the BMA [presumably GMC is intended]. The use of this title therefore is not acceptable unless the member holds such qualification. That is, members must use the prefix 'Mr' [and not 'Dr'] before their names unless they are registered medical practitioners, even though they might, for example, possess a 'Doctorate in Osteopathy', 'Doctorate in Acupuncture', etc. issued by any professional organisation.

Those practitioners who hold a recognised non-medical doctorate e.g. a doctorate in philosophy can use the title 'Dr' but must explain after it the type of doctorate it is.

Unwise massage

Situation 1   Unwise massage

Kate visited a masseur to seek help with a nagging back pain. Following the treatment she is considerably worse and has now sought the advice of her GP, who has told her that she has a slipped disc which has been caused or aggravated by the massage which was entirely inappropriate for her condition. Does she have any remedy?

If Kate visited a masseur who is a member of one of the respected organisations which have a code of conduct she may have some redress through the organisation. She would have to establish that the masseur should have realised that her condition contraindicated massage. If she discovers that the masseur is not affiliated to any self-regulating organisation she may find that she is without remedy; there is no register from which to get the masseur struck off and, if she were to consider litigation, she might find that the masseur is uninsured. There is no point in suing a defendant who would be unable to pay the compensation.

Unsuccessful remedial work

Situation 2   Unsuccessful remedial work
Following a manual handling incident, Martha was referred to a practitioner in remedial massage. After several months of attendance, she had been told that remedial massage was not an appropriate treatment for the injury she had sustained.

Whoever referred Martha to the inappropriate therapy would have to take some responsibility for such a referral if, at the time, it was apparent that her injury required a different form of treatment. However if, after a few sessions, the therapist herself should have been aware that her treatment was not suitable, she should have told Martha accordingly. If Martha has suffered harm, over and above the original injury, she may have some claim for compensation from both the referrer and the therapist, depending upon the facts.

CONCLUSIONS

Whilst there are areas of physiological therapies which are well regulated through self-devised schemes, some of which are now state registered, there is concern that many hundreds of people may be offering massage and other services to an ill-informed public who are vulnerable to any deficiencies and shortcomings in the services offered to them. This may be an important area for government concern.

Questions and Exercises

1. How can the well trained and registered members of a physiological or massage organisation protect themselves from those who have no training?
2. Devise a leaflet designed to advise clients on their rights in relation to treatment by a member of the opposite sex.
3. Is express consent always obtained from a client, or is it assumed that the mere presence of the client in the treatment room implies consent? What would be safer practice in obtaining consent? (see Chapter 9)

35

Psychotherapy and other counselling

DEFINITION

Psychotherapy literally means the treatment of mental disorder by psychological means. Some therapists however might not consider evidence of mental disorder necessary but that their treatment can develop any individual's full potential.

BACKGROUND

There are many different philosophies and theories of treatment which come under the umbrella of the main organisations in this field and it would be inappropriate to trace the history of each in a work of this kind. It is also difficult to distinguish between those which are seen as part of orthodox health care and those which are properly described as complementary. Clinical psychologists, for example, would probably be seen as part of orthodox medicine and health care. They are well-recognised members of the multi-disciplinary team in psychiatric care, trained, on government purchased courses, following a degree in psychology, to a standard approved for chartered membership status of the British Psychological Society (BPS). They are in short supply and numerous unfilled vacancies exist for their services within the NHS.

Psychotherapists and counsellors are increasingly employed within the NHS, but many practising in more specialist areas, would probably look to private practice for their income, rather than rely upon referrals from registered medical practitioners within the NHS.

The justification for including a chapter on this field in a work of this nature is that many of the different forms of psychotherapy have not received full recognition from practitioners of orthodox medicine, and that it is a growing area of popularity so an explanation of the ways in which it provides self-regulation are of significance to the rights of the consumer. In addition, its practice gives rise to many issues of a legal nature.

Umbrella organisations

There are several umbrella organisations which are described below covering a comprehensive range of therapies.

The United Kingdom Council for Psychotherapy

From the Foster Report of 1971 to the launch of the first National Register of Psychotherapists in 1993, the profession of psychotherapy has changed from a state of fragmentation to a cohesive structure containing approximately seventy psychotherapy organisations arranged in eight Sections and representing every known variety of psychotherapy.[1]

The National Register is organised by the United Kingdom Council for Psychotherapy (UKCP). The declared aim of the UKCP is to achieve statutory regulation for psychotherapy. The eight sections of the UKCP are shown in Box 35.1.

Box 35.1 Psychotherapy Sections of the UKCP

1. Analytical (3 member organisations)
2. Behaviour and Cognitive (1 member organisation)
3. Experiential Constructivist (2 member organisations)
4. Family, Couple, Sexual and Systemic (5 member organisations)
5. Humanistic and Integrative (23 member organisations)
6. Hypnotherapy (5 member organisations)
7. Psychoanalytic and Psychodynamic (28 member organisations)
8. Psychoanalytically based therapy with children (2 member organisations)

Each organisation and its members, who are in the Register maintained by the UKCP, must comply with the ethical guidelines drawn up by the UKCP (see below).

It is impossible in a work of this kind, to look in depth at the 70 member organisations of the UKCP and just two will be considered to show the nature of the organisation and how it runs. The two selected are the British Association of Psychotherapists and the British Psychodrama Association (see below). The British Association for Counselling will also be considered.

The British Confederation of Psychotherapists

Another umbrella for psychotherapists with overlapping membership with the UKCP is the British Confederation of Psychotherapists. BCP was set up as an association of psychoanalysts, analytical psychologists, psychoanalytic psychotherapists and child psychotherapists with the purpose of promoting the maintenance of appropriate standards in the selection, training, practice and professional conduct of psychoanalytic psychotherapists.

To be admitted to membership organisations must meet the standards required by the Confederation on the selection, training, qualification and admission to full or associate membership of an appropriate professional association. Each institution has a Code of Ethics which aims to protect the public by setting out the appropriate standards for professional conduct. Each Code also establishes disciplinary procedures to ensure that practitioners observe the requirements of the Code of the institution. The Confederation published a Register of member organisations and their members. Members of the public are encouraged to take the advice of a responsible professional when seeking a referral to psychoanalytic psychotherapy.

At present members may belong to both the UKCP and the BCP, but this is seen as a transitional time for the BCP, since its aim is to secure a single membership organisation specifically for those practising in the field of psychoanalysis.

Sample organisations

British Association of Psychotherapists (BAP)

BAP is a member of the UKCP within section 7 and is also a member of the British Confederation of Psychotherapists (BCP). The BAP was formed in 1951 to bring together for mutual support and stimulation psychotherapists with various theoretical viewpoints who share a psychodynamic orientation. In 1963 two separate parallel training programmes were established following a Psychoanalytic and Jungian theoretical basis. It was established as a limited company in 1977 and charitable status was achieved in 1979.

The aims of the BAP are shown in Box 35.2.

Box 35.2   Aims of the British Association of Psychotherapists

- to promote the knowledge and skills of psychotherapy and the education, training and competence of psychotherapists
- to establish and maintain standards of professional competence and conduct
- to promote mutual understanding and co-operation between the various disciplines of psychotherapy
- to provide for the selection, training and qualification of students entering this profession
- to establish and maintain alone or, if appropriate, in association with other bodies a register of persons recognised as competent to practise as professional psychotherapists
- to improve the professional skill of those already qualified and of others concerned with the promotion of mental health
- to represent the views of psychotherapists on matters of professional development and practice and on issues relating to mental health
- to promote the practice of psychotherapy so as to bring it within the reach of a wider section of the community

---

The British Psychodrama Association

Psychodrama is a method of group psychotherapy and is defined by J L Moreno as

the science which explores the truth by dramatic methods. It deals with interpersonal relations and private worlds.[2]

The British Psychodrama Association in its Code of Ethics and Practice covers topics such as:

- confidentiality
- remuneration
- contract
- boundaries
- professional conduct and
- society.

Appendices cover guidelines for child protection issues and also guidelines on the ethical issues of videotaping, audio recording or filming of psychodrama, and subsequent viewing or broadcasting.

The Association has also prepared a Code of Ethics and Practice for the Supervision of Psychodramatists and a Code of Ethics and Practice for Trainees, Trainers and Training Organisations. The Association employs an external moderator, part of whose role is to be available to facilitate and adjudicate on any matter raised by an aggrieved member of the association.

The British Association for Counselling (BAC)

The British Association for Counselling (BAC) was founded to bring together the commitment and resources of a wide range of people through individual and organisational membership. Its functions are shown in Box 35.3.

Box 35.3 Functions of British Association for Counselling

- has developed Codes of Ethics and Practice for counsellors, counselling skills, trainers in counselling and counselling skills and the supervision of counsellors
- operates an accreditation scheme for individual counsellors, supervisors, trainers, and counsellor training courses
- runs an information office responsible for the publication of directories
- produces publications about counselling
- publishes a quarterly journal
- maintains a film and video library about counselling
- liaises with a network of local affiliated groups

Divisions within the British Association of Counselling include:

- Association for Counselling at Work
- Association for Pastoral Care and Counselling

- Association for Student Counselling
- Counselling in Education
- Counselling in Medical Settings
- Personal/Sexual/Relationship/Family Counselling
- Race and Cultural Education in Counselling

All members of the BAC are required to abide by its Code of Ethics and Practice for counsellors. The introduction states that:

Whilst this code cannot resolve all ethical and practice related issues, it aims to provide a framework for addressing ethical issues and to encourage optimum levels of practice. Counsellors will need to judge which parts of this code apply to particular situations. They may have to decide between conflicting responsibilities.

BAC also has a Complaints Procedure which can lead to the expulsion of members for breaches of its Code of Ethics and Practice.

REGISTRATION ISSUES

Opposition to control

Not all therapists working in this field are content to see the development of registers or wish to see state regulation. For example the Independent Practitioners Network acts as a network for counsellors, psychotherapists, educators and growth and allied practitioners. It does not distinguish

between more or less qualified or 'registered' members, since we recognise that there are many routes to being a good practitioner. The structure is horizontal and multi-centred rather than vertical and pyramidal. Our aim is to provide intending clients with a context of basic security within which they can make their own decisions about which practitioner is valuable for them. Rather than using a central code of practice, each peer group creates and circulates its own.

The network consists of units of about five to ten practitioners 'who are willing to stand by each other's work' and who take responsibility for supporting each other's good practice and the good practice of other groups in the network, and for addressing any problems and conflicts in their own work. Part of the philosophy of the network is that 'no organisation has the right or the ability to decide who should practise therapy, facilitation or equivalent skills'.

National registers

In 1971 the Foster Report recommended that there should be a Statutory Register of Psychotherapists. This has not yet been achieved in relation to the whole diverse field of practitioners working in this area. In 1975 however, the British Confederation of Psychotherapists launched its national register. It maintains a register of organisations and their members which enables it to provide to the public the names of those who are appropriately trained and are members of professional associations to which, for the public protection, they are accountable for their work and for their professional conduct.

The BCP publishes a brochure *Finding a Therapist* which is an appendix to the Register and also a separate publication.

The United Kingdom Council for Psychotherapy has maintained since 1993 a National Register for Psychotherapists. The registers of both the BCP and the UKCP are usually available in public libraries. A register is also kept by the United Kingdom Register for Counsellors.

Self-regulation or statutory regulation

A statutory regulation working body has been set up with representatives from:

* British Confederation of Psychotherapists
* British Psychology Society
* Royal College of Psychiatrists
* United Kingdom Council for Psychotherapy
* United Kingdom Register for Counsellors

The task of the working party is to consolidate the structures which support self-regulation and to explore the implications of statutory registration.

The existence of these national registers does not prevent any person calling themselves a psychotherapist. The UKCP and the other organisations are now seeking to move towards statutory regulation.

This would have the effect of protecting the public as well as regulating the practice of psychotherapists from other European Union countries who wished to move to the United Kingdom. The mutual recognition of qualifications can only occur between European Union Countries where legal control of an occupation exists. In the absence of a legal framework, any European Union national can practise in this country. The United Kingdom Council for Psychotherapy continues to be active in the attempts to found a European Association for Psychotherapy that can establish the boundaries of the profession in the European Union.[3]

PROFESSIONAL STATUS AND STANDARDS

An example of training requirements

Full membership of the BAP is dependent upon successful completion of the professional training programme set by the BAP together with fulfilling the conditions for full membership set by the Council of BAP and approval by the Council. BAP itself offers four part-time training programmes covering:

* psychoanalytic psychotherapy with adults
* Jungian analytic psychotherapy with adults
* psychoanalytic psychotherapy with adults for child psychotherapists
* psychoanalytic psychotherapy with children and adolescents.

Definitions of standards of competence

In the Ethical Guidelines of the UKCP it is a requirement that members should 'maintain their ability to perform competently and to take the necessary steps to do so'. This would incorporate into professional standards the Bolam test discussed in Chapter 3 together with the necessity of ongoing professional development of the kind required statutorily by the United Kingdom Central Council for Nursing, Health Visiting and Midwifery (UKCC) of its registered practitioners.

In addition each organisation which is a member of the UKCP or the BAC would have its own additional requirements. For example BAP members are required to ensure that they maintain a satisfactory standard of professional competence and the Association provides ongoing professional development for full members.

Rules on professional misconduct

Whilst each institution associated with the BCP and the UKCP has its own Code of Ethics, these Codes must comply with the requirements of the BCP and the UKCP and any changes to these Codes must be notified to the umbrella organisations thus ensuring a continuing process of accountability. Failure by any individual to comply with the relevant Code could lead to striking off from the Register kept by the BCP and the UKCP. The ethical guidelines of the United Kingdom Council for Psychotherapy cover the topics shown in Box 35.4.

Box 35.4   Ethical guidelines of the UKCP

1. Aim of the Guidelines
2. Code of Ethics: qualification, terms, conditions and methods of practice, confidentiality, professional relationships, relationship with clients, research, publication, practitioner competence, insurance, detrimental behaviour
3. Advertising
4. Code of Practice: each member organisation of the UKCP will have its own Code of Practice approved by the appropriate UKCP section
5. Complaints procedure
6. Sanctions: suspension or removal from a member organisation automatically leads to the deletion of the member from the UKCP register
7. Monitoring complaints

The British Association of Psychotherapists requires its members to conform to the Code of Ethics which is contained in the Bye-laws. It emphasises the requirements shown in Box 35.5.

Box 35.5   Main requirements of the Code of Ethics of BAP

- always acting in the best interest of the patient maintaining the relationship with the patient on a professional basis
- not exploiting the patient in any way
- treating all knowledge of the patient confidentially and not passing it on without his or her prior consent, unless the safety of the patient or others is threatened
- ascertaining that responsibility for the patient's medical welfare is held by a medically qualified person
- refraining from claiming to possess qualifications which are not possessed
- refraining from direct advertising or from permitting direct advertisements for the purpose of obtaining patients

---

Insurance cover and professional indemnity

The UKCP as part of its ethical guidelines requires members to ensure that their professional work is adequately covered by appropriate indemnity insurance. Similarly a requirement of BAP is that members have sufficient malpractice insurance to meet any legal claim that may be made against them in their professional role. However good practice would indicate that it is also advisable for practitioners to have insurance cover for injuries to visitors on the premises and other basic public liability cover. One area of concern in relation to possible litigation is that of false memory syndrome where high awards have been made in the USA (see below).

One of the main insurance brokers in providing cover for those who work in the field of psychotherapy and osteopathy is Devitts. They have over 15 years experience in obtaining insurance cover for these specific therapies. The main organisation they use for cover is the Royal Sun Alliance. The premiums are based upon the level of training and members of organisations which are accredited or approved through the BAC or one of the other recognised associations will obtain lower premiums. Those seeking cover who are not members of the main organisations will have their applications scrutinised very carefully.

Cover is also provided for legal expenses in connection with any claim and also in respect of any disciplinary proceedings brought by the association of which the therapist is a member.

LAWS RELATING TO THE THERAPY

False memory syndrome

Of recent concern to those working in this field are legal actions in relation to allegedly false accusations of sexual or other abuse. In the United States a father won $500 000 from therapists who had helped his daughter 'remember' his attacks on her. Gary Ramona said after the eight week trial in Napa, California:

I'm delighted the jury saw the same thing that I did – that my daughter's so-called suppressed memories are the result of drugs and quackery. These people have destroyed my life.[4]

His daughter Holly had begun consulting a therapist for treatment for bulimia and depression and had been told by the therapist that 80% of bulimia patients had been sexually abused.

The difficulties for lawyers, social workers, doctors and family members in distinguishing false memories from memories of incidents which actually took place are immense. Research such as that carried out by Professor Loftus, a psychologist at University of Washington, which was reported to the American Association for the Advancement of Science,[5] showed the existence of phenomenon which she described as 'imagination inflation', where just getting subjects to imagine incidents was enough to lead them to believe that they had experiences they would not otherwise believe that they had had.

The British False Memory Society has been established to provide support for those who see themselves as the victims of false memories and to educate persons who are involved in the syndrome. They have prepared a video to this end.

The fact remains, however, that there are cases of abuse and that psychotherapists do provide support and help to those who have been victims of abuse. The concern of these therapists is that many actual victims may be reluctant to come forward and seek help because they fear that they may not be believed.

The most famous case of recovered memory was that of Eileen Franklin Lipsker who claimed to remember seeing her father rape and murder her eight year old friend, some twenty years after the event. Ms Lipsker recovered the memory at the age of 28 while watching her daughter at play. Her father was arrested as the result of her recovered memory and was tried, convicted of murder and sentenced to life imprisonment.[6]

SITUATIONS WITH LEGAL SIGNIFICANCE
Ending the treatment

Situation 1   Ending the treatment
A client who had become emotionally entangled with her psychotherapist was advised by him that the sessions should now be ended and he was of the view that he could no longer be of assistance. She felt very aggrieved by this having been in therapy with him for over four years and had understood that the recommended time for the therapy to last was well over eight years. She was prepared to bring legal action.

There are two possible causes of action for the client in situation 1 if compensation is required:

● to seek an action for breach of contract, or
● to sue for negligence.

Alternatively, if she is not anxious to obtain compensation she could seek to bring a complaint.

Her chances of succeeding with a breach of contract will depend upon the nature of the agreement with the psychotherapist and any provision relating to the ending of the contract. Ways in which a contract can be ended are discussed in Chapter 4. It is unlikely that the courts will see the contract as persisting without the right of either party to end it on giving notice.

Any claim in negligence will depend for its success on the client being able to show that by ending the treatment the therapist is in breach of the duty of care and as a result harm has occurred to the client. Most Associations would have recommended practice on how any therapist should bring a treatment situation to an end. It may well be that this particular therapist has failed to comply with what would be regarded as the reasonable standard of care in bringing the client/therapist relationship to an end.

Complaints procedures have been established by both the UKCP and the BCP and all their member organisations. Confirmation of justification of the complaint could lead to the psychotherapist being removed from his specific organisation and, if that is a member of the UKCP or the BCP, from those organisations as well.

If of course the psychotherapist is not a member of any recognised organisation, and at present there is nothing to prevent any person setting themselves up as a psychotherapist and taking clients, then the client has little redress other than through the laws of contract and negligence which, as can be seen above, might be difficult to use successfully.

An intimate relationship

Situation 2 An intimate relationship

After three years of therapy, a more intimate relationship developed between the therapist and the client, both of whom were married to other partners. When the therapist advised the client that the relationship must end she protested and threatened to report the therapist for rape, on the grounds that in the therapeutic relationship she had not had the mental capacity to give consent to the sexual relationship, that the therapist had abused his professional position and that he had exploited her vulnerability.

Situation 2 is unfortunately not unknown. Most associations in their Code of Ethics and professional practice attempt to ensure high standards of professional practice by their members. The client would therefore have a good case to bring before the association which could hold professional conduct proceedings to look into the allegations. As far as any allegation of rape is concerned, it would have to be shown that there was no consent by the client to the sexual intercourse. The burden would be on the prosecution to show this beyond all reasonable doubt. Much would depend upon the mental condition of the client at the time as evidenced by other people and the awareness of the therapist as to her lack of capacity to give consent.

The Prevention of Professional Abuse Network (POPAN) is an organisation which exists to protect clients against abuse by therapists and will provide advice and support.

It was set up in 1990 to bridge a serious gap in counselling and support services. It is a company limited by guarantee and a registered charity. POPAN provides information, support and advocacy. It arranges mutual support groups and promotes increased public and professional knowledge about the existence of abuse in the health care field and understanding its effects. It also campaigns to raise professional and ethical standards of behaviour and the improvements in health care policies and practice. POPAN is funded by grants from the Department of Health and the Mental Health Foundation and donations from supporters.

Confidentiality and children at risk

All the approved organisations for psychotherapy recognise the duty of confidentiality owed by the therapist to the client. However, this duty is usually seen as being subject to an exception where the safety of another person is at risk. Thus in situation 3 the

Situation 3   Confidentiality and children at risk
A therapist is informed by a client that she was abused by her father and fears that her nieces and nephews are now subject to abuse. She refuses to involve the authorities or inform her sister, whose children are at risk, because she wants to keep her relationship with her father secret. The therapist is concerned for the safety of the children.

psychotherapist could, if she had sufficient information to provide reasonable grounds for fear over the safety of the children, pass this information on to the Area Child Protection Committee. This disclosure could come under the exception to the duty of confidentiality under the heading 'public interest' (see chapter 10). However this might irrevocably harm the work that she is doing with the client. Clearly the best practice would be to discuss with the client her feelings about the protection of the children. It may be that the client would then be prepared to make these disclosures herself in the best interests of the children or agree that the psychotherapist can do so. The sensitive issue of confidentiality is explored by Christopher Bollis and David Sundelson[7] in their book, *The New Informants*.

Fixation

Situation 4   Fixation
A therapist is aware that the client is completely obsessed with her to the extent of watching her door and following her wherever she goes. She has advised the client that this conduct could result in the sessions ending and the client has pleaded with her not to stop the sessions and promises that she will end this behaviour. However the situation does not change and the stalking continues.

In Chapter 5 the new legislation of protection from harassment is discussed. There is now a remedy both in the criminal law and in civil law for anyone who is persistently harassed. An injunction can be obtained. It is recommended that organisations of members who are vulnerable to stalking and other forms of harassment should devise procedures for their members on the action which should be taken.

Confidentiality and supervision

Situation 5   Confidentiality and supervision
A counsellor receives supervision from a colleague. During the supervision she gives out details from which the supervisor is able to identify the client, and thereby becomes aware that this client had suffered from sexual abuse as a child. Unknown to the counsellor, the supervisor passes this information on to another person, without any lawful justification. When the client discovers that the supervisor received this confidential information she wishes to sue the counsellor for breach of confidentiality. Will she succeed in her action?

As can be seen from Chapter 10, the duty of confidentiality is clear and arises from a variety of sources. Certain exceptions are recognised. Does this situation fall into any of the exceptions?

There appears to be no consent from the client.

If supervision is essential for good counselling practice then possibly the supervision could be justified, somewhat indirectly, as being in the interests of the client. However it does not follow that supervision should justify the passing on of confidential information. The difficulty is that although the supervision session would consider the issue of child abuse, what should not have taken place is the additional information given to the supervisor from which the client was identified.

There is no evidence from the few facts given here that any of the other exceptions to the duty of confidentiality apply here.

The conclusion must be that the client has suffered as a result of an unjustified breach of confidentiality. Both the counsellor and the supervisor are responsible. Both could be successfully sued by the client. (This is unlikely because the publicity from any court proceedings could cause the client further harm.) What might be a more appropriate remedy would be disciplinary action taken by the professional body against both counsellor and supervisor.

This could take account of the fact that the misconduct of the supervisor was far worse than that of the counsellor. The supervisor is in breach of the Code of Ethics and Practice for supervisors of counsellors set by the BAC both in passing on information obtained from the counsellor and also in failing to ensure that the counsellor worked in a way to protect the personal identity of the client.

Marital discord

Situation 6   Marital discord
As a result of psychotherapy which took place over two years the Hamptons' marriage has ended. The wife blames the end of the marriage on her husband's therapist and is threatening to sue her. Will she succeed?

Two legal questions arise?

- Does the therapist owe a duty of care to the partner of her client?
- Is there a contract between the therapist and the partner?

The second question is easily answered: in contract law the only parties who can sue for breach of contract are those who are parties to the contract because of the doctrine of privity (see Chapter 4). Therefore, assuming the husband paid for the sessions and the agreement was intended to create legal relations, he could sue for breach of contract but not his wife.

On the first question the therapist certainly owes a duty of care to her client, but does this extend to the spouse of the client? When a solicitor allowed a beneficiary to witness a will, which therefore excluded the beneficiary from inheriting under the will, the solicitor was liable to the beneficiary[8]. However it could be said that in this case the solicitor was also failing in his duty to his client, because he failed to take care that the client's wishes were properly executed.

Even if a duty of care to the wife can be established, it is even more difficult to define what the standard of the psychotherapist should be and whether this particular psychotherapist fell below this reasonable standard of care. Even if a breach can be shown, can it be established that the breach actually caused the end of the marriage? Were there not other causative factors? Maybe the psychotherapist brought to light a situation which would have occurred any way. The case is fraught with difficulties and legal action would clearly seem to be contraindicated.

CONCLUSIONS

The move towards state regulation for the numerous organisations which are active in the field of psychotherapy and related areas is growing apace and major developments have taken place in the last few years in developing a cohesive structure. The attitude of the Labour Government elected in 1997 will be essential in any progress towards state regulation. If it is achieved it will open up a new era in relationships across the European Community. There are strong voices, however, against any further regulation of the different professions.

Questions and Exercises

1. Do you consider that the duty of confidentiality between a psychotherapist and client should be stronger than that owed by other therapists to their clients – because of the nature of the disclosures?
2. In view of the strong feeling against registration and uniformity felt by some psychotherapists, do you consider that a convincing case could be made against any form of self-regulation?
3. What protection, if any, do you consider that the law should give to the clients of psychotherapists over and above that which is available from the general principles of the civil and criminal law (see Chapters 3, 4 and 5)?

REFERENCES

1. Pokorny MR 1997 Foreword to the National Register of Psychotherapists 1997. UKCP, London
2. British Psychodrama code of ethics and practice 1996
3. Pokorny MR 1997 Foreword to the National Register of Psychotherapists 1997. UKCP, London
4. Hiscock J Father wins rape memory damages. Sunday Telegraph 15 May 1994
5. Hawkes N False memories can be created by imagining events. The Times 15 February 1997
6. MacIntyre B Californian wins damages in false memory incest case. The Times 16 May 1994, p 12
7. Bollis C, Sundelson D 1995 The new informants. Karmac Books, London
8. Ross v. Caunters [1979] 3 All ER 580

36

Reflexology

DEFINITION

This therapy is based on the principle that there are 'reflexes' or 'responsible zones' in the feet and hands which correspond to each and every part and organ of the body. When pressure and manipulation are applied to these areas, it brings about the normal functioning of all the organs and glands in the body, it improves the nerve function and blood supply and it induces a state of relaxation.

BACKGROUND

History

The origins of reflexology can be traced to practice in Egypt, Persia, China and Japan more than 5000 years ago. It developed in the West with the work of Dr William Fitzgerald, an American physician, specialising in ear, nose and throat complaints, who discovered the existence of 10 zones of communication passing vertically through the body. He discovered that the effect of applying pressure to certain areas of the fingers was to induce anaesthesia in areas of the head and face so that he could carry out surgery.

His work was taken up by Dr Shelby Riley and by the latter's physical therapist, Eunice Ingham, who undertook extensive research into plotting the pathways of the reflexes and working on the feet. She also found that by working on these reflexes she could achieve a healing effect. In 1938 she published *Stories the Feet can Tell* and founded the National Institute of Reflexology. The International Institute of Reflexology was formed in 1974 by Eunice Ingham in response to the demand for tuition. It was established to promote her methods, known as the Ingham method.

A student of Eunice Ingham, Doreen Bailey, returned to England and introduced reflexology in the UK in the 1960s.

Techniques and applications

Different techniques are used including:

- Traditional reflexology
- Reflex zone therapy
- Metamorphic technique
- Morrell method
- Holistic multidimensional reflexology
- Vaxuflect reflexology.[1]

Reflexology is used for migraine, sinus problems, back problems, poor peripheral circulation and stiffness and tension. It is also used as a preventative measure to maintain the body in a state of good health.

Research

Research evidence on its effectiveness is building up. For example research on use of reflexology in premenstrual syndrome (PMS) is quoted by Adam Jackson.[2] He reports on a randomised controlled study of premenstrual symptoms treated with ear, hand and foot reflexology. Each woman was asked to keep a diary beginning two months before the treatments and continuing through the period of treatment and for two months afterwards.

The results of the reflexology treatments were quite dramatic. Total reduction of PMS symptoms in the treatment group was 46% during the treatment period, but this remained much the same at 41% in the eight weeks following the treatment. The reduction in the placebo group was less than half that observed in the treatment group. Furthermore, over 83% of the treatment group experienced at least 30% reduction in symptoms whereas only 24% of the placebo group experienced the same reduction.

Contraindications identified by Pamela Griffiths are shown in Box 36.1.

Box 36.1 Contraindications for use of reflexology

- Some individuals might find the intensity of the therapy unacceptable
- Not generally used for diagnosis, except in preventive health care
- In conditions such as diabetes and hyper/hypothyroidism the therapist must work closely with the doctor
- Not suitable in the first trimester of pregnancy
- Should be used cautiously with patients in depressive or manic states
- Should be used with care in epilepsy and in acute conditions

---

REGISTRATION AND TRAINING

There is no single governing body for training at present but several different courses exist, many being affiliated with the British Register of Health Practitioners or the Association of Reflexologists.

The Association of Reflexologists was founded in 1984 and aims to monitor and maintain standards of professional practice. It is not affiliated to any one school but full membership is only available to reflexologists who have trained on a course accredited by the Association, who have been in practice for a year and who agree to be bound by the Association's rules and ethical code. It keeps a register of members and publishes a quarterly journal *Reflexions*. Members use the letters OMAR or MAR. About 70 courses in the UK have been accredited by the Association.

The British Reflexology Association was founded in 1985 to act as a representative body for persons practising the method of reflexology as a profession and for students training in the method. It has four categories of membership: fellow, ordinary, associate, and student. It issues an official newsletter *Footprints*. A council of ten members acts as the governing body of the Association. The official teaching body of the British Reflexology Association is the Bayly School of Reflexology, which is affiliated to the Institute of Complementary Medicine. Graduates from the Bayly School may apply for membership after a minimum of one year in practice. They can then use the title 'Registered Reflexologist' and use the letters MBRA.

The International Federation of Reflexologists was formed in 1980s by a group of professional reflexologists who felt that training standards and levels of professional competence were not high enough. It keeps a register of professional therapists and has a list of accredited schools which all teach to a centrally agreed syllabus. All therapists take a separate course in anatomy and physiology in addition to reflexology.

Definitions of standards of competence and rules on professional misconduct are laid down by the national associations and misconduct can result in loss of membership.

SITUATIONS WITH LEGAL SIGNIFICANCE
Post session crisis

Situation 1   Post session crisis

Following her first reflexology session, a client reported to the reflexologist that she was experiencing 'flu like symptoms, feeling light headed, lethargic, with difficulties in sleeping, and with changes in blood pressure. The reflexologist reassured the client and explained that these symptoms were commonly seen as part of a healing crisis due to the detoxification of the body. Subsequently the client visited her doctor who said that she was suffering from glandular fever. She now wishes to sue the reflexologist.

The client would have to show that the reflexologist failed to follow a reasonable standard of care and as a result she has suffered harm. The harm would presumably be the delay in the diagnosis of the glandular fever. However it may be difficult to establish what would have been the reasonable standard the reflexologist should have followed. Expert evidence would be required on the extent to which the reflexologist failed to ensure that the client did not cease to obtain advice from a registered medical practitioner.

Contraindicated

Situation 2 Contraindicated
A client failed to tell the reflexologist when she first met her that she suffered from epilepsy. Had the reflexologist been aware of that she would not have treated her. Unfortunately during a session, the client suffered from a grand mal seizure and fell off the treatment couch, fracturing her pelvis. She was unable to work for several months and, as a self-employed person, had no sick pay. She is now claiming compensation from the therapist.

The outcome from any litigation in this situation will depend very much upon the facts which can be established. If the therapist in her checklist whilst taking the client's history, actually asked about epilepsy and the client denied this then the client would not have a case. If the reflexologist failed to ask the client, and reasonable practice would have required such an inquiry, then clearly there is fault. The importance of getting such information in writing is clear. Thus if the reflexologist had a printed list of information and questions for the client to check before treatment began, which included epilepsy, this would support the therapist in showing that she followed the correct practice and is therefore not accountable for the client's harm.

All in the family

Situation 3 All in the family
Mavis attended a 10 week course on reflexology, for one night a week. After the course she agreed to give her niece a session. She knew that the niece was pregnant but had not been told of any contraindications about this in her course. Unfortunately whilst Mavis was working on the ankles, the niece experienced a sharp pain and started to miscarry. She is now claiming compensation from Mavis for the loss of a much wanted baby. Mavis is not insured and is wondering if she could recover the compensation from the instructor.

In law, there can be liability for negligent advice. However it must be established that the person receiving the information, to the knowledge of the giver of the information, was relying upon that advice. In this case the liability of the instructor would depend upon the understanding between her and the course participants. If the instructor had explained that the course was not intended to provide a training in reflexology and the students would not be qualified at the end of the course to carry out treatments on other persons, then the instructor should not be liable for the harm caused to Mavis' niece. If on the other hand, such information was not made clear, and the students were justified in expecting the course to make them practitioners of reflexology, then there could be liability on the part of the instructor if she was negligent in failing to warn of the contraindications.

It would have to be shown that the lecturer was directly responsible for the harm: there may have been some contributory negligence in that Mavis may have been expected to read some books which would have warned about treating a pregnant woman. There is also arguably contributory negligence on the part of the niece in submitting herself to treatment when pregnant to someone with such brief and incomplete training.

CONCLUSION

Whilst there is a developing body of anecdotal evidence which supports the work of reflexology, there is general agreement that at present how it works is not understood. It is nevertheless described along with aromatherapy as 'one of the most favoured complementary therapies with nurses in the United Kingdom'.[3] Evaluating results by using accepted scientific methods has been slow to develop, practitioners pointing to the therapy being so closely tailored to the needs of the individual as to make traditional research methods difficult to apply. However if there is to be support for reflexology within the NHS, objective evidence as to its clinical effectiveness will become essential.

Questions and Exercises

1. Since an organisation exists which provides registered status for a reflexologist is there any additional value in obtaining state registration?
2. Devise a leaflet which includes both information about reflexology and a check list for clients to be read and completed before the first treatment takes place.
3. A reflexologist has difficulty in obtaining information from general practitioners about her client's state of health and medical history, even though the client has given consent to the information being made available. What action should the reflexologist take? (Refer to Chapter 10 and the section on access to health records).

REFERENCES

1. Griffiths P 1995 Reflexology In: Rankin-Box D The nurses handbook of complementary therapies. Churchill Livingstone, Edinburgh; also reprinted 1996 in Complementary Therapies in Nursing and Midwifery 2: 13–16
2. Jackson A 1995 Nursing Times 91(13): 64 (quoting Oleson T and Flocco W 1993 Randomised controlled study of premenstrual symptoms treated with ear, hand and foot reflexology. Obstetrics and Gynaecology 82: 906–11
3. Trevelyan J, Booth B 1994 Complementary medicine for nurses, midwives and health visitors. Macmillan, London

Shiatsu

DEFINITION

Shiatsu literally means 'finger pressure' and has been in existence for thousands of years, possibly even before acupuncture. It involves the pressing on specific points on the meridians to stimulate or sedate the flow of vital energy in the body. In Shiatsu, palms, fingers, thumbs, knuckles, elbows, knees and feet can be used to exert pressure. In contrast, in acupressure, which may be used by some practitioners in acupuncture, only finger pressure is used. Shiatsu is seen as an holistic therapy in that the practitioner helps to balance the energy flow of the client.

BACKGROUND

The modern development of shiatsu developed from the work of Master Shizuto Masunga who advocated a way of treatment based on the Five Elements Theory (fire, earth, metal, water and wood) and the division between two complementary energy forces: Yin (negative) and Yan (positive) (see Chapter 16 on acupuncture).

REGISTRATION AND TRAINING

The Shiatsu Society was set up in 1981 to facilitate communication within the field of Shiatsu and to make the benefits of this form of healing more widely recognised across the country. It permits membership to anyone over the age of 18 years who is studying Shiatsu, either as a special interest or with the intention of becoming a fully qualified Shiatsu practitioner. The Society compiles a Practitioners Register of qualified therapists, who have passed both the theory and practical examinations set by the Shiatsu Society's independent assessment panel.

REGULATORY MATTERS

Rules on professional misconduct

The Shiatsu Society has prepared a Code of Conduct and Ethics for its register of qualified practitioners. The main topics are shown in Box 37.1.

Box 37.1   Code of Conduct and Ethics of the Shiatsu Society

- Introduction
- Complaints procedures
- Appeals procedures
- The Rules
- Teaching
- Shiatsu and Medicine
- Members to be aware of and abide by the law in respect of children, venereal disease, animals, herbs and insurance
- Advertisement
- Surroundings
- Schools

Insurance cover and professional indemnity

In the third year of training students of the Shiatsu Society are required to take out professional indemnity insurance. This enables students to work on members of the public under the guidance of a Registered Teacher. The Society provides professional indemnity insurance cover for shiatsu practitioners which is available to all current members on the Register.

Definitions for purchasing contracts

The Shiatsu Society emphasises that shiatsu must not be offered as an alternative to orthodox medicine but as complementary to it.

SITUATIONS WITH LEGAL SIGNIFICANCE

Brittle bones

Situation 1   Brittle bones

Unknown to the Shiatsu practitioner the client suffered from brittle bones. During the session, the client shrieked out and the therapist realised that she had probably caused a fracture. The client is blaming her for her lack of skill. A letter advising that litigation is proceeding has now been sent by the client's solicitor.

The therapist's liability will depend upon whether any reasonable Shiatsu practitioner would have ascertained whether the client was suffering from specific disorders before the treatment started; whether there were any harmless tests which could have been carried out to ensure that treatment would be safe; and whether certain questions were asked but the client did not answer them honestly. If the therapist can show that she did all that was reasonable action for compensation would fail since the fracture occurred without any negligence on her part.

Abortion wanted

Situation 2   Abortion wanted

A Shiatsu practitioner was asked to provide treatment for an unmarried girl of 27 years. The client was asked if she was pregnant and she replied 'definitely not'. Treatment then commenced and pressure was placed upon points which would have been avoided in the case of a pregnant woman. The client appeared to be in some discomfort following the session and the therapist suggested that she should sit quietly and have a drink. Subsequently, the client rushed to the toilet. The therapist was later informed that the client had miscarried and is worried about being involved in an illegal abortion.

Under the Abortion Act 1967 (as amended), an abortion is only lawful if the requirements of the Act are satisfied. Except in an emergency situation two registered medical practitioners must be of the opinion formed in good faith that an abortion is justified under one of four conditions. The termination must be carried out by a registered medical practitioner (or another health professional acting under his or her direction[1]) in a place registered for such purposes.

However to commit an offence under the Act the termination must have been wilfully carried out. Here the therapist was not aware that the client was pregnant; she had asked the correct questions and there appears to be no reason why she should have realised that the client had misinformed her. She lacked the mental element (*mens rea*) (see Chapter 5) necessary for committing an unlawful termination.

Whether the client has committed an offence will depend upon whether her actions come under the provisions of the Offences Against the Person Act 1861, section 58, which makes it an offence for any woman being with child to unlawfully administer to herself any poison or noxious thing with intent to procure her miscarriage. Could Shiatsu be described as the administration of a noxious thing and was it unlawfully administered? The answer would probably be negative to both questions. However there is no decided case. Nor would a prosecution against the client succeed under the Infant Life Preservation Act 1929 which makes it a criminal offence to destroy the life of a child capable of being born alive. It would appear to be too early a stage in the pregnancy for the child to be capable of being born alive.

Post session vulnerability

Situation 3   Post session vulnerability

Following an acupressure session, the client arose too fast, became dizzy and fell onto the floor. This caused a slipped disc. She is now attending an osteopath and has asked the therapist to refund her the fees the osteopath is charging.

To establish liability of the therapist, the client would have to show that the therapist was at fault, and as a consequence the client has suffered harm. Should the therapist have told the client to get up slowly? Should the therapist have helped the client to her feet? Is there anything else that a reasonable therapist in acupressure would have done which this therapist failed to do? If any of these questions can be answered affirmatively and it can be shown that as a consequence of this failure the client suffered harm, then there may be liability. Expert evidence would be necessary to establish the reasonable standard of care of an acupressure therapist.

CONCLUSION

Shiatsu, like other therapies which are holistic in nature, is growing in popularity as people seek to maintain their health and personal well-being. As cynicism with the capability of orthodox medicine to resolve chronic conditions grows, so shiatsu, along with yoga and acupuncture is growing in popularity as the answer to many stress-related disorders. This being so, and as it is a direct (although non-invasive) therapy with several contraindications, it is likely that the amount of litigation and compensation claims arising will also increase.

Questions and Exercises

1. You discover that a person, who has attended a few of your Shiatsu sessions, but has not been professionally qualified, is now intending to set up in practice in the neighbourhood. Do you have any right of legal action?
2. A person on the register of the Shiatsu Society must work in a complementary role to orthodox medicine, not in an alternative role. How would you implement this if you are aware that a client is not consulting her general practitioner over her medical condition?
3. Design an information leaflet for clients which sets out the nature of the treatment, any possible risks attached to it and any information the client should give you before the treatment commences.

REFERENCE

1. Royal College of Nursing v. Department of Health and Social Security [1981] 1 All ER 545

38

Yoga

DEFINITION

The meaning of yoga is 'union' or 'joining' and it means the joining of the individual soul with the divine or absolute. Yoga, which originally came from India, is therefore more than a complementary therapy: it is a philosophy about life and personal development covering physical, mental and spiritual health.

BACKGROUND

The exact origins of yoga are not known but there is evidence from archaeology that it dates back at least 5000 years. Ill health is seen as imbalances or blockages in the flow of 'prana', a form of energy. Prana flows along channels known as 'nadis' and is concentrated in centres of energy known as 'chakras'. Physical posture and breathing exercises are intended to purify the body to enable the prana to flow effectively. Some postures (known as 'asanas', which means a seat or platform) improve the balance, develop specific muscles, and stimulate the energy of the body. Meditation is used to increase sensitivity to the needs of the body and the mind.

Research carried out by the Yoga Biomedical Trust between 1983–4 showed that, of the cases reported, the percentage of yoga practitioners who claimed that yoga had benefited the condition was over 90% in the following ailments: back pain, arthritis or rheumatism, anxiety, nerve or muscle disease, heart disease, duodenal ulcers, cancer and alcoholism.

There are several organisations which promote the teaching of yoga.

The British Wheel of Yoga was founded in the early sixties and is now the largest yoga organisation in the UK with approximately 4500 members. It is listed under the Movement and Dance Division of the Central Council of Physical Recreation. It has published leaflets describing the benefits of yoga in a range of conditions including stress and relaxation, pregnancy, and multiple sclerosis.

409

The leaflet on multiple sclerosis points out some of the dangers including:

The individual should avoid shaking of the limbs as this could cause tremors; ... the practice of Tratakam may need to be avoided, particularly candle gazing as in some cases it can influence double vision ... The mantra which includes the high 'eee-eee' should also be avoided since this particular sound seems to affect the optic nerve, which is normally beneficial. Multiple sclerosis sufferers have however been known to experience temporary loss of vision and for this reason this chant should be omitted from the practice.

The Yoga for Health Foundation was established 25 years ago and is a registered charity. It permits any person to become a member on payment of a subscription. Membership includes a quarterly magazine, newsletters, membership of Ickwell Bury centre and free advice on the yoga approach to problems. It has some 4000 members and has trained about 500 teachers.

REGISTRATION AND TRAINING

The main organisations providing training and standard setting for teachers of yoga are:

- the Iyengar Yoga Institute
- the British Wheel of Yoga (BWT)
- The Yoga Biomedical Trust (YBT) and
- the Yoga for Health Foundation.

Lists of members who practise in small groups or on an individual basis are available from the organisations.

YBT was formed in 1983 to promote yoga therapy as a healing science. It is a registered charity. It works with members of the medical profession and with medical scientists in all aspects of its programme, including training and research.

BWT runs a diploma course. Entry is only open to those who have practised Yoga in classes acceptable to BWT for at least two years. The course covers 600 hours study comprising a minimum of 150 hours of personal tuition plus 450 hours of study time. The basic course takes about four years to complete. Eight assessments have to be undertaken before the student can apply for the teaching diploma.

The Yoga for Health Foundation provides training schemes for members of the Foundation including those who wish to be instructors. The training scheme covers the philosophy and psychology of yoga, the anatomy and physiology of yoga and pranayama and asana.

Definitions of standards of competence

The title YBT Yoga Therapy Practitioner is only applied to yoga therapists who have trained with YBT and have satisfied YBT examiners. On gaining sufficient credits for the Diploma in Yoga therapy a certificate is awarded. From 1997–8 qualified YBT therapists will be required to attend a given number of advanced workshops/review sessions with YBT. An association of YBT Yoga Therapists is in the process of being set up.

The British Wheel of Yoga standards are laid down in association with its education committee in conjunction with the tutors on the diploma course. It is itself the accrediting body for other organisations such as the Scottish Yoga Teachers Association.

Rules on professional misconduct

The YBT uses the rules set down by the Institute of Complementary Medicine in relation to professional conduct and discipline.

The handbook of B.K.S. Iyengar Yoga Teachers' Association sets out the rules relating to the teaching syllabus, the principles of teaching, the constitution of the organisation, guidelines for the teaching of asanas and pranayama and employers' liability and public/products liability insurance. An appendix covers the aims and objects of Ramamani Iyengar Memorial Yoga Institute. The qualifications of a disciple from the Iaitiriya Upanishad is published by B.K.S. to remind members of the basis of the art of Yoga and sets out 20 stipulations the first three of which are:

- Bow down to the Lord Naryana
- The Guru is Brahama, the Guru is Vishnu, the Guru is Mahesvar (the creator, the preserver and the destroyer) – the Guru is the Universal Spirit, therefore pay homage to the Guru
- Speak the truth.

The Yoga for Health Foundation has stated that the question of professional misconduct has not arisen.

Insurance cover and professional indemnity

YBT qualified therapists are self-employed and make their own insurance arrangements. However, on qualifying with YBT, they are eligible to appear on the British Register of Complementary Practitioners, which gives them an automatic significant reduction in premiums paid to the Reliant Financial Services Ltd (operating for Sun Alliance International).

Members of B.K.S. Iyengar are also covered by an insurance policy negotiated on their behalf.

Yoga for Health Foundation has insurance cover with a ceiling of £2 million for all its qualified teachers.

DEFINITIONS FOR PURCHASING CONTRACTS

Referral to The Yoga Biomedical Trust (YBT) in Great Ormond Street are now being made from NHS departments and General Practitioners and YBT's qualified yoga therapy practitioners are co-operating with local GPs to provide treatment for a range of chronic conditions. There appear to be no standard terms for such contracts laid down by the various associations and individual practitioners agree their own terms.

SITUATIONS WITH LEGAL SIGNIFICANCE

Yoga must be practised under supervision particularly where the client is pregnant, has recently been in a road accident or had surgery, or is suffering from any major illness or disorder. The British Wheel of Yoga for example in its publication on yoga and pregnancy emphasises that Yoga postures should be learned and practised under the supervision of a reliable teacher and not learned from books or cassettes.

Failure to inform the instructor

Situation 1   Failure to inform the instructor
Jane arrived late for her first yoga class and therefore missed the instructor's opening remarks about the dangers of carrying out certain exercises in pregnancy. She took part in all the exercises and that night she miscarried. This was her first pregnancy after 10 years of marriage. Is the instructor liable?

The instructor owes a duty of care to those she is instructing (see Chapter 3 on negligence). If the instructor failed to ascertain whether this was the first class Jane attended, if there was any likelihood of Jane being pregnant and if so give her the appropriate warning, then there may be evidence of the instructor's breach of the duty of care. The British Wheel of Yoga publication on yoga and pregnancy states that 'if you are new to Yoga and particularly if this is your first pregnancy, do consult your doctor and Yoga teacher before commencing study'. Failure to ensure that each student has a copy of this or a similar leaflet may be seen as a breach of the duty of care.

However for Jane to obtain compensation she must also prove that it was as a result of this failure by the instructor that the miscarriage occurred. There may have been other causes of the miscarriage, not linked to yoga. In addition it could be argued that there is an element of contributory negligence by Jane in attending a class of yoga without first checking on whether such activity could be harmful during pregnancy. The existence and the extent of any contributory negligence will depend upon Jane's knowledge and what she had been told by other people about care during pregnancy.

B.K.S. Iyengar in its members' handbook gives specific warnings about teaching pregnant students. It also provides a declaration form to be signed by students that they are not suffering any of the diseases in a list of 12 set out on the form.

A bad neck

Situation 2   A bad neck
Ralph had been attending yoga for some months when he was injured in a car accident, the car behind having driven into him causing him a whiplash injury. He was not treated in the A&E department. He went to the yoga class hoping that it would bring some relief to his pain. Unfortunately, however, one of the neck exercises exacerbated the condition and he is now concerned about loss of feeling in his arm and hands. Can he obtain compensation?

As discussed in situation 1, the instructor has a duty of care to the students and if a reasonable instructor would have stated that particular care should be taken if anyone has been involved in an accident or is suffering from any disability, then failure to give that advice could be seen as evidence of a breach of the duty of care. However specific problems arise here. Should the advice be given at every session? Had Ralph heard the advice at the first session, but then forgot it when it became specifically relevant to him? Should advice be given in writing at each session or a notice pinned to the wall? These questions would, in the event of court action proceeding, be answered by a yoga expert as to what would be the reasonable standard of care by an instructor.

However Ralph will still have to prove causation, i.e. that it was the failure by the instructor which has led to his additional harm. His failure to obtain treatment following the road accident may have contributed to the additional suffering rather than any yoga exercise.

Heart attack

Situation 3   Heart attack

Mary who had been practising yoga for over 20 years informed her instructor that she had had a bad night and considerable discomfort in her chest which she considered to be indigestion. The instructor advised her to carry out only the exercises which she felt comfortable with. Whilst undergoing an exercise known as 'the cobra' Mary had a massive heart attack and, despite attempts to resuscitate her, she was pronounced dead on arrival at hospital.

Her husband is now blaming the instructor for failing to realise that Mary had a heart condition, for permitting her to undertake the exercises, and for not advising her to seek medical advice or go straight to hospital. What is the legal liability of the instructor?

Situation 3 raises issues in relation to the duty of care and the standard of care owed to the class by the instructor. It may well be that the instructor gave Mary the correct advice and that it is not the responsibility of the instructor to diagnose medical conditions. All that has been said in situations 1, and 2 in relation to the definition of the standard of care and causation applies here.

In addition a possible defence which could be brought on behalf of the instructor is the defence of voluntary assumption of risk (volenti non fit injuria). This means that where a person undertakes an activity which could cause harm there is an understanding that he or she does it at his or her own risk (see Chapter 3). To establish this defence, it must be shown that the person harmed knew of the risks, agreed to run the risk of harm arising, and that the harm which arose was the same as that which was foreseen. This is a different defence than that of an exclusion of liability which would not be maintainable under the Unfair Contract Terms Act 1977 (see Chapter 3) if personal injuries or death arise from negligence.

Advice from the help column

Situation 4   Advice from the help column
A yoga therapist is concerned about whether one of the persons attending his classes should continue to do so following a serious abdominal operation and sent a letter to the newsletter of a yoga organisation asking for advice. The client's GP had washed his hands of the situation by saying 'I do not know what you do in Yoga – ask the instructor'. In the reply printed in the journal, the columnist suggested various exercises which should be safe. The client is now complaining that his abdominal problems have been aggravated by the exercises and is claiming compensation. Could there be any liability on the columnist of the newsletter?

There can be liability for giving advice. It depends if a duty of care is created between the giver of the advice and the person seeking to rely upon it. Can it be said that in this situation a special relationship exists between the columnist and the person seeking advice? The answer is that there could be and it would not be possible for the columnist to exclude liability for any harm caused by his negligent information if personal injury or death arose from reliance on that negligent information. Liability for loss or damage of property could be excluded (see Chapter 3 on negligence). The question to be decided therefore is whether the advice given in the column was reasonable. This would be tested against the reasonable standard of yoga practice. The client might also have a complaint against the GP. Should a GP just brush off a question about the advisability of taking part in Yoga? Perhaps it could be argued that the GP was justified in expecting the yoga instructor to be sufficiently informed as to when the practice of certain exercises would be contraindicated. Perhaps the instructor should not have relied upon the columnist. Such questions would be answered by experts in the field of yoga therapy.

CONCLUSIONS

The growth of interest in yoga since the 1960s in the UK has been remarkable. There is no sign that its popularity is diminishing. As a philosophy of life, it can be seen as specially relevant to the stress and anxieties of modern existence. Work groups in lunch time and evening sessions for all classes and ages of people are growing in popularity. There is good research evidence of the effects of yoga exercises on heart rate and respiration and in managing a wide range of disabilities. There may be further demand for referrals to yoga classes to be available within the NHS.

There is an inherent incompatability between the philosophy of yoga practitioners and other complementary therapists. Yoga is not seen as a therapy and thus the development of NVQs and professionalism is considered by some as alien to its philosophy.

Questions and Exercises

1. Design a leaflet which could be given to all students attending a yoga class, explaining to them any specific dangers of which they should be aware and what information they should be giving to the instructor.
2. A student who has been attending yoga classes for over five years now wishes to take her own classes. Is there any reason in law, why she would not be able to approach the local authority and offer to take yoga evening classes on their behalf?

REFERENCE

1. Hedley Byrne & Co v. Heller & Partners [1963] 2 All ER 575

Holistic medicine

DEFINITION

'Holistic' means whole and many therapies which are discussed in the preceding chapters in this Section, e.g. homeopathy and acupuncture are based on a philosophy of looking at the health and fulfilment of the whole person, and a consultation will be preceded by a lengthy interview identifying any imbalance. Chinese traditional medicine is an example of one of the main holistic therapies.

Some therapies, not immediately seen as treating the whole person, may have an holistic form. Thus one type of massage is called 'Holistic'.

It places treatment within a holistic framework: the therapist will emphasise the importance of looking at her or his client's lifestyle, as well as offering a massage for a particular problem.[1]

Similarly aromatherapy may be of an holistic type, where the oils and massage are used to treat the whole person and a wide range of mental, physical and spiritual concerns.

HOLISTIC ORGANISATIONS

There are organisations designed to encourage orthodox health professionals to practise holistically.

Holistic Nurses Association

This was formed to provide a forum which promotes and encourages research and education amongst nurses wishing to practise holistically. Its definition of holistic nursing is shown in Box 39.1.

Box 39.1   Definition of Holistic Nursing[2]

Holistic Nursing recognises that health proceeds from a balance of our physical, emotional, spiritual, psychological and social needs.
   Our wholeness is dependant upon our relationship to each other, our environment and that which gives our life meaning.
   Holistic Nursing begins with an open mind and willingness to explore the potential for personal growth, health and well-being for ourselves and others.

The Holistic Nurses Association has three levels of membership:

- Full membership for those registered with the UKCC
- Student membership for student nurses
- International membership for nurses, health visitors and midwives.

British Holistic Medical Association

This was formed in 1983 and recognises that whole care is based on the following principles:

- responding to a person as a whole – spiritual, mental and physical aspects
- responding with a range of approaches
- encouraging self-help and personal responsibility
- recognising that any carer is also a whole person who needs support and the chance to grow.

M Webbern, Director of the British Holistic Medical Association described the work of the Association in an article in *Complementary Therapies in Medicine*.[3]

The Association of General Practitioners of Alternative Medicine

This Association provides support and encourages training for GPs who are involved in these non-conventional therapies. It announced in the summer of 1997 that it is making a development fund appeal to set up a college/headquarters/clinic to provide a postgraduate training in natural medicine for GPs with the aim of eventually making treatment by natural means available to everyone throughout the UK. It would also provide research facilities into the healing, prevention and cure of disease by natural means.[4]

RESEARCH

One problem identified by Caroline Stevensen[5] in carrying out research into holistic therapies is the choice of appropriate outcome measures. As part of a research design validated standardised measures of outcome are required. She suggests that

In some instances, holistic complementary therapy research may lend itself more appropriately to the non-statistical format where the whole person can be taken into account as well as addressing the needs of the clinicians concerned.

LEGAL ISSUES

One problem which arises from the perspective of the lawyer is in identifying the standard of the duty of care which applies in holistic therapies. If it is alleged that harm has occurred, how is the relevant standard of care determined. This is a common theme in the section on situations with a legal significance in the specialist chapters. Again and again the problems of determining the standard of care of an individual practitioner in terms of the *Bolam* test is raised. Thus in homeopathy clients presenting superficially with the same health problem will be treated in different ways, depending upon what the therapist has identified in the original interview. This renders it virtually impossible to determine with any certainty what the standard of care of a reasonable competent practitioner would be in any given situation.

REFERENCES

1. Trevelyan J, Booth B 1994 Complementary Medicine for Nurses, Midwives and Health Visitors. Macmillan, London
2. Taken from a leaflet issued by the Holistic Nursing Association
3. Webbern M 1996 British Holistic Medical Association Complementary Therapies in Medicine 4(1): 67–8
4. News item. Caduceus Summer Issue No 36 1997
5. Stevensen C 1995 Research Issues, chapter 5 In: The nurses handbook of complementary therapies, Rankin-Box D (ed). Churchill Livingstone, Edinburgh

Postscript

SECTION CONTENTS

40

In conclusion

The Labour Party whilst in opposition declared its intention to introduce complementary therapies into the NHS as part of a comprehensive and effective National Health Service,[1] setting up an Office of Complementary Medicine. The NHS Confederation has endorsed this rhetoric in its Report,[2] calling for complementary medicine to be more tightly regulated and seeking a government review of its effectiveness, training and regulation procedures. At the time of writing, it is too early to see whether these plans are to be implemented and it will hinge on the EU reaction to the Lannoye Report. More legislation may be forthcoming, providing state registration to some of the larger organisations which have made progress in self-regulation.

It is true that many therapies will of necessity remain outside any revised statutory framework since this is not relevant or appropriate to their needs, either in terms of the protection of the general public or the protection of the standards of their practice. Indeed it has been forcibly and cogently argued by Stone and Matthews[3] that statutory regulation is an unrealistic and unworkable goal for many complementary therapies, the interests of which are far better served by voluntary self-regulation. However the failure of such therapies to develop research on their clinical effectiveness may have a major adverse effect on their availability to clients through NHS or on private health insurance.

Inevitably, as I have researched for this book and been aware of the enthusiasm and the successes which individual therapists have claimed, I have had the realisation that at this moment in time we may be in a stage of knowledge comparable to that which existed before Harvey and his identification of the circulation of blood. Perhaps in the 21st century, the scientific basis of the energy fields will be identified and healing, acupuncture, telepathy – all the diverse therapies will be linked through a new understanding. A law of human energy will be defined and a scientific explanation will be provided for the numerous successes which now take place. Perhaps, too, a law of influence will be discovered to explain how homeopathy and similar therapies work. If this were to occur, modern orthodox medicine would have to incorporate the new knowledge into its syllabus and core of learning.

In the meantime, in the absence of scientific proof and the absence of state regulation, we must ensure that our existing legal framework firstly provides protection against the minority who may abuse or exploit their position or cause harm and secondly safeguards the rights and liberties of individuals to follow ideologies and theories of personal health and fulfilment.

423

Whatever changes the future brings, it is hoped that this book will provide therapist, client, and health manager alike with an understanding of the foundation of the laws which currently apply to their practice and their rights, so that as changes take place, their knowledge can advance and they can take a more informed part in the debate on the nature of the forms of regulation which are appropriate for a diverse and flourishing part of our health care.

REFERENCES

1. Facilitation not prescription. Labour Party press release June 1994
2. NHS Confederation 1977 Complementary Medicine in the NHS
3. Stone J, Matthews J 1996 Complementary medicine and the law. Oxford University Press, Oxford

Addresses

Action for Victims of Medical Accidents
Bank Chambers 1 London Road
Forest Hill London SE23 3TP
(Tel 0181 291 2793)

Aromatherapy Organisations Council
3 Latymer Close Braybrooke
Market Harborough Leicester LE16 8LN
(Tel 01858 434242)

Aromatherapy Trade Council
PO Box 52
Market Harborough Leicester LE16 8ZX

The Arts Council
105 Piccadilly London W1V 0AU

Association for Dance Movement Therapy
c/o The Art Therapies Department
Springfield Hospital Glenburnie Road
London SW17 7DJ

Association of Physical and Natural Therapists
27 Old Gloucester Street
London WC1N 3XX
(Tel 0966 181588 or 01453 765178)

Association of Professional Astrologers
Secretary: Maureen Ravenhall
80 High Street Wargrave
Berks. RG10 8DE
(Tel 01734 404424)

Association of Reflexologists
27 Old Gloucester Street
London WC1N, 3XX
(Tel 0990 673320)

Association of Systematic Kinesiology
39 Browns Road Surbiton
Surrey KT5 8ST
(Tel 0181 399 3215)

Ayurvedic Company of Great Britain Ltd
50 Penywern Road London SW5 9SX
(Tel 0171 370 2255/6)

Ayurvedic Medical Association UK
59 Dolverton Road
South Croydon CR2 8PJ
(Tel 0181 657 6147)

Bach Flower Centre
Mount Vernon Bakers Lane
Brightwell-cum-Sotwell
Wallingford Oxon OX10 0PZ
(Tel 01491 834678)
(Fax 01491 825022)

Bates Association of Great Britain
Friars Court 11 Tarmount Lane
Shoreham-by-Sea
West Sussex BN43 6RQ

The Bayly School of Reflexology
Monks Orchard Whitbourne
Worcester WR6 5RB
(Tel and Fax 01886 821207)

British Acupuncture Council
Park House 206–8 Latimer Road
London W10 6RE
(Tel 0181 964 0222)
(Fax 0181 964 0333)

British Alliance of Healing Associations
26 Highfield Avenue Herne Bay
Kent CT6 6LM
(Tel 01227 373804)

British Association for Art Therapists Ltd
11a Richmond Road, Brighton, Sussex
BN2 3RL

British Association for Autogenic Training and Therapy
c/o Mrs J Bird 18 Holtsmere Close
Garston
Watford Herts WD2 6NG

British Association for Counselling
1 Regent Place Rugby
Warwickshire CV21 2PJ
(Tel 01788 550899)
(Information line 01788 578328)
(Fax 01788 562189)

British Association for Dramatherapists
41 Broomhouse Lane Hurlingham
London SW6 3DP

British Association of Psychotherapists
37 Mapesbury Road London NW2
4HJ
(Tel 0181 452 9823)
(Fax 0181 452 5182)

British College of Acupuncture
8 Hunter Street London WC1N 1BN
(Tel 0171 833 8164)

British College of Naturopathy and Osteopathy
(Tel 0171 435 7830)

British Complementary Medicine Association
9 Soar Lane Leicester LE3 5DE
(Tel 0116 2425406)

British Confederation of Psychotherapists
37 Mapesbury Road London NW2
4HJ
(Tel 0181 830 5173)

British Holistic Medical Association
Rowland Thomas House
Royal Shrewsbury Hospital South
Shrewsbury
Shropshire SY3 8XF

British Homeopathic Association
27a Devonshire Street London W1N
1RJ
(Tel 0171 935 2163)

British Hypnosis Research
Southpoint 8 Paston Place
Brighton BN2 1HA
(Tel 01273 693622)

British Hypnotherapy Association
1 Wythburn Place London W1H 5W1
(Tel 0172 262 8852/723 4443)

British Massage Therapy Council
Greenbank House 65a Adelphi Street
Preston PR1 7BH
(Tel 01772 881063)

British Medical Acupuncture Society
Newton House Newton Lane Lower
Whitley
Warrington Cheshire WA4 4JA
(Tel 01925 730727)

British Psychodrama Association
8 Rahere Road Cowley Oxford OX4
3QG
(Tel and Fax 01865 715055)

British Rebirth Society
18 Woodfield Road Redland Bristol
BS6 6JQ

British Reflexology Association
Administration Office Monks Orchard
Whitbourne Worcester WR6 5RB
(Tel and Fax 01886 821207)

British School of Osteopathy
275–287 Borough High Street
Southwark London SE1 1JE
(Tel 0171 407 0222)

British Society for Music Therapy
25 Rosslyn Avenue East Barnet EN4
8DH
(Tel 0181 368 8879)

British Society of Dowsers
Sycamore Barn Hastingleigh
Ashford Kent TN25 5HW
(Tel and Fax 01233 750253)

**British Society of Experimental
and Clinical Hypnosis**
c/o: Department of Psychology
Grimsby General Hospital
Scartho Road Grimsby DN33 2BA
(Tel 01472 879238)

**British Society of Medical and
Dental Hypnosis**
73 Ware Road Hertfort
Herts. SG13 7ED
(Tel 0181 905 4342)

British Wheel of Yoga
1 Hamilton Place Boston Road
Sleaford Lincs NG34 7ES
(Tel 01529 306851)

**Centre for Complementary
Medicine**
North West School of Nursing and
Health Studies

Stockport College of FE and
HE Wellingtom Road South Stockport
Cheshire SK1 3UQ
(Tel 0161 958 3191)

**Centre for the Study of
Complementary Medicine**
51 Bedford Place
Southampton Hampshire SO1 2DG

Charity Commission
St Albans House 57/60 Haymarket
London SW1Y 4QX
(Tel 0171 210 4477)
(Fax 0171 210 4545)

College of Healing
Runnings Park Croft Bank
West Malvern Worcs WR14 4DU
(Tel 01684 566450)
(Fax 01684 892047)

**College of Integrated Chinese
Medicine**
40 College Road Reading RG6 1QB
(Tel 01734 263366)

**Confederation of Healing
Organisations**
Suite J 113 High Street
Berkhamstead HP4 2DJ
(Tel 01442 870660)

**Council for Complementary and
Alternative Medicine**
Park House 206–8 Latimer Road
London W10 6RE
(Tel 0181 968 3862)

Council for Music in Hospitals
340 Lower Road Little Bookham
Surrey KT23 4EF

European Therapy Studies Institute
7 Chapel Road Worthing
East Sussex BN11 1EG

The Faculty of Homoeopathy
The Royal London Homoeopathic
Hospital
Great Ormond Street
London WC1R 3HR

Federation of Holistic Therapists
38a Portsmouth Road Woolston
Southampton SO19 9AD
(Tel 01703 422695)
(Fax 01703 447968)

**General Council and Register of
Naturopaths**
Registered Office: Frazer House
6 Netherall Gardens London NW3
5RR
Secretary: Szewiel M
Goswell House 2 Goswell Road
Street Somerset BA16 0JG
(Tel 01458 840072)
(Fax 01458 840075)

**General Council and Register of
Osteopaths**
56 London Road Reading Berkshire
RG1 4SJ

**Greater World Christian Spiritual
Association**
3 Conway Street London W1P 5HA
(Tel 0171 436 7555)

Guild of Naturopathic Iridologists
94 Grosvenor Road
London SW1V 3LF
(Tel 0171 834 3579)

Holistic Nurses Association
Membership Secretary: Nicky Baker
Trevaunance Barton Hill Road
Torquay TQ2 8LA
(Tel 01803 326542)

Hygeia College of Colour Therapy
Brook House Avening
Tetbury Glos GL8 8NS
(Tel 01453 832150)

Independent Practitioners Network
London contact: Alan Hancock
AMAP Organisation
91 Fortess Road London NW5 1AG
(Tel 0171 284 4143)

Inner Sound
8 Elms Avenue London N10 2JP
(Tel 0181 444 4855)

Institute of Allergy Therapies
Llangwyryfon Aberystwyth Dyfed
SY23 4EY
(Tel and Fax 01974 241376)

**Institute for Complementary
Medicine**
15 Tavern Quay
London SE16 1QZ
(Tel 0171 237 5165)

**International Association of
Clinical Iridologists**
853 Finchley Road London NW1 8LX
(Tel 0181 458 7781)

**International Association of Colour
Therapy**
PO Box 3 Potters Bar EN6 3ET
(Tel 01707 876928)

Iyengar Yoga Institute
223a Randolph Avenue
London W9 1NL
(Tel 0171 624 3080)

Kinesiology Federation
PO Box 83 Sheffield S7 2YN
(Tel and Fax 0114 281 4064)

Live Music Now
38 Wigmore Street London W1H 9DF

**London and Counties Society of
Physiologists**
330 Lytham Road Blackpool FY4 1DW
(Tel 01253 408443)

**London School of Acupuncture
and Traditional Chinese Medicine**
36/7 Featherstone Street
London EC1Y 8QX

**Massage Therapy Institute of Great
Britain**
PO Box 2726 London NW2 4NR
(Tel 0181 208 1607)

**National College for Hypnotherapy
and Psychotherapy**
12 Cross Street
Nelson Lancashire

**National Federation of Spiritual
Healers**
Old Manor Farm Studio Church Street
Sunbury-on-Thames Middlesex TW16
6RG
(Tel 01932 783164)

**National Institute of Medical
Herbalists**
56 Longbrook Street Exeter Devon
EX4 6AH
(Tel 01392 426022)

**National School of Hypnotherapy
and Psychotherapy**
The Central Register of
Advanced Hypnotherapists
28 Finsbury Park Road
London N4 2JX
(Tel 0171 359 6991)

Northern College of Acupuncture
124 Acomb Road York YO2 0EY
(Tel 01904 785120)

Osteopathic Information Service
PO Box 2074 Reading
Berkshire RG1 4YR
(Tel 01734 512051)

Owl College of Hypnosis
2 Buchanan Street Leigh
Greater Manchester WN7 1XT

The Performing Rights Society
29–33 Berners Street London W1P
4AA

Phonographic Performance Ltd
Ganton House 14–22 Ganton Street
London W1V 1LB

**Prevention of Professional Abuse
(POPAN)**
1 Wyvil Court Wyvil Road
London SW8 2TG
(Tel 0171 622 6334)

Radionic Association
Baerlein House Goose Green
Deddington Banbury Oxon OX15 0SZ
(Tel 01869 338852)

Register of Chinese Herbal Medicine
PO Box 400 Wembley HA9 9NZ
(Tel 0181 904 1357)

Reiki Association
68 Howard Road Westbury Park
Bristol B56 7UX
(Tel 01981 550829)
(Fax 0117942 0275)

**Research Council for
Complementary Medicine**
60 Great Ormond Street
London WC1N 3JF
(Tel 0171 833 8897)

Royal College of Nursing
Special Interest Group in
Complementary Medicine RCN 20
Cavendish Square London W1M 0AB

School of Phytotherapy
Bucksteep Manor Bodle Street Green
Hailsham Sussex BN27 4RJ
(Tel 01323 833812/4)
(Fax 01323 833869)

Shiatsu Society
31 Pullman Lane Godalming
Surrey GU7 1XY
(Tel and Fax 01483 860771)

Society of Homoeopaths
2 Artizan Road Northampton NN1
4HU
(Tel 01604 21400)
(Fax 01604 22622)

Spirtualists Association
10 Belgrave Square
London SW1X 8P11

Therapy Training College
8–10 Balaclava Street
Kings Heath Birmingham B14 7SG
(Tel 0121 444 5435)

Society of Teachers of the Alexander Technique
London House 266 Fulham Road
London SW10 9EL
(Tel 0171 351 0828)

United Kingdom Council for Psychotherapy
167–69 Great Portland Street
London W1N 5FB
(Tel 0171 436 3002)
(Fax 0171 436 3013)

UK Training College of Hypnotherapy and Counselling
10 Alexandra Street
London W2 5NT
(Tel 0171 221 1796/727 2006)

World Federation of Healing
6 Whitworth House Buckhurst House
Bexhill-on-Sea East Sussex TN40
1UA
(Tel 01424 214457)

World Federation of Hypnotherapists
Belmont Square 46 Belmont Road
Ramsgate Kent CT11 7QG
(Tel 01843 587929)

Yoga Biomedical Trust
Royal London Homoeopathic Hospital
60 Great Ormond Street
London WC1N 3HR
(Tel 0171 833 7267)

Yoga for Health Foundation
Ickwell Bury
Ickwell Green
Near Biggleswade SG18 9EF
(Tel 01767 627271)

Yoga Therapy Centre
Royal London Homoeopathic Hospital
Trust
60 Great Ormond Street
London WC1N 3HR
(Tel 0171 833 7267)

Bibliography for complementary medicine

LAW BOOKS

Atiyah P S *The sale of goods* 9th edn. (by John Adams), Pitman Publishing, London. 1995

Bond H J, Kay P *Business Law* 2nd edn, Blackstone Press, London. 1995

Clarkson C M V, Keating H M *Criminal Law: Text And Materials* 3rd edn, Sweet And Maxwell, London. 1994

Clayton P *Law For The Small Business* 6th edn, Kogan Page, London. 1988

Griffiths M *The Law Of Purchasing And Supply* 2nd edn. Pitman Publishing, London. 1996

Koffman L, MacDonald E *The Law Of Contract* 2nd edn, Tolley Publishing Company, Croydon. 1995

Male J M *Landlord And Tenant (M&E Handbooks)* 4th edn, Pitman Publishing, London. 1995

Middleton F, Lloyd S *Charities The New Law,* Jordans, Bristol. 1992

Moore V *Planning Law* 5th edn, Blackstone Press, London. 1995

Read P A (ed) *Commercial Law Textbook: Sale Of Goods, Consumer Credit And Agency,* HLT Publications, London. 1995

Richards P *Law Of Contracts* 2nd edn, Pitman Publishing, London. 1995

Walker R, Ward R *English Legal System* 7th edn, Butterworth, London. 1994

BOOKS ON COMPLEMENTARY THERAPIES.

Arcier M *Aromatherapy,* Hamlyn, London. 1992

A to Z of alternative therapy, Blitz, Leicester. 1994

Auteroche B *et al. Acupuncture and moxibustion: A guide to clinical practice,* Churchill Livingstone, New York. 1992

Bates W H *The Bates method for better eyesight without glasses,* Holt, Reinhart and Winston, New York. 1919 (reprinted) Thorsons, London. 1995

Boyd H *Introduction to homoeopathic medicine* 2nd edn, Beaconsfield Publishers, Bucks. 1989

Brook E *A Woman's book of herbs,* The Women's Press, London

Buckman R, Sabbagh K *Magic or medicine? an investigation into healing,* Pan Books, London. 1994

Campbell E, Brenna J H *Dictionary of mind, body and spirit: ideas, people and places* (revised edn), Aquarian Press, London. 1994

Davidson I *Here and now: An approach to christian healing through Gestalt,* Darton Longman and Todd, London. 1991

Davis P *Aromatherapy – an A – Z,* C W Daniel, Saffron Walden. 1988

Ernst E (ed) 1996 Complementary Medicine: an objective appraisal. Butterworth Heinemann, Oxford

Feldenkrais M *Awareness through movement,* Penguin Arkana, London. 1990

Fulder S *The handbook of complementary medicine,* Coronet Books, 1989

Graham H *Time, energy, and the psychology of healing,* Jessica Kingsley, London. 1990

Graham H *The magic shop: an imaginative guide to self-healing,* Rider, London. 1992

Hall D *Iridology,* Piatkus, London. 1994

Hulke M (ed) *The encyclopedia of alternative medicine and self-help,* Hutchinson, 1978

Harland M, Finn G *The Barefoot homoeopath,* Hyden House, Hampshire. 1991

Kaptchuk T *The web that has no weaver,* Congdon and Weed, New York. 1983

La Tourelle M, Courtney A *Thorsons introductory guide to kinesiology,* Thorsons, London. 1992

Maciocia G *The foundations of chinese medicine,* Churchill Livingstone, Edinburgh. 1989

Macpherson H, Kaptchuk E J (eds) *Acupuncture in practice,* Churchill Livingstone, Edinburgh. 1997

McNief S *Art as medicine: creating a therapy of the imagination,* Shambhala, London. 1992

Micozzi M (ed) *Fundamentals of complementary and alternative medicine,* Churchill Livingstone, New York. 1996

Mills S *The essential book of herbal medicine,* Penguin Arkana, Harmondsworth. 1993

Nuffield Institute of Health *Researching and evaluating complementary therapies: the state of the debate.* May 1995 (Report can be obtained from the Nuffield Institute for Health, 71–5 Clarendon Road, Leeds LS2 9PL (Tel. 0113 233 6983)

Price S, Price L *Aromatherapy for health professionals,* Churchill Livingstone, Edinburgh. 1995

Radionic Association *Introduction to Radionics,* Radionic Association, Banbury. 1980

Rankin-Box D (ed) *The nurse's handbook of complementary therapies,* Churchill Livingstone, Edinburgh. 1995

Rowlands B *The Which? guide to complementary medicine,* Which? Books, 1997

Roy M *The principles of homoeopathic philosophy,* Churchill Livingstone, Edinburgh. 1994

Sayre-Adams J, Wright S *The theory and practice of therapeutic touch,* Churchill Livingstone, Edinburgh. 1995

Sharma U *Complementary medicine today: practitioners and patients* (revised edn), Routledge, London. 1995

Shepherd D *Homoeopathy for the first aider,* C W Daniel, Saffron Walden. 1992

Speight P *Homoeopathy: a home prescribed,* C W Daniel, Saffron Walden. 1992

Stanway A *Alternative medicine,* Bloomsbury, London. 1985

Tiran D *Aromatherapy in midwifery practice,* Baillière Tindall, London. 1996

Tisserand R, Balacs A *Essential oil safety: a guide for health care,* Churchill Livingstone, Edinburgh. 1995

Train D, Mack S (eds) *Complementary therapies for pregnancy and childbirth,* Ballière Tindall, London. 1995

Trevelyan J, Booth B *Complementary medicine for nurses, midwives and health visitors,* Macmillan, London. 1994

Vithoulkas G *Homoeopathy,* Thorsons, Wellingborough. 1985

Wells R, Tschudin V (eds) *Wells' supportive therapies in health care,* Baillière Tindall, London. 1994

Which? *Which? Way to Health* 1992. Alternative medicine November 45–9 London Consumers Association

Wilkes E *A national survey of the use of complementary therapies in hospice care*. Unpublished report 1994 (Trent Palliative Care Unit, Sykes House, Little Common Lane, Abbey Lane, Sheffield)

GOVERNMENT AND OFFICIAL PUBLICATIONS

Cameron-Blackies G, Mouncer Y *Complementary therapies in the NHS* Birmingham National Association of Health Authorities and Trusts (NAHAT) 1993 Research Paper No 10

British Medical Association *Complementary Medicine: New approaches to good practice,* OUP/BMA, Oxford. 1993

Charity Commissioners *So you want to start a charity CC21* Charity Commissioners for England and Wales, 1996

European Commission 1989 *Council Directive (89/48/EC)* Official Journal European Community No L. 19/16–23

European Commission 1990 *Proposal for a council directive on the liability of the suppliers of services Presented to the Commission of the EC Com (90) 482. Final – syn 308 (from Denise R-B article in BJN May 1992*

Woodham A *Health Education Authority guide to complementary medicine and therapies,* Health Education Authority, London. 1994

Sources of further information

Alternative Health Information Bureau, 12 Upper Station Road, Dalett, Hertfordshire WD7 88X (Tel 01923 469496 fax 01923 857670) produces a bimonthly magazine on research in complementary therapies.

   Note During 1993–4 Nursing Times published a series of articles on complementary medicine covering 14 different therapies. 1995 Nursing Times started a new series on lesser known therapies.

   Acumedic Ltd London publishes specialist books on acupuncture. Acupuncture Research Centre Research Reports Available from FTCM 122A Acomb Road York YO2 4EY

Mintel Market Intelligence report complementary medicines London

Mintel Market Intelligence 1995 18–19 Long Lane London EC1A 9HE

MORI *Survey on complementary therapies,* MORI, London. 1989

RCCM *Medical attitudes to complementary medicine public usage of complementary medicine* examples of resource packs provided by Research Council for Complementary Medicine, 60 Great Ormond Street, London WC1N 3JF (Tel. 0171 833 8897)

Richardson J *Complementary therapy in the NHS: a service evaluation of the first year of an outpatient service in a local district general hospital,* Health Services Research and Evaluation Unit, London 1995 (90pp £15 The Lewisham Hospital NHS Trust Lewisham High Street London SE13 6LH (service provided acupuncture, homeopathy and osteopathy to 883 patients in its first year))

Robinson J (ed). *The alternative and complementary health compendium,* Millenium Profiles, Bognor Regis. 1996 (£15.99 + £2 p&p Millenium Profiles, Eurocommunica, 4 Bersted Mews, Bersted Street, Bognor Regis, W. Sussex PO22 9RR)

Thomas K, Fell M, Parry G, Nicholl J *National survey of access to complementary health care via general practice,* Sheffield Centre for Health and Related Research, Sheffield. 1995 (50pp £6.50 available from SCHARR, Regent Court, 30 Regent Street, Sheffield SI 4DA (Tel. 0114 282 5202))

Glossary

Acceptance	an agreement to the terms of an offer which leads to a binding legal obligation, i.e. a contract.
Accusatorial	a system of court proceedings where the two sides contest the issues (contrast with inquisitorial).
Act	of Parliament, statute.
Actionable per se	a court action where the plaintiff does not have to show loss, damage or harm to obtain compensation, e.g. an action for trespass to the person.
Actus reus	the essential element of a crime which must be proved to secure a conviction, as opposed to the mental state of the accused (*mens rea*).
Adversarial	the approach adopted in an accusatorial system.
Advocate	a person who pleads for another: it could be paid and professional, such as a barrister or solicitor, or it could be a lay advocate either paid or unpaid.
Arrestable offence	an offence defined in section 24 of the Police and Criminal Evidence Act 1984 which gives to the citizen the power of arrest in certain circumstances without a warrant.
Balance of probabilities	the standard of proof in civil proceedings.
Bench	the magistrates, Justices of the Peace.
Bolam test	the test laid down by Judge McNair in the case of Bolam *v.* Friern HMC on the standard of care expected of a professional in cases of alleged negligence.
Burden of proof	the duty of a party to litigation to establish the facts, or in criminal proceedings the duty of the prosecution to establish both the *actus reus* and the *mens rea*.
Cause of action	the facts that entitle a person to sue.
Certiorari	an action taken to challenge an administrative or judicial decision (literally: to make more certain).
Civil action	proceedings brought in the civil courts.

Common law	law derived from the decisions of judges, case law, judge made law.
Conditional fee system	a system whereby client and lawyer can agree that payment of fees is dependent upon the outcome of the court action.
Conditions	terms of a contract (see warranties).
Constructive knowledge	knowledge which can be obtained from the circumstances.
Continuous service	the length of service which an employee must have served in order to be entitled to receive certain statutory or contractual rights.
Contract	an agreement enforceable in law.
Contract for services	an agreement, enforceable in law whereby one party provides services, not being employment, in return for payment or other consideration from the other.
Contract of service	a contract for employment.
Counter-offer	a response to an offer which suggests different terms and is therefore counted as an offer not an acceptance.
Damages	a sum of money awarded by a court as compensation for a tort or breach of contract.
Declaration	a ruling by the court, setting out the legal situation.
Dissenting judgment	a judge who disagrees with the decision of the majority of judges.
Distinguished (of cases)	the rules of precedent require judges to follow decisions of judges in previous cases, where these are binding upon them. However in some circumstances it is possible to come to a different decision because the facts of the earlier case are not comparable to the case now being heard, and therefore the earlier decision can be 'distinguished'.
Ex gratia	as a matter of favour e.g. without admission of liability, of payment offered to a claimant.
Expert witness	evidence given by a person whose general opinion based on training or experience is relevant to some of the issues in dispute.
Frustration (of contracts)	the ending of a contract by operation of law, because of the existence of an event not contemplated by the parties when they made the contract e.g. imprisonment, death, blindness.

Re F ruling	a professional who acts in the best interests of an incompetent person who is incapable of giving consent, does not act unlawfully if he follows the accepted standard of care according to the Bolam test.
Guardian ad litem	a person with a social work and child care background who is appointed to ensure that the court is fully informed of the relevant facts which relate to a child and that the wishes and feelings of the child are clearly established. The appointment is made from a panel set up by the local authority.
Hierarchy	the recognised status of courts which results in lower courts following the decisions of higher courts (see precedent). Thus decisions of the House of Lords must be followed by all lower courts unless, they can be distinguished (see above).
Inquisitorial	a system of justice whereby the truth is revealed by an inquiry into the facts conducted by the judge, e.g. coroner's court.
Invitation to treat	the early stages in negotiating a contract, e.g. an advertisement, or letter expressing interest. An invitation to treat will often precede an offer which when accepted leads to the formation of an agreement which, if there is consideration and an intention to create legal relations, will be binding.
Judicial review	an application to the High Court for a judicial or administrative decision to be reviewed and an appropriate order made: e.g. declaration.
Justice of the Peace	a lay magistrate i.e. not legally qualified who hears summary (minor) offences and sometimes indictable (serious) offences in the magistrates court in a group of three (bench – see above).
Mens rea	the mental element in a crime (contrasted with *actus reus*).
Offer	a proposal made by a party which if accepted can lead to a contract. It often follows an invitation to treat.
Plaintiff	one who brings an action in the civil courts.
Plea in mitigation	a formal statement to the court aimed at reducing the sentence to be pronounced by the judge.
Practice direction	guidance issued by the head of the court to which they relate on the procedure to be followed.

Precedent	see hierarchy.
Prima facie	at first sight, or sufficient evidence brought by one party to require the other party to provide a defence.
Privity	the relationship which exists between parties as the result of a legal agreement.
Professional misconduct	conduct unworthy of a nurse, midwife or health visitor.
Proof	evidence which secures the establishment of a plaintiff's or prosecution's or defendant's case.
Prosecution	the pursuing of criminal offences in court.
Quantum	the amount of compensation, or the monetary value of a claim.
Reasonable doubt	to secure a conviction in criminal proceedings the prosecution must establish beyond reasonable doubt the guilt of the accused.
Rescission	where a contract is ended by the order of a court, or by the cancellation of the contract by one party entitled in law to do so.
Statute law	law made by Act of Parliament.
Stipendiary magistrate	a legally qualified magistrate who is paid (i.e. stipend).
Strict liability	liability for a criminal act where the mental element does not have to be proved; in civil proceedings liability without establishing negligence.
Subpoena	an order of the court requiring a person to appear as a witness (subpoena ad testificandum) or to bring records/documents (subpoena duces tecum).
Summary judgment	a procedure whereby the plaintiff can obtain judgment without the defendant being permitted to defend the action.
Tort	a civil wrong excluding breach of contract. It includes: negligence, trespass (to the person, goods or land), nuisance, breach of statutory duty and defamation.
Trespass to the person	a wrongful direct interference with another person. Harm does not have to be proved.
Ultra vires	outside the powers given by law (e.g. of a statutory body or company).
Vicarious liability	the liability of an employer for the wrongful acts of an employee committed whilst in the course of employment.

Volenti non fit injuria	to the willing there is no wrong; the voluntary assumption of risk.
Ward of court	a minor placed under the protection of the High Court, which assumes responsibility for him or her and all decisions relating to his or her care must be made in accordance with the directions of the court.
Warranties	terms of a contract which are considered to be less important than the terms described as conditions: breach of a condition entitles the innocent party to see the contract as ended, i.e. repudiated by the other party, breach of warranties entitles the innocent party to claim damages.
Wednesbury principle	the court will intervene to prevent or remedy abuses of power by public authorities if there is evidence of unreasonableness or perversity. Principle laid down by the Court of Appeal in the case of Associated Provincial Picture House Ltd *v.* Wednesbury Corporation [1948] 1 KB 233.
Without prejudice	without detracting from or without disadvantage to. The use of the phrase prevents the other party using the information to the prejudice of the one providing it.
Writ	a form of written command, e.g. the document which commences civil proceedings.

Index

C

National College for Hypnotherapy and
  Psychotherapy, 429
National Consumer Council
  Guide to Patients' Rights, on healing, 306
  report on Consumer Protection Act 1987, 198
National Disability Council, 116
National Federation of Spiritual Healers,
  305–306, 429
National Health Service, 119–123
  access to complementary medicine, 4–6
  Alexander Technique, 242
  aromatherapy, 252
  art, 260
  chiropractic, 284
  complaints, 176–179
  contracts, 45
  healing, 306
  and homeopathy, 329
  independent contracting with, 111–112
  Labour Party policy, 423
  litigation authority, 37
  local bargaining by staff, 111
  Management Executive, consent forms, 141
  records, 206
  yoga, referrals, 411
  see also entries beginning NHS...
National Health Service Act 1977, 120
  representations on social services, 179
National Institute of Medical Herbalists,
  317–318, 429
National Institute of Reflexology, 399
National Lottery, 270
National Occupational Standards, healing, 304
National Poisons Unit, 321
National Register of Psychotherapists, 386
National School of Hypnotherapy and
  Psychotherapy, 429
National Spiritualist Church, 308
Natural Therapeutic and Osteopathic Society,
  369
Nature Cure Association of Great Britain, 358
Naturopathy, 357–363
Nausea
  acupuncture for, 239–240
  essential oils and pregnancy, 247–248
  herbal medicines for, 317
Necessaries, contracts for, 44
Necessity, compulsory treatment, 138–139
Neck
  acupuncture for, 233
  injury, yoga case, 412–413
Needles, dirty, 234–235, 238–239
Negligence, 19–38
  of accreditation of training courses, 168–169
  breach of confidentiality, 146–147
  death resulting from, 72–73
  health and safety at work, 193–194, 199
  and palmistry, 270–271
  in providing information, 285–286

teaching, 172
time limits, 181
Negligent advice, 33
Negligent misrepresentation, 47
Nelsons, Bach flower remedies, 273–274
Neonates, aromatherapy, 248
Nervous shock see Post traumatic stress disorder
Nervous system, kinesiology, 353
Neurohypnotism, 340
Neurosurgery, paralysis from, 140–141
New Age, British Astrological and Psychic
  Society, 268–269
New informants (Bollis and Sundelson), 395
New intervening cause of harm, 25
Newsletter advice, yoga case, 414
New Woman, campaign on labelling, 251
NHS *see* National Health Service
NHS agreements, 121, 122
NHS Confederation Report, 102–103, 423
NHS trusts, 121–122
  health and safety regulations enforcement,
    192
  records, 206
No fault liability, 36
Non-fatal offences against the person, 70–71
Non-medicinal products, 251
Northern College of Acupuncture, 429
Northern Institute of Massage, 381
Norway, side-effects of acupuncture, 236
Norwich Union, 126
Notice of dangers, 222–223
Notice of ending contracts, 52
  of employment, 108–109
Notifiable diseases, 152–153
'No win – no fee' (conditional fees), 34–35, 438
Nuclear magnetic resonance, magnetic
  properties of water, 326
Nurses, Midwives and Health Visitors Act 1979,
  76
Nursing
  complementary therapies, 8
  Complementary Therapies in Nursing Forum,
    89–90
  holistic, 417–418
  hypnotherapy, 341–342
  reflexology, 403
  Therapeutic Touch, 306
  UKCC, 91
Nursing home care, local authorities, 123–124
Nursing law and ethics, 18
Nutritional therapies, 365–368
  insurance band, 60
Nuts, allergy therapy case, 366–367

O

Oakely, Dr, University College, London,
  Hypnosis Unit, 341

Q